The Cardiology Intensive Board Review Question Book

The Cardiology Intensive Board Review Question Book

Edited by

Leslie Cho, M.D.
Assistant Professor of Medicine
Department of Cardiology
Loyola University Medical Center
Mayfield, Illinois

Brian P. Griffin, M.D.
Director, Cardiovascular Training Program
Department of Cardiovascular Medicine
The Cleveland Clinic Foundation
Cleveland, Ohio

Eric J. Topol, M.D.
Provost and Chief Academic Officer
Chairman, Department of Cardiovascular Medicine
The Cleveland Clinic Foundation
Cleveland, Ohio

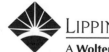 LIPPINCOTT WILLIAMS & WILKINS
A **Wolters Kluwer** Company
Philadelphia · Baltimore · New York · London
Buenos Aires · Hong Kong · Sydney · Tokyo

Acquisitions Editor: Ruth W. Weinberg
Developmental Editor: Erin McMullan
Supervising Editor: Mary Ann McLaughlin
Production Editor: Brooke Begin, Silverchair Science + Communications
Manufacturing Manager: Colin Warnock
Cover Designer: Kevin Kall
Compositor: Silverchair Science + Communications
Printer: Maple Press

Library of Congress Cataloging-in-Publication Data

The cardiology intensive board review question book / editors, Leslie Cho, Brian P. Griffin, Eric J. Topol.-- 1st ed.
    p. ; cm.
  Includes bibliographical references.
  ISBN 0-7817-4229-3
  1. Cardiology--Examinations, questions, etc. I. Cho, Leslie. II. Griffin, Brian P., 1956- III. Topol, Eric J., 1954-
  [DNLM: 1. Cardiovascular Diseases--Examination Questions. 2. Cardiovascular Diseases--drug therapy--Examination Questions. 3. Heart--physiology--Examination Questions. WG 18.2 C2687 2003]
  RC669.2 .C375 2003
  616.1'2'0076--dc21

2002040641

10 9 8 7 6 5 4 3 2 1

*To the Cardiovascular Disease Fellows
at The Cleveland Clinic Foundation,
past, present, and future*

Contents

Contributing Authors.. ix

Preface.. xi

1. Arrhythmia 1
Robert A. Schweikert and Walid I. Saliba

2. Valvular Heart Disease 31
Maran Thamilarasan

3. Acute Myocardial Infarction.. 71
Deepak L. Bhatt

4. Coronary Artery Disease.. 105
Debabrata Mukherjee

5. Pharmacology 159
Michael A. Militello and Jodie M. Fink

6. Aorta and Peripheral Vascular Disease 187
Craig R. Asher and Monica B. Khot

7. Congestive Heart Failure... 221
Gary S. Francis and Leslie Cho

8. Adult Congenital Heart Disease 241
Sasan Ghaffari and Raymond Q. Migrino

9. Physiology/Biochemistry 265
Marc S. Penn

10. Hypertension... 273
Matthew G. Deedy

11. Pericardial Disease 289
Monvadi B. Srichai and Wael A. Jaber

12. Common Echocardiographic Images in Cardiovascular Medicine............... 315
Brian P. Griffin

Index 339

Contributing Authors

Craig R. Asher, M.D.
Staff Cardiologist
Department of Cardiovascular Medicine
The Cleveland Clinic Foundation
Cleveland, Ohio

Deepak L. Bhatt, M.D.
Director, Interventional Cardiology
  Fellowship
Department of Cardiovascular Medicine
The Cleveland Clinic Foundation
Cleveland, Ohio

Leslie Cho, M.D.
Assistant Professor of Medicine
Department of Cardiology
Loyola University Medical Center
Mayfield, Illinois

Matthew G. Deedy, M.D.
Associate Staff
Clinical Section
Department of Cardiovascular Medicine
The Cleveland Clinic Foundation
Cleveland, Ohio

Jodie M. Fink, Pharm.D.
Pharmacotherapy Outcomes Specialist
Department of Pharmacy
The Cleveland Clinic Foundation
Cleveland, Ohio

Gary S. Francis, M.D.
Professor of Medicine
Department of Cardiology
The Cleveland Clinic Foundation
Cleveland, Ohio

Sasan Ghaffari, M.D., F.A.C.C.
Staff Cardiologist
Department of Cardiovascular Medicine
The Cleveland Clinic Foundation
Cleveland, Ohio

Brian P. Griffin, M.D.
Director, Cardiovascular Training Program
Department of Cardiovascular Medicine
The Cleveland Clinic Foundation
Cleveland, Ohio

Wael A. Jaber, M.D.
Staff Cardiologist
Department of Cardiovascular Medicine
The Cleveland Clinic Foundation
Cleveland, Ohio

Monica B. Khot, M.D.
Staff Cardiologist
Department of Cardiology
Indiana Heart Physicians
Beech Grove, Indiana

Raymond Q. Migrino, M.D.
Associate Staff
Department of Cardiology
The Cleveland Clinic Foundation
Cleveland, Ohio

Michael A. Militello, Pharm.D.
Affiliate Professor of Clinical Pharmacy
University of Toledo College of Pharmacy
Cardiology Clinical Specialist: Pharmacist
Department of Pharmacy
The Cleveland Clinic Foundation
Cleveland, Ohio

Debabrata Mukherjee, M.D.
Assistant Professor of Internal Medicine
Department of Cardiology
University of Michigan Medical School
Ann Arbor, Michigan

Marc S. Penn, M.D., Ph.D.
Director, Experimental Animal Laboratory
Departments of Cardiovascular Medicine and Cell Biology
The Cleveland Clinic Foundation
Cleveland, Ohio

Walid I. Saliba, M.D.
Associate Staff
Department of Cardiovascular Medicine
The Cleveland Clinic Foundation
Cleveland, Ohio

Robert A. Schweikert, M.D.
Associate Staff
Department of Cardiovascular Medicine
Section of Electrophysiology and Pacing
The Cleveland Clinic Foundation
Cleveland, Ohio

Monvadi B. Srichai, M.D.
Fellow in Cardiovascular Medicine
The Cleveland Clinic Foundation
Cleveland, Ohio

Maran Thamilarasan, M.D.
Associate Staff Cardiologist
Department of Cardiovascular Medicine
The Cleveland Clinic Foundation
Cleveland, Ohio

Preface

This book of questions on cardiovascular disease is aimed at providing a review of common topics addressed on the Cardiovascular Board examination and recertification examination. We have included subjects, images, and tracings that are important not only for examinations, but are also very relevant to clinical practice. The questions are presented in two formats that are commonly used in examinations: the single best answer format and the format in which a list of topics must be appropriately matched with another list. The correct answers with short explanations are given at the end of each chapter. A more complete discussion of the topics in this book is available in Topol, *Textbook of Cardiovascular Medicine*, to which this book is complementary. A more succinct discussion of these topics is available in the *Manual of Cardiovascular Medicine*, edited by Drs. Marso, Griffin, and Topol.

We would like to thank all of those who have made this book possible, including the contributors; our colleagues; the cardiovascular disease fellows at The Cleveland Clinic Foundation; and the Graphics group, Cardiovascular Disease Department, The Cleveland Clinic Foundation, without whose help the making of this book would be impossible. Finally, we would like to thank our families for their support in all our endeavors. We hope you enjoy the book and find it useful.

Leslie Cho, M.D.
Brian P. Griffin, M.D.
Eric J. Topol, M.D.

The Cardiology
Intensive Board Review
Question Book

CHAPTER 1

Arrhythmia

Robert A. Schweikert and Walid I. Saliba

QUESTIONS

NOTES

1. Which of the following antiarrhythmic medications would be the best choice for treatment of a patient with AFib and significant renal insufficiency?

   A. propafenone
   B. sotalol
   C. dofetilide
   D. flecainide

2. Which of the following antiarrhythmic drugs is not at least partially cleared by hemodialysis?

   A. disopyramide
   B. procainamide
   C. sotalol
   D. amiodarone

3. Which of the following antiarrhythmic medications has active metabolites?

   A. amiodarone
   B. sotalol
   C. dofetilide
   D. flecainide

4. A patient arrives at the emergency department with symptomatic narrow complex tachycardia. The patient is hemodynamically stable. The decision is made to administer IV adenosine. Under which of the following circumstances should the dosage of adenosine be reduced?

   A. The patient is taking theophylline.
   B. The patient is taking dipyridamole.
   C. The patient has significant valvular regurgitation.
   D. The patient has a significant left-to-right shunt.

1

5. Which of the following antiarrhythmic drugs increases serum digoxin levels?

A. flecainide
B. propafenone
C. quinidine
D. all of the above

6. Which of the following medications is contraindicated for use with dofetilide?

A. digoxin
B. diltiazem
C. verapamil
D. propranolol

7. Which of the following antiarrhythmic drugs is the least negative inotrope?

A. dofetilide
B. sotalol
C. amiodarone
D. flecainide

8. Which of the following antiarrhythmic drugs may be more likely to have proarrhythmia at increased heart rates?

A. sotalol
B. flecainide
C. quinidine
D. dofetilide

9. Which of the following statements is *true* regarding antiarrhythmic drugs with reverse-use dependence?

A. Antiarrhythmic drugs with reverse-use dependence have greater efficacy for arrhythmia prevention than termination and have less risk for ventricular proarrhythmia after AFib termination (at slower sinus rates) than during AFib.
B. Antiarrhythmic drugs with reverse-use dependence have less efficacy for arrhythmia prevention than termination and have greater risk for ventricular proarrhythmia after AFib termination (at slower sinus rates) than during AFib.
C. Antiarrhythmic drugs with reverse-use dependence have greater efficacy for arrhythmia prevention than termination and have greater risk for ventricular proarrhythmia after AFib termination (at slower sinus rates) than during AFib.
D. Antiarrhythmic drugs with reverse-use dependence have less efficacy for arrhythmia prevention than termination and have less risk for ventricular proarrhythmia after AFib termination (at slower sinus rates) than during AFib.

10. Which of the following is *true* regarding the Cardiac Arrhythmia Suppression trials (CAST I and II)?

A. The treatment drugs increased mortality for patients without heart disease.
B. All class IC antiarrhythmic drugs were found to increase mortality.
C. The treatment drugs effectively suppressed PVCs.
D. The antiarrhythmic drugs studied were flecainide, propafenone, and moricizine.

11. Which of the following antiarrhythmic drugs is the most potent sodium channel blocker?

    A. flecainide
    B. lidocaine
    C. disopyramide
    D. procainamide

12. The serum concentration or drug effect of which of the following medications is *not* increased in the presence of amiodarone?

    A. digoxin
    B. cyclosporine
    C. warfarin
    D. none of the above

13. Which of the following antiarrhythmic drugs is *not* a Vaughan Williams class III drug?

    A. sotalol
    B. ibutilide
    C. mexiletine
    D. dofetilide

14. Which of the following antiarrhythmic drugs is approved by the FDA for acute pharmacologic conversion of AFib to sinus rhythm?

    A. procainamide
    B. amiodarone
    C. ibutilide
    D. all of the above

15. Which of the following effects is expected when administering adenosine to a patient with recent cardiac transplantation (denervated heart)?

    A. no effect
    B. diminished effect
    C. enhanced effect
    D. delayed effect

16. For which of the following antiarrhythmic drugs is proarrhythmia *not* dose related?

    A. dofetilide
    B. quinidine
    C. sotalol
    D. ibutilide

17. Which of the following is not typically a "short RP" regular narrow QRS tachycardia?

    A. orthodromic atrioventricular reentrant tachycardia (AVRT)
    B. atrioventricular nodal reentrant tachycardia (AVNRT)
    C. permanent junctional reciprocating tachycardia (PJRT)
    D. nonparoxysmal junctional tachycardia

18. A patient presents with regular narrow QRS tachycardia. An esophageal electrode shows a 1:1 atrial to ventricular relationship during tachycardia.

The VA interval is measured as 55 msec. Which of the following is the most likely diagnosis?

A. orthodromic AVRT
B. atrial tachycardia
C. AVNRT
D. PJRT

19. A 17-year-old patient who is known to have Wolff-Parkinson-White syndrome presents with a regular narrow complex tachycardia with a cycle length of 375 msec (160 bpm) that occurred with a sudden onset. You note that there is a 1:1 atrial to ventricular relationship and that the RP interval is 100 msec. The best initial treatment is

A. IV procainamide
B. atropine
C. IV verapamil
D. catheter ablation

20. A 25-year-old patient presents with the sudden onset of tachycardia and is found to have a regular narrow QRS tachycardia with a cycle length of 340 msec (176 bpm). An ECG appears to show P waves visible just after each QRS complex. You place an esophageal electrode and confirm a 1:1 atrial to ventricular relationship with a VA interval of 110 msec. During the tachycardia, there is spontaneous development of LBBB, and a slower tachycardia with a VA interval of 150 msec is now seen. What is the most likely diagnosis for the second tachycardia?

A. AVNRT
B. orthodromic AVRT using a right-sided accessory pathway
C. orthodromic AVRT using a left-sided accessory pathway
D. VT with 1:1 VA conduction

21. A 65-year-old man presents after an arrest while eating at a local restaurant. On arrival, paramedics documented VF, and he was successfully resuscitated. He has a history of MI and CHF. Serum electrolytes are remarkable only for mild hypokalemia. MI is ruled out by ECG and serial blood tests of myocardial enzymes. Subsequent evaluation includes cardiac catheterization, which shows severe three-vessel CAD and severe LV systolic dysfunction. A nuclear myocardial perfusion scan shows a large area of myocardial scar without significant viability in the territory of the left anterior descending coronary artery. The decision is made to treat the CAD medically. Which of the following is the best management strategy for his arrhythmia?

A. PO amiodarone
B. ICD implantation if an EP study shows inducible VT or VF
C. ICD implantation
D. beta-blocker medication

22. A 55-year-old woman has CAD and moderately severe LV systolic dysfunction (LVEF, 34%). Routine ambulatory Holter monitoring shows asymptomatic frequent ventricular ectopy with PVCs and occasional runs of nonsustained VT. Which of the following statements about the management of this patient is *true*?

A. Implantation of an ICD is indicated.

B. Implantation of an ICD is indicated if an EP study shows inducible VT.

C. Treatment with amiodarone is indicated, and if the arrhythmia recurs, then an EP study is indicated.

D. No treatment is indicated unless the arrhythmia becomes symptomatic.

23. Which of the following is *false* regarding ICDs?

A. ICDs are programmable devices with antibradycardia and antitachycardia capabilities.

B. Biphasic shocks require more energy for cardioversion and defibrillation than monophasic shocks.

C. ICDs may terminate VT with cardioversion shocks or antitachycardia pacing.

D. The use of MRI is contraindicated for the patient with an ICD.

24. All of the following are *true* statements about the ICD implantation procedure *except*

A. The right-chest site is preferred over the left-chest site for ICD systems with an "active can," in which the ICD pulse generator acts as one component of the shocking electrode system.

B. Implantation of an ICD system is similar to implantation of a pacemaker system.

C. The incidence of postoperative infection is generally 1% to 4%.

D. The incidence of operative mortality is less than 1%.

25. A patient arrives at the emergency department after experiencing multiple shocks from his ICD. The shocks were not preceded by any symptoms. He is noted to be in sinus rhythm on presentation, and, while on the monitor, he receives several more shocks from the ICD without any arrhythmias noted. Which of the following is the most appropriate initial step in the management of this patient?

A. Immediately arrange for a programmer for interrogation and reprogramming of the ICD.

B. Arrange for urgent surgery in the EP lab.

C. Initiate antiarrhythmic drug therapy.

D. Place a "donut" magnet over the ICD site.

26. All of the following patients have indications for ICD implantation *except*

A. a 35-year-old man with hypertrophic cardiomyopathy with clinical features indicating high risk for sudden cardiac death

B. a 17-year-old girl with congenital long-QT syndrome and recurrent syncope despite optimal medical therapy

C. a 60-year-old man with CAD, prior MI, LV dysfunction, and incessant sustained VT

D. an 80-year-old man with leukemia in remission and CAD who survived an episode of cardiac arrest with documented VF

27. Which of the following is most important for successful resuscitation of an adult patient with out-of-hospital cardiac arrest?

A. IV epinephrine

B. early DC-shock defibrillation

C. IV antiarrhythmic drugs

D. early intubation

28. Which of the following rhythms documented at the time of resuscitation from cardiac arrest carries the poorest prognosis for long-term survival?

    A. asystole
    B. electromechanical dissociation (EMD) or pulseless electrical activity (PEA)
    C. VF
    D. VT

29. Which of the following rhythm disturbances is most commonly documented for an adult with out-of-hospital sudden cardiac death resuscitated within the first 4 min after arrest?

    A. asystole
    B. EMD or PEA
    C. monomorphic VT
    D. VF

30. Which of the following may be responsible for multiple ("cluster") shocks from an ICD?

    A. recurrent VT
    B. AFib with rapid ventricular response
    C. lead malfunction
    D. all of the above

31. Which of the following treatments is *not* useful for a patient with frequent episodes of vasovagal syncope?

    A. dual-chamber pacemaker implantation
    B. midodrine
    C. beta-blocker medications
    D. diuretics

32. Which of the following statements about syncope are *true*?

    A. A carefully performed initial evaluation (history, physical examination, basic hematologic or biochemical studies, and an ECG) may provide an etiology for syncope in 50% to 60% of cases.
    B. The majority of syncopal episodes occur in patients without cardiac or neurologic disease.
    C. Neurally mediated syncope is the most common cause of syncope.
    D. All of the above are true.

33. Which of the following treatment options has been most consistently shown to be effective for the primary prevention of sudden cardiac death in patients with CAD and recent MI?

    A. D-sotalol
    B. beta-blocker medications
    C. amiodarone
    D. dofetilide

34. Which of the following is the most common condition associated with sudden cardiac death in the United States?

    A. hypertrophic cardiomyopathy
    B. CAD
    C. valvular heart disease
    D. dilated cardiomyopathy

35. A 55-year-old man is referred for recurrent syncope. The episodes consist of a prodrome of weakness and nausea followed by loss of consciousness. Physical examination is unremarkable. ECG and exercise treadmill stress test were normal. Which of the following is the most appropriate next step?

    A. EP study
    B. signal-averaged ECG
    C. head-upright tilt table testing
    D. ambulatory Holter monitoring

36. Which of the following is the most common type of response during vaso-vagal syncope?

    A. predominantly cardioinhibitory (decreased heart rate)
    B. predominantly vasodepressor (decreased BP)
    C. combination of cardioinhibitory and vasodepressor
    D. none of the above

37. A 25-year-old man is referred for evaluation of an abnormal ECG that was found at the time of a routine examination. The ECG shows a short PR interval with ventricular preexcitation consistent with the Wolff-Parkinson-White pattern. He has not had any symptoms such as palpitations, light-headedness, near syncope, or syncope. You order an ambulatory Holter monitor, which shows intermittent ventricular preexcitation. What is the most appropriate next step in the evaluation of this patient?

    A. exercise test
    B. catheter ablation
    C. EP study
    D. none of the above

38. A 40-year-old woman presents to the emergency department with tachycardia. An ECG shows regular narrow complex tachycardia at 160 bpm. Atrial activity is difficult to discern in the tracing, but during tachycardia, there appears to be an "r prime" in lead V1 that is not present on an ECG during sinus rhythm recorded a few months earlier. Which of the following is the most likely diagnosis?

    A. AVNRT
    B. AVRT
    C. atrial tachycardia
    D. atrial flutter

39. Which of the following statements is *false* regarding multifocal atrial tachycardia (MAT)?

    A. *MAT* is defined as an atrial arrhythmia with at least three distinct P-wave morphologies, an irregular PR interval, and an irregular ventricular response.
    B. MAT can be confused with AFib.
    C. DC cardioversion is effective in the treatment of MAT.
    D. The initial treatment for MAT is correction of the underlying condition.

40. Which of the following statements about head-upright tilt table testing is *true*?

    A. The specificity of the test is approximately 80%.
    B. The sensitivity of the test is approximately 80%.
    C. The reproducibility of the test is approximately 80%.
    D. All of the above are true.

41. Patients with an implanted pacemaker may safely use all of the following equipment *except*

    A. cellular phones
    B. weapon detectors
    C. arc welding equipment
    D. microwave ovens
    E. electric power tools

42. An 80-year-old man with chronic AFib of 15 years' duration is admitted with recurrent episodes of dizziness and a recent episode of syncope. He has normal LV function and no evidence of CAD. In-hospital telemetry confirms the presence of slow ventricular rate and frequent pauses (4 sec) that correlate with his lightheadedness. His medications consist of warfarin sodium (Coumadin). The most appropriate course of action includes which of the following?

    A. reassuring the patient and instructing him to come back if he has recurrence of syncope
    B. prolonged monitoring with a loop recorder
    C. EP testing to evaluate for ventricular arrhythmia
    D. permanent pacemaker implant
    E. ICD implant

43. A decision was made in the previous case to proceed with a permanent pacemaker. Which would be the most suitable pacing modality?

    A. dual-chamber system programmed to DDDR
    B. dual-chamber system programmed to DDDR with mode switching
    C. dual-chamber system programmed to DDIR
    D. single-chamber system in the ventricle programmed to VVIR
    E. single-chamber system in the atrium programmed to AAIR

44. Which one of the following is *true* about "pacemaker syndrome"?

    A. Symptoms usually include fatigue, dizziness, and hypotension.
    B. It occurs equally in atrial-based and ventricular-based pacing systems.
    C. It does not occur in patients who have 1:1 ventriculoatrial conduction.
    D. It can be treated with fludrocortisone.
    E. It is treated by increasing the VVI baseline pacing rate.

45. In hypertrophic cardiomyopathy, dual-chamber pacing has been associated with all of the following *except*

    A. increased LV systolic dimension
    B. increased LV diastolic dimension
    C. reduced MR
    D. changed activation of the septum activation
    E. reduced LV outflow gradient

46. Of the following patients, who is the most likely to carry the diagnosis of sick sinus syndrome (SSS)?

    A. a 65-year-old woman with a resting sinus arrhythmia varying from 70 to 85 bpm
    B. a 30 year old with sinus pauses 1.5 sec in duration
    C. a 20-year-old athletic man with sinus bradycardia at 25 bpm while sleeping
    D. a 73-year-old man with chronic AFib and a ventricular rate of 40 bpm during peak treadmill test
    E. a 70 year old with sinus bradycardia and AV block secondary to a beta-blocker overdose

47. A 76-year-old patient with dilated cardiomyopathy and LBBB on baseline TTE is undergoing evaluation for syncope. Placement of a catheter near his bundle during EP testing is most likely to

    A. induce AFib
    B. induce VT
    C. perforate the atrium
    D. perforate the ventricle
    E. induce CHB

48. A 25-year-old patient with a history of depression is brought to the emergency room after ingesting some of her mother's prescription medications, including diltiazem and metoprolol. Her pulse rate is 25 bpm, and her BP is 90/50. Her ECG shows sinus bradycardia and high-grade AV block. In preparation for temporary pacemaker placement, which of the following is most likely to be effective?

    A. IV calcium gluconate
    B. isoproterenol infusion
    C. IV atropine
    D. IV magnesium sulfate
    E. IV glucagon

49. Which of the following is the EP mechanism of typical atrial flutter most likely related to?

    A. intraatrial reentry
    B. ectopic automatic atrial focus
    C. triggered activity secondary to delayed afterdepolarization
    D. triggered activity secondary to early afterdepolarization
    E. none of the above

50. A young patient is admitted to the intensive care unit with amitriptyline overdose. Three hours after gastric lavage, he develops hypotension and wide complex tachycardia that is recurrent despite cardioversion. Appropriate management includes which of the following?

    A. IV bretylium
    B. temporary pacemaker with overdrive pacing
    C. IV calcium gluconate
    D. administration of sodium-containing solution
    E. IV magnesium sulfate

51. Which of the following mechanisms is believed to cause sudden death related to the use of terfenadine?
    A. Na^+ channel blockade with increase in QRS duration
    B. K^+ channel blockade with increase in the QT interval
    C. Ca^{2+} channel blockade with no change in the QRS or QT intervals
    D. myocardial ischemia secondary to coronary spasm
    E. none of the above

52. A 50-year-old man with chronic obstructive pulmonary disease related to chronic smoking presents to the emergency room with palpitations. ECG shows narrow QRS tachycardia at 165 bpm. His BP is 125/60. Expiratory wheezes are heard on lung examination. His medications include albuterol inhaler and theophylline. The most appropriate initial treatment includes which of the following?
    A. adenosine IV bolus
    B. digoxin loading over 6 hours
    C. verapamil IV bolus
    D. propafenone IV bolus
    E. immediate cardioversion

53. An 80 year old undergoes dual-chamber pacemaker placement for CHB. Excellent ventricular and atrial capture thresholds were obtained at the time of the implant. The pacemaker programmed parameters are as follows: mode DDD; lower rate, 70 bpm; upper rate, 130 bpm; atrial sensitivity, 0.25 mV (most sensitive setting); ventricular sensitivity, 1.00 mV; AV delay, 175 msec; pace/sense configuration, bipolar. The next day, the following rhythm strip was recorded (Fig. 1).

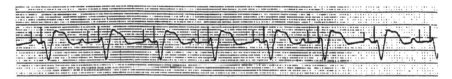

FIGURE 1

This rhythm strip shows
    A. normal pacemaker function for the programmed parameters
    B. atrial noncapture
    C. ventricular noncapture
    D. atrial undersensing
    E. ventricular undersensing

54. As related to the previous case, the most appropriate corrective action is to
    A. reassure the patient and schedule a follow-up in 6 months for reevaluation
    B. increase the energy output on the atrial channel to assure atrial capture
    C. change the atrial sensitivity setting
    D. suspect a pulse generator defect and replace it with a new one
    E. obtain a CXR to document atrial-lead dislodgment and reposition the lead

55. A 55-year-old woman returns to the clinic after a recent dual-chamber pacemaker placement. She reports frequent palpitations and fatigue. These episodes last for several minutes before stopping. A Holter monitor recorded the following rhythm (Fig. 2):

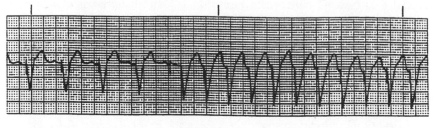

FIGURE 2

The pacemaker is programmed to mode DDD; lower rate, 80 bpm; upper rate, 150 bpm; AV delay, 200 msec; postventricular atrial RP, 150 msec. The latter part of this rhythm strip shows

A. VT induced by the pacemaker
B. initiation of atrial tachycardia with atrial tracking
C. pacemaker-mediated tachycardia
D. pacemaker function failure with inappropriate rapid ventricular pacing
E. artifact

56. A 60-year-old man is having a transtelephonic pacemaker check. He has recently undergone a pacemaker upgrade from a single-chamber–ventricular to a dual-chamber system. He is reporting the same "old" symptoms he had with the VVI system. The following rhythm was recorded (Fig. 3):

Free Running

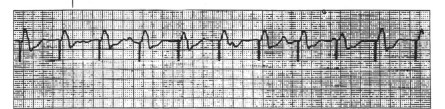

Magnet

FIGURE 3

Which of the following is *true*?

A. A CXR should be obtained to check atrial-lead position.
B. The rhythm strip shows normal dual-chamber pacemaker function.
C. The pacemaker is programmed to VVI mode.
D. Underlying rhythm is AFib with expected auto mode switch response to VVI.
E. None of the above is true.

57. An 82-year-old man receives a dual-chamber pacemaker for SSS. Routine transtelephonic check (without and with magnet) shows the following strips (Fig. 4):

Free Running

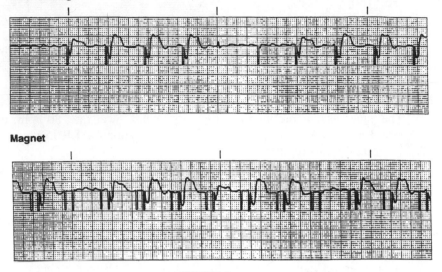

Magnet

FIGURE 4

Which of the following is *true*?

A. The pacing mode is VVI secondary to automatic mode switch.
B. There is consistent atrial capture on the magnet strip.
C. There is consistent ventricular capture.
D. Ventricular sensing cannot be determined by the available strips.
E. Atrial sensing cannot be determined by the available strips.

The following tracings (Figs. 5 through 8) are obtained during EP evaluation of AV conduction in different patients. HRA (*high right atrium*) and HBE (*His bundle electrogram*) are the intracardiac electrograms, recording from the high right atrium and the His bundle regions, respectively. Which of the following is *true* for these tracings?

58.

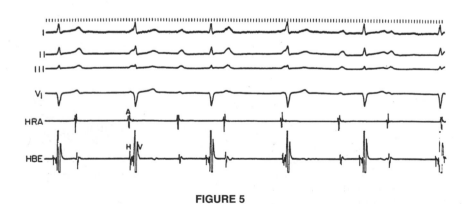

FIGURE 5

59.

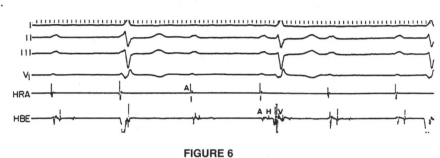

FIGURE 6

60.

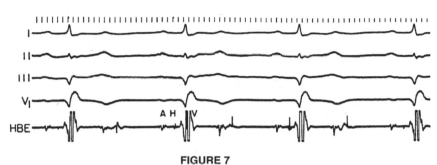

FIGURE 7

61.

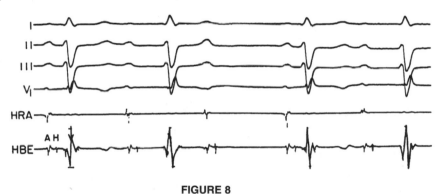

FIGURE 8

A. CHB at the level of the AV node
B. CHB at the infra-Hisian (below the His bundle) level
C. second-degree AV block at the AV node level
D. second-degree AV block at an infra-Hisian level
E. first-degree AV block

62. A 38-year-old woman with congenital CHB undergoes a dual-chamber permanent pacemaker. A 12-lead ECG obtained after the procedure shows NSR with atrial tracking (A sense–V pace behavior). The ventricular-paced complex has an RBBB morphology. Further evaluation should include

A. obtaining a portable anteroposterior CXR to evaluate lead position
B. obtaining a two-view (anteroposterior and lateral) CXR to evaluate lead position
C. repeating the 12-lead ECG
D. requesting a pacemaker interrogation
E. reassuring the patient without ordering further tests

NOTES

63. Which of the following is *true* regarding EP testing of the conduction system?

    A. It is indicated in patients with symptomatic third-degree heart block to identify the level of block.
    B. An abnormal sinus node recovery time is an indication for pacemaker placement.
    C. A normal sinus node recovery time rules out the diagnosis of SSS.
    D. Patients with evidence of infra-Hisian block during EP testing should be considered for permanent pacing.
    E. Ambulatory ECG is less reliable than EP testing in evaluating SSS.

64. Which of the following statements is *true* regarding Brugada's syndrome?

    A. It is characterized by ST elevation and an IRBBB pattern in the right precordial leads.
    B. The EKG manifestations can be exacerbated by sotalol.
    C. It is the leading cause of death in young men in the Middle East.
    D. AFib is the most frequently reported arrhythmia.
    E. It is effectively treated with beta-blockers.

65. In patients with long-QT syndrome

    A. EP testing is indicated to evaluate for inducible ventricular arrhythmias.
    B. The mechanism of torsades de pointes (TdP) is believed to be related to early afterdepolarization.
    C. Sotalol is effective for the treatment of the associated ventricular tachyarrhythmias.
    D. Hyperkalemia increases the risk of TdP.
    E. Cardiac arrest typically occurs at rest.

66. A 75-year-old man is admitted with upper GI bleeding. His ECG shows sinus rhythm at 90 bpm, with a PR of 220 msec, RBBB, and left anterior fascicular block. He had one episode of near syncope 2 days before this admission. His current hematocrit is 20. You are consulted regarding the need for a pacemaker. Which of the following is *true*?

    A. You should proceed with permanent pacemaker placement in the setting of bifascicular block.
    B. You should proceed with ICD placement.
    C. You should perform EP testing to evaluate the AV conduction system.
    D. You should reassure the patient and suggest no further testing.
    E. You should prescribe beta-blockers to slow down the sinus rate.

67. Which of the following criteria is most helpful in differentiating SVT from VT in a patient presenting with wide complex tachycardia?

    A. The patient is older than 65 years.
    B. The tachycardia rate is greater than 160 bpm.
    C. The patient is awake with a BP of 110/65 mm Hg.
    D. There is an RS pattern in V2.
    E. There is AV dissociation.

68. A 76-year-old man walks into the emergency room reporting palpitations and dizziness. A 12-lead ECG shows wide complex tachycardia at a rate of 160 bpm. His BP is 110/50 mm Hg. He reports that he recently sustained an MI. He has not had any similar symptoms before. Which of the following should be included in further evaluation and treatment of his arrhythmia?

A. verapamil, 10-mg IV bolus, to treat SVT with aberrancy, as the patient is hemodynamically stable
B. immediate DC cardioversion
C. procainamide, 15 mg/kg IV over 30 to 60 min
D. immediate cardiac catheterization and angioplasty, as needed
E. digoxin, 1 mg IV over 6 hours in four divided doses

69. A 55-year-old man had a pacemaker initially implanted 8 years ago over the left prepectoral area. Two months earlier, his old pacemaker reached end-of-life, and he underwent replacement of the pacemaker using the existing leads. He is presenting now with dull pain, swelling, and mild erythema over the pacemaker pocket site that started 1 week earlier, together with low-grade fever. He reports some purulent drainage from the incision site. Blood cultures were drawn. The best course of action is

A. to prescribe PO antibiotics for 2 weeks
B. to admit the patient for IV antibiotics and pacemaker system extraction
C. to prescribe long-term suppressive PO antibiotics, as the pacemaker and leads system are too old to be extracted
D. to remove the recently implanted pulse generator on the left, leaving the old leads in place, and implant a new pacemaker system on the right prepectoral area
E. to incise and drain the pacemaker pocket and allow it to heal with secondary intention with daily change of dressing

70. Which of the following is a *correct* statement concerning external cardioversion of AFib?

A. Acute MI is a contraindication to cardioversion, as it results in further myocardial damage.
B. A nonsynchronized shock should be delivered, because the rhythm is irregular.
C. Inadequate synchronization may occur with peaked T waves, low-amplitude signal, and malfunctioning pacemakers.
D. Digoxin therapy should be discontinued for 48 hours before elective cardioversion.
E. Patients with pacemakers should not undergo cardioversion because of the risk of pacemaker damage.

71. In patients with Wolff-Parkinson-White syndrome, with which of the following is acute pharmacologic treatment of AFib best achieved?

A. diltiazem
B. lidocaine
C. verapamil
D. procainamide
E. adenosine

72. A 75-year-old patient with a history of ischemic cardiomyopathy develops worsening heart failure symptoms during episodes of AFib despite a controlled ventricular rate. Which of the following is included in a reasonable trial of pharmacologic therapy?

A. flecainide
B. sotalol
C. verapamil
D. disopyramide
E. amiodarone

73. Which of the following is *true* regarding the use of digoxin in AFib?

    A. It is superior to placebo for the acute conversion of AFib.
    B. It controls ventricular rate during exercise in most patients.
    C. It can control ventricular rate at rest in many patients.
    D. It effectively maintains sinus rhythm after cardioversion.
    E. Because of its hepatic clearance, it is safe to use in patients with renal insufficiency.

74. Which of the following patients does *not* need anticoagulation with warfarin?

    A. a 71-year-old man with dilated cardiomyopathy and paroxysmal AFib
    B. a 74-year-old woman with chronic AFib who had ablation of the AV junction and a single-chamber permanent pacemaker
    C. a 40-year-old woman with paroxysmal AFib and hypertrophic cardiomyopathy
    D. a 35-year-old woman with mitral stenosis who underwent elective cardioversion 1 week ago
    E. a 45-year-old man with paroxysmal AFib and no structural heart disease

75. Which of the following statements regarding flecainide as a treatment of AFib is *true*?

    A. It may contribute to an increase in the digoxin level.
    B. It may be used without an AV nodal blocking agent because of its potent effect on the AV conduction system.
    C. It has been shown to be effective and safe for use in patients with hypertrophic cardiomyopathy.
    D. It has no effect on the acute conversion of AFib but only on maintenance of sinus rhythm postcardioversion.
    E. It is used for the treatment of AFib but not atrial flutter.

76. Which of the following mechanisms is responsible for AFib occurring in the immediate postoperative period after a maze procedure?

    A. change in the atrial refractory period as a result of the surgical manipulation
    B. autonomic imbalance as a result of the surgical intervention
    C. misplacement of a suture line
    D. an incomplete or omitted suture line
    E. inhibition of atrial natriuretic peptide secretion as a result of the surgical manipulation

77. Characteristics of arrhythmogenic RV dysplasia include all the following *except*

    A. fatty infiltration of the RV
    B. fatty infiltration of the right atrium
    C. monomorphic VT
    D. abnormal signal-averaged ECG
    E. it may be detected by cardiac MRI

78. Concerning the cardiac AP, all of the following are true *except*

A. The AP duration in the atrium is shorter than that in the ventricle.

B. Myocytes located within the ventricular myocardium (so-called M cells) have longer AP duration than those located in the endocardial region.

C. Phase 3 (repolarization) is predominantly mediated by the Na^+ outward current.

D. The transient outward current that mediated phase I of the AP is more prominent in atrial than ventricular myocytes.

E. In atrial and ventricular myocytes, phase 0 of the AP (depolarization) is mediated by the Na^+ inward current.

79. Which of the following statements is *not* true concerning anticoagulation and AFib?

A. In patients with chronic AFib, anticoagulation for 3 weeks is indicated before cardioversion.

B. If AFib has been present for less than 2 days, anticoagulation for 3 weeks is not considered necessary before cardioversion.

C. In patients with chronic AFib, if no atrial thrombi are detected by TEE, cardioversion may be performed while maintaining anticoagulation during and for at least 4 weeks after the procedure.

D. Patients with chronic AFib in whom pharmacologic conversion with ibutilide is planned need not be anticoagulated.

E. An international normalized ratio of 2:3 is considered an adequate anticoagulation level.

80. The following tachycardia was induced during EP testing of a 36-year-old woman with recurrent palpitations (Fig. 9).

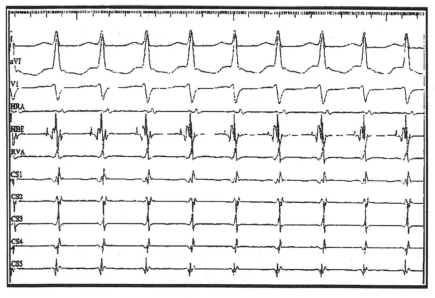

FIGURE 9

Which of the following is the most likely diagnosis?

A. AVNRT

B. orthodromic reentrant tachycardia

C. antidromic reentrant tachycardia

D. VT

E. idiopathic left VT

ANSWERS

1. A. Propafenone. Sotalol and dofetilide are primarily excreted by the renal route and should be used cautiously, if at all, in patients with significant renal insufficiency. Flecainide primarily undergoes hepatic elimination (approximately 70%) but has 25% renal elimination. The route of elimination for propafenone is 99% hepatic.

2. D. Amiodarone.

3. A. Amiodarone. Sotalol, dofetilide, and flecainide do not have significant active metabolites. Amiodarone is metabolized to the active metabolite, desethyl amiodarone.

4. B. The patient is taking dipyridamole. Dipyridamole potentiates the effect of adenosine by interfering with metabolism; therefore, a reduced dose of adenosine is recommended. An increased dose of adenosine is recommended in the presence of methylxanthines such as theophylline, which antagonizes the effect of adenosine (blocks receptors), and other factors such as slow circulation time, valvular regurgitation, and left-to-right shunts that reduce the effectiveness of adenosine.

5. D. All of the above. Several antiarrhythmic drugs may elevate digoxin serum concentrations, including quinidine, amiodarone, flecainide, propafenone, and calcium channel blockers.

6. C. Verapamil. Verapamil may increase serum levels of dofetilide due to interference with renal excretion and hepatic metabolism.

7. A. Dofetilide. Amiodarone has a mildly negative inotropic effect. Flecainide and sotalol have a moderately negative inotropic effect. Dofetilide does not have significant inotropic effects.

8. B. Flecainide. Flecainide is a class IC antiarrhythmic drug, and these agents exhibit "use dependence." This refers to the property of increased drug effect at increased heart rates. Sotalol and dofetilide are class III antiarrhythmic drugs that exhibit "reverse use dependence"—that is, greater drug effect at slower heart rates.

9. C. Antiarrhythmic drugs with reverse use dependence have greater efficacy for arrhythmia prevention than termination and have greater risk for ventricular proarrhythmia after AFib termination (at slower sinus rates) than during AFib. Antiarrhythmic drugs with use dependence, such as sotalol and dofetilide, have greater antiarrhythmic effect at slower heart rates. Consequently, drug efficacy is enhanced at the relatively slower rates in sinus rhythm, making these drugs more effective for prevention of AFib than those drugs with use dependence. Likewise, for proarrhythmia, the antiarrhythmic drugs with reverse-use dependence are more likely to produce ventricular proarrhythmia after conversion to sinus rhythm at the relatively slower sinus rate or with a postconversion pause.

10. C. The treatment drugs effectively suppressed PVCs. CAST studied the concept that PVC suppression in the postinfarction period would reduce the

incidence of sudden cardiac death. Patients without heart disease were, therefore, excluded from these studies. CAST I studied flecainide, encainide, and moricizine versus placebo. Demonstration of effective suppression of PVCs by one of the drugs was necessary before a patient could be randomized to drug or placebo treatment. Propafenone, another class IC antiarrhythmic drug, was not studied. CAST I was prematurely terminated by the safety committee after only a 10-month average follow-up due to significantly increased incidence of arrhythmic death and nonfatal cardiac arrests in the flecainide and encainide treatment groups. CAST II was a continuation of the study with only moricizine versus placebo, but this study was also terminated early due to an increased incidence of cardiac arrest in the moricizine treatment group.

11. A. Flecainide. All of these drugs are class I antiarrhythmic medications and have sodium channel–blocking properties to various degrees. The class IC agents, such as flecainide, have the most potent sodium channel–blocking effects, and the class IB agents, such as lidocaine, have the least potent sodium channel–blocking effects.

12. D. None of the above. Amiodarone increases serum digoxin and cyclosporine concentrations and enhances warfarin effect.

13. C. Mexiletine is not a Vaughn Williams class III drug. Mexiletine is a class IB antiarrhythmic drug.

14. C. Ibutilide. Ibutilide is the only antiarrhythmic drug approved by the FDA for acute pharmacologic conversion of AFib to sinus rhythm.

15. C. Enhanced effect. Patients with denervated hearts are supersensitive to the effects of adenosine.

16. B. Proarrhythmia with quinidine is idiosyncratic and not dose related. The other drugs listed have dose-related proarrhythmia.

17. C. PJRT. Regular narrow QRS tachycardias can be grouped into two categories based on the timing of the atrial and ventricular relationship during the arrhythmia—that is, the position of the P wave relative to the QRS or R wave. Tachycardias that have a shorter RP than PR interval are termed *short RP tachycardias,* and tachycardias that have a longer RP than PR interval are termed *long RP tachycardias.* Orthodromic AVRT is an accessory pathway–mediated reentrant tachycardia that uses the AV node as the antegrade limb and the accessory pathway as the retrograde limb of the arrhythmia circuit. The P wave, representing the retrograde activation of the atria, is generally seen just after the QRS complex within the ST segment and is, therefore, a short RP tachycardia. AVNRT in its typical form uses the AV-nodal slow pathway for the antegrade limb and the AV-nodal fast pathway for the retrograde limb of the arrhythmia circuit. The P wave, representing the retrograde activation of the atria, is, therefore, within or shortly after the QRS complex and is, therefore, a short RP tachycardia. Nonparoxysmal junctional tachycardia is an automatic or triggered arrhythmia that originates in the AV junction. The P wave may be just before, within, or just after the QRS complex. The permanent form of junctional reciprocating tachycardia is a special type of orthodromic AVRT that involves a posteroseptal accessory pathway with decremental (AV nodal-like) conduction properties. This decremental retrograde conduction property results in delay in the retro-

grade activation of the atria during the tachycardia, and, consequently, the P wave is seen well beyond the QRS/ST segment and closer to the next QRS complex (a long RP interval).

18. C. AVNRT. Atrial tachycardia and PJRT are long RP tachycardias and, therefore, would not have such a short VA interval. PJRT is a special type of orthodromic AVRT that involves a posteroseptal accessory pathway with decremental (AV nodal-like) conduction properties and, hence, has a long RP (long VA) interval. Due to the time required to reach the accessory pathway for the retrograde portion of the arrhythmia circuit, orthodromic AVRT generally has a VA interval longer than 70 msec. Therefore, a VA interval shorter than 70 msec excludes orthodromic AVRT and makes AVNRT the most likely diagnosis.

19. C. IV verapamil. A sudden onset of a regular narrow complex tachycardia with a cycle length of 375 msec and an RP interval of 100 msec is a short RP tachycardia (the PR interval would be 375 msec – 100 msec = 275 msec, so the RP is shorter than the PR). This patient most likely presents with orthodromic AV reentrant tachycardia, a reciprocating tachycardia circuit that involves antegrade conduction through the AV node and retrograde conduction through the accessory pathway (however, AV node reentrant tachycardia is also possible). As the AV node is a necessary component of the arrhythmia circuit, AV nodal blockade effectively terminates this type of tachycardia. Although not listed as an option in this exercise, vagal maneuvers, such as Valsalva, coughing, or carotid sinus massage, may be quite effective and avoid the potential risks associated with administration of medications. Verapamil and other drugs that block AV conduction, such as beta-blockers and adenosine, may be quite useful for termination of AV reentrant tachycardia. This should not be confused with the management of AFib in the setting of Wolff-Parkinson-White syndrome, in which administration of AV nodal blocking drugs, such as verapamil, is contraindicated. In that situation, IV procainamide or DC cardioversion is the correct management. A precautionary note regarding the use of adenosine for regular narrow QRS tachycardia in patients with Wolff-Parkinson-White syndrome: Adenosine may precipitate AFib and result in a very rapid ventricular response (preexcited tachycardia). Atropine has no role in the treatment of these types of arrhythmia. Catheter ablation is not generally an acute treatment option for this arrhythmia, although this approach may be an excellent option for chronic treatment (cure).

20. C. Orthodromic AVRT using a left-sided accessory pathway. A regular narrow QRS tachycardia that has VA interval prolongation with the development of bundle branch block is most consistent with an orthodromic AVRT using an accessory pathway ipsilateral to the bundle branch. During AVRT, the antegrade limb of the circuit is the AV node and His Purkinje/bundle branch system, and the retrograde limb is the accessory pathway. Block in a bundle branch ipsilateral to an accessory pathway creates a larger circuit, as the antegrade limb must now use the contralateral bundle branch, and, therefore, the VA interval increases. This results in an increase in the tachycardia cycle length (a slower tachycardia). Of note, a slower tachycardia with bundle branch block itself does not necessarily have the same significance. Other types of tachycardia may slow due to a change in conduction of other components of the tachycardia circuit, such as the conduction through the AV node (A-H interval). Thus, it is important to demonstrate VA

interval prolongation during bundle branch block to implicate an ipsilateral accessory pathway participating in AV reentrant tachycardia.

21. C. ICD implantation. Cardiac arrest with VT or VF in the absence of reversible causes (e.g., MI, severe electrolyte or metabolic disorders) is a class I indication for ICD implantation. ICD implantation for such patients is superior to amiodarone drug therapy, as demonstrated in the Antiarrhythmics Versus Implantable Defibrillator (AVID) trial. The Canadian Implantable Defibrillator Study examined a similar population of patients and, although not statistically significant, showed a strong trend for the superiority of ICDs. Demonstration of inducible VT or VF in these types of patients is not necessary.

22. B. Implantation of an ICD is indicated if an EP study shows inducible VT. The Multicenter Automatic Defibrillator Implantation Trial (MADIT) evaluated patients with CAD, ischemic cardiomyopathy with an LV EF of less than 35%, and nonsustained VT. This study showed that for patients with inducible VT at baseline EP study and after administration of IV procainamide, treatment with an ICD was superior to treatment with antiarrhythmic drugs. This is a class I indication for ICD implantation.

23. B. Biphasic shocks require less energy for cardioversion and defibrillation than monophasic shocks. All of the modern ICDs use biphasic-shock waveforms for cardioversion and defibrillation. All of the other statements about ICDs are true.

24. A. Modern ICD systems employ the pulse generator as a component of the shocking electrode configuration ("active can"). In general, the left-chest site for the pulse generator results in lower energy requirements for cardioversion and defibrillation.

25. D. Place a "donut" magnet over the ICD site. The patient is having inappropriate or spurious shocks from the ICD, most likely due to detection of electrical noise from a malfunction of the ICD lead. It is imperative that further shocks be prevented immediately, not only for patient comfort, but also to prevent induction of life-threatening ventricular arrhythmias (including ventricular arrhythmia storm) due to the ICD shocks. The most effective action at this point is placement of a magnet over the ICD site. This prevents the ICD from delivering any therapies. It would not be optimal to delay the prevention of further shocks while waiting for an ICD programmer. Of note, unlike pacemakers, ICDs do not have an asynchronous pacing response to application of a magnet.

26. C. A 60-year-old man with CAD, prior MI, LV dysfunction, and incessant sustained VT would not be a candidate for ICD implantation. Incessant VT is a contraindication to ICD implantation. An ICD in this situation would lead to an excessive number of shocks. Better control of the arrhythmia would be necessary before ICD implantation could be considered. An ICD may be indicated for some patients with certain familial or inherited conditions with a high risk for life-threatening ventricular tachyarrhythmias, such as congenital long-QT syndrome or hypertrophic cardiomyopathy. Patients who survive a cardiac arrest due to VF without reversible causes are candidates for ICD implantation, even with comorbid conditions such as cancer, unless the life expectancy is 6 months or shorter.

27. B. Early DC-shock defibrillation. The two most crucial factors that determine the value of out-of-hospital resuscitation for patients who experience sudden cardiac death are citizen-bystander cardiopulmonary resuscitation and early DC-shock defibrillation.

28. A. Asystole. EMD or PEA and, in particular, asystole tend to be found in increasing proportions as the time since arrest increases. This is likely due to degeneration of prolonged VF. When VF is the documented rhythm at the time of resuscitation, the long-term survival is approximately 25%. When EMD or PEA is the documented rhythm, the long-term survival rate drops to approximately 6%, and it drops even further, to approximately 1%, when asystole is documented.

29. D. VF. The initial rhythm documented in a patient who undergoes sudden cardiac death is dependent on the time elapsed since the arrest. Most episodes of sudden cardiac death (approximately 65% to 85%) that are documented electrocardiographically are due to malignant ventricular arrhythmias such as VF. Monomorphic VT is uncommonly documented as a cause of out-of-hospital sudden cardiac death, perhaps due to degeneration of unstable VT to VF. Asystole and EMD or PEA are found in greater proportions as the time since arrest increases, as these rhythms are likely the result of prolonged VF.

30. D. All of the above. Multiple ICD shocks in a short period ("cluster shocks") may occur from all of the conditions listed. The absence of symptoms is not a reliable method of discriminating between these causes.

31. D. Diuretics. The treatment of vasovagal syncope is generally focused on volume maintenance and expansion (fluids, salt supplementation, mineralocorticoids) and vasoconstriction (midodrine). Diuretics are, therefore, to be avoided, as the relative hypovolemia produced by these drugs may exacerbate episodes of vasovagal syncope. Beta-blocker medications may be useful for suppressing the triggering events of the vasovagal episodes. Cardiac pacing for patients with frequent vasovagal syncopal episodes has recently been shown to be effective for suppression of these episodes in a randomized clinical trial, the North American Vasovagal Pacemaker Study.

32. D. All of the above are true. A carefully performed initial evaluation has been reported to provide an etiology for syncope in 50% to 60% of cases. This evaluation includes a detailed medical history (including history from witnesses to the event), physical examination, basic hematologic and biochemical studies, and an ECG. Neurally mediated syncope is the most common cause of syncope, particularly in the absence of structural heart disease.

33. B. Beta-blocker medications. Several randomized trials of the use of beta-blocker medications for patients after MI have shown efficacy for the prevention of sudden cardiac death (including propranolol, timolol, metoprolol, and acebutolol). Trials of amiodarone in this setting have provided mixed results. Two large randomized trials, the European Myocardial Infarct Amiodarone Trial (EMIAT) and the Canadian Amiodarone Myocardial Infarction Arrhythmia Trial (CAMIAT), examined the use of amiodarone in patients after MI and did not show a reduction in overall mortality with the use of amiodarone. The Polish Amiodarone trial showed that amiodarone improved survival only in

patients with preserved LV function after MI. The Survival with Oral D-sotalol (SWORD) trial studied the use of the D-isomer of sotalol (D-sotalol) in patients with recent MI and LV dysfunction. This study found worse survival in the group treated with D-sotalol that in the group treated with placebo. The Danish Investigations of Arrhythmias and Mortality on Dofetilide (DIAMOND) studies showed that dofetilide had a neutral effect on total mortality compared with placebo in the treatment of post–MI patients with LV dysfunction.

34. B. CAD. CAD is the predominant disease process associated with sudden cardiac death in the United States, accounting for 64% to 90% of cases. The other cardiomyopathies, such as dilated and hypertrophic cardiomyopathies, together account for approximately 10% to 15% of cases of sudden cardiac death.

35. C. Head-upright tilt table testing. Syncope in the absence of structural heart disease is most likely neurally mediated (vasovagal). The head-upright tilt table test is the most appropriate test to evaluate for this condition. This test initiates the vasovagal episode by maximizing venous pooling, sympathetic activation, and circulating catecholamines. In general, the test involves at least 30 min of 70-degree head-up tilt angle without a saddle support. An addition of a catecholamine challenge with isoproterenol is sometimes used. Among symptomatic patients, the sensitivity of the head-upright tilt table test is approximately 85%. The specificity of the head-upright tilt table test is good, with the frequency of an abnormal tilt table test in control subjects being 0% to 15%. In the absence of structural heart disease, EP study, ambulatory Holter monitoring, and the signal-averaged ECG are low yield.

36. C. Combination of cardioinhibitory and vasodepressor. Vasovagal syncopal episodes may be classified according to the response of the BP and heart rate during an episode. Predominant cardioinhibition involves an episode in which the drop in heart rate is the prevailing event, whereas a vasodepressor response involves an episode in which the drop in BP is the prevailing event. Most vasovagal syncopal episodes are of the mixed variety. Note that the same patient may have any of these types of vasovagal responses with each episode.

37. D. None of the above. No further evaluation or treatment is indicated for an asymptomatic patient with intermittent ventricular preexcitation. In an asymptomatic patient with a manifest accessory pathway (i.e., Wolff-Parkinson-White pattern by ECG), the main concern is risk stratification. With such patients, there may be an increased risk of sudden cardiac death due to very rapid ventricular response across the accessory pathway during AFib. Demonstration of intermittent preexcitation by ambulatory Holter monitoring or by exercise treadmill testing indicates that the accessory pathway does not support very rapid 1:1 AV conduction, and, hence, the likelihood of sudden cardiac death from AFib would be low.

38. A. AVNRT. An "r prime" in lead V1 during regular narrow complex tachycardia that is not present during sinus rhythm indicates the inscription of the P wave in the terminal QRS, and this is very specific for AVNRT.

39. C. DC cardioversion is not an effective treatment for MAT. The other statements about MAT are true. If correction of the underlying condition is not effective or not possible, then treatment with calcium channel blockers and supplementation with potassium or magnesium may be effective. Treatment

with beta-blocker medications may be problematic for patients with chronic pulmonary disease.

40. D. All of the above are true. All of the statements about head-upright tilt table testing are true.

41. C. Arc welding equipment may not be safely used. Normally functioning electrical power tools and home appliances usually have no effect on modern pacemakers. However, arc welding produces a strong electromagnetic field, which may result in pacemaker inhibition or noise reversion, and should be avoided in pacemaker-dependent patients. Other potential sources of interference include MRI imaging, lithotripsy, and betatron radiation.

42. D. Permanent pacemaker implant. This patient has evidence of symptomatic bradycardia on Holter monitoring, which constitutes a class I indication for permanent pacemaker placement. He has AV conduction system disease with no obvious reversible causes, which is most probably due to idiopathic fibrosis (Lev's disease). Prolonged monitoring will probably show more episodes of bradycardia, which was already seen during telemetry and which places this elderly patient at risk for syncope and injury. EP testing for ventricular arrhythmia is not indicated in view of the absence of structural heart disease. Likewise, ICD is not indicated.

43. D. Single-chamber system in the ventricle programmed to VVIR. This patient is in chronic AFib, and, therefore, physiologic pacing in the atrium cannot be achieved. Furthermore, conversion and long-term maintenance of sinus rhythm in this situation are very unlikely. Therefore, there is no indication for placement of an atrial lead. DDDR with mode switching and DDIR will behave like a VVIR system in this patient, at the expense, however, of an additional lead (atrial) and a more expensive dual-chamber pacemaker.

44. A. Pacemaker syndrome is caused by pacing the ventricle asynchronously, which results in AV dissociation or VA conduction. Symptoms consist of fatigue, dizziness, dyspnea, and weakness, with or without hypotension. The mechanism is believed to be related in part to atrial contraction against a closed AV valve and release of atrial natriuretic peptide. It occurs with ventricular pacing and is, therefore, worsened by increasing pacing rate and relieved by allowing intrinsic conduction (if present) by lowering the pacing rate, programming rate hysteresis, or upgrading to a dual-chamber system. Therapy with fludrocortisone and other volume-expansion modalities is not helpful.

45. B. Dual-chamber pacing in hypertrophic cardiomyopathy alters activation of the septum and has been shown echocardiographically to increase the LV end-systolic dimension without changing the LV end-diastolic dimension. It also reduces the LV outflow gradient; this can persist for up to 2 months after discontinuation of pacing. MR was also shown to decrease, a finding that is also related to change in septal activation.

46. D. A 73-year-old man with chronic AFib and a ventricular rate of 40 bpm during peak treadmill test. The 73-year-old man with AFib and slow ventricular rate during exercise is the classic example of SSS. This usually indicates degenerative disease of the cardiac conduction system involving the AV node as well as the sinus node. The finding of sinus arrhythmia varying by 15 bpm in an older patient, the profound nocturnal bradycardia in young

athletes, and the sinus pauses in young patients are related mostly to a high vagal tone and do not indicate sinus node disease.

47. E. Induce CHB. Patients with true complete LBBB are at risk for developing transient CHB during catheter manipulation in the septal region of the tricuspid valve. This is due to transient traumatic block of the right bundle branch.

48. E. IV glucagon. This patient has an overdose of diltiazem and metoprolol. These drugs slow sinoatrial and AV conduction. Calcium and magnesium have no effect in reversing these bradycardic effects. Isuprel and atropine are not likely to overcome the beta-blockade of metoprolol. IV glucagon acts on a specific receptor. This results in an increase in intracellular cyclic adenosine monophosphate, which enhances both sinoatrial and AV node conduction despite the presence of beta-blockade.

49. A. Intraatrial reentry. The mechanism of typical atrial flutter has been shown to be related to a reentrant circus movement, most commonly in the right atrium along the tricuspid valve, involving the posterior cavotricuspid isthmus. Radiofrequency ablation of this isthmus is an effective treatment. Early afterdepolarizations are related to conditions that prolong repolarization, such as arrhythmia in the long-QT syndrome. Delayed afterdepolarizations are usually related to digoxin toxicity.

50. D. Administration of sodium-containing solution. Amitriptyline has sodium channel blocking properties and induced QRS widening and VT. Increasing the extracellular sodium concentration by the administration of sodium-containing solution decreases the association of this drug with the sodium channel.

51. B. K^+ channel blockade with increase in QRS duration. Like other QT-prolonging drugs, terfenadine (a nonsedating H_1-receptor blocker) has K^+ channel–blocking properties, which delay myocardial repolarization and predispose to a specific form of polymorphic VT: TdP. Exacerbating factors include, among others, baseline QT prolongation, concomitant ingestion of other QT-prolonging drugs, and hypokalemia.

52. C. Verapamil IV bolus. Adenosine is commonly used to terminate SVT. However, this patient is on theophylline, which is an effective blocker of adenosine receptor. Propafenone might be poorly tolerated by this patient because of its associated beta-blocking activity, which might increase airway resistance. Digoxin shortens the refractory period of the atrium and might potentially accelerate an atrial tachycardia. Immediate cardioversion is not needed, as the patient appears hemodynamically stable, and it would be reasonable to attempt pharmacologic therapy initially with verapamil.

53. D. This rhythm shows evidence of atrial undersensing. The pacemaker is programmed to DDD. In this mode, an appropriately sensed P wave should cause inhibition of the atrial spike; a ventricular spike is then delivered after the programmed AV interval or inhibited by an intrinsic R wave. In this strip, the P wave is present in each complex. However, in complexes 2, 4, 6, and 8, an atrial spike follows the intrinsic P wave because the intrinsic P wave was not appropriately sensed by the pacemaker.

54. E. Obtain a CXR to document atrial-lead dislodgment and reposition the lead. Atrial undersensing occurring early after implantation commonly

results from lead dislodgment. Other possibilities include inappropriate programmed sensitivity and lead maturation process, which usually occurs at 2 to 4 weeks postimplant. This event occurred very early postimplant, making lead maturation an unlikely possibility. Atrial sensitivity is already programmed to the most sensitive setting available on most pacemakers. In this case, CXR confirmed lead dislodgment, and the lead was repositioned, with adequate pacing and capture thresholds confirmed on follow-up.

55. C. Pacemaker-mediated tachycardia. In this strip, there is evidence of atrial undersensing (fifth complex) with loss of AV synchrony. This causes retrograde P-wave conduction, which is sensed by the pacer (because of short programmed PVARP), and results in ventricular pacing, causing a pacemaker-mediated tachycardia or endless-loop tachycardia. Acute treatment of this condition includes the application of a magnet to inhibit atrial sensing, thereby breaking the tachycardia loop. The spontaneous termination of these episodes in this patient are most probably related to intermittent atrial undersensing, which interrupts the tachycardia loop. Further prevention of these episodes includes reprogramming the PVARP, AV delay, or atrial sensitivity. Pacemaker-mediated tachycardia is an abnormal consequence of normal pacemaker function.

56. A. A CXR should be obtained to check atrial-lead position. On the magnet mode, there are AV sequential spikes, with capture of the ventricle by the atrial stimulus. So, the programmed mode is DDD. In the nonmagnet mode, there is no atrial sensing, with only ventricular pacing. This strongly suggests that the recently placed atrial lead has dislodged into the ventricle. A CXR will be diagnostic. The other possibility is swapping of the atrial and ventricular leads, but one might expect atrial capture with the second stimulus in the magnet mode, which is not the case.

57. A. The initial rhythm strip shows background AFib with VVI pacing, most probably related to automatic mode switch. The absence of atrial pacing suggests adequate atrial sensing (of the fibrillation), which resulted in the mode switch behavior. Atrial pacing cannot be determined in the presence of AFib. There is adequate ventricular sensing, as determined on the nonmagnet strip (th complex); however, there is intermittent ventricular capture noted.

58. A. CHB at the level of the AV node. In this tracing, there are background NSR with CHB and a narrow escape rhythm that is junctional in origin. This is apparent in the HBE tracing, in which the atrial deflections are completely dissociated from the H-V deflections. Therefore, the atrial impulse entering the AV node is not conducting down to the His bundle (A is not followed by His potential), indicating that the level of block is at the level of the AV node.

59. B. CHB at the infra-Hisian (below the His bundle) level. In this tracing, there is background NSR with CHB and a relatively wide escape rhythm. In the HBE tracing, each atrial deflection is followed by an initial His deflection and a third, smaller deflection, H', indicating that there is conduction delay within the His bundle itself. This is suggestive of significant His-Purkinje conduction disease. Therefore, the atrial impulse enters the AV node, conducts down to the His bundle (normal AH interval), where it encounters conduction delay (HH'), and then fails to propagate to the ventricle, indicating that the level of block is at or below the level of the bundle of His. There is obvious AV dissociation with a ventricular escape rhythm.

60. D. Second-degree AV block at an infra-Hisian level. In this tracing, the surface ECG shows NSR with 2:1 AV block. The HBE tracing shows constant AH with 2:1 block below the level of the His bundle.

61. D. Second-degree AV block at an infra-Hisian level. In this tracing, the surface ECG shows NSR with second-degree type I AV block (Wenckebach). Because the QRS is wide, this type of block is usually localized either to the AV node or within or below the His bundle. In this situation, the HBE tracing shows progressive prolongation in the HV interval before it blocks in a 3:2 conduction pattern. Therefore, the conduction delay is not at the level of the AV node but at or below the His bundle. As opposed to Wenckebach in the AV node, which is usually benign in nature, this type of infra-Hisian block indicates His-Purkinje conduction system disease and is an indication for pacemaker placement, as it may progress to CHB.

62. B. Obtaining a two-view (anteroposterior and lateral) CXR to evaluate lead position. The presence of an RBBB-paced QRS complex pattern suggests that the ventricular lead is in the LV. The lead may enter the LV through an atrial or VSD or via perforation of the interventricular septum. It may also be inadvertently introduced into an artery and passed retrogradely through the aortic valve. Another possibility is placement into one of the LV branches of the coronary sinus. Although sometimes an apical position in the RV in a rotated heart can potentially give an RBBB paced pattern, a two-view CXR should be obtained to rule out LV positioning. A single-view portable AP will not distinguish an LV from an apical RV placement. If LV placement is confirmed on the lateral radiograph, repositioning of the lead is indicated.

63. D. Patients with evidence of infra-Hisian block during EP testing should be considered for permanent pacing. Patients with symptomatic CHB do not need EP testing because the decision for a permanent pacemaker is already made. The sensitivity and specificity of sinus node recovery time is approximately 70%, making this test less than ideal; in most cases, the decision as to whether to implant a pacemaker in cases of suspected sinus node dysfunction depends on symptoms and correlation with ambulatory monitoring rather than results of EP testing. Patients with infra-Hisian block tend to have an unpredictable course and should be considered for permanent pacing.

64. A. Brugada's syndrome has been described worldwide but is most common in Asian countries and is the leading cause of death in young men in part of Thailand. It is characterized by ST-segment elevation and an IRBBB pattern in the right precordial leads. These features can be induced with sodium channel blockers such as flecainide or ajmaline. (Sotalol is a potassium channel blocker.) It is believed to be related to a mutation in the sodium channel gene. It is associated with a high incidence of sudden cardiac death resulting from VF. Risk assessment and therapy appear to be poorly defined at this time, but the implantation of an ICD has been advocated.

65. B. The pathognomic arrhythmia associated with long-QT syndrome is TdP. The mechanism is believed to be related to early afterdepolarization and triggered activity. Sotalol causes QT prolongation and is contraindicated in patients with long QT. Hypokalemia, not hyperkalemia, is associated with an increase of TdP in this situation. EP testing is of no value and is not indicated for the risk stratification of patients with long-QT syndrome. Cardiac arrest occurs typically with vigorous activity and infrequently during sleep.

66. C. You should perform EP testing to evaluate the AV conduction system. The patient had an episode of near syncope, which could be related to his GI bleeding, but the possibility of intermittent heart block in the setting of bifascicular block cannot be ruled out. This is a class I indication for EP testing to evaluate AV conduction. If there is evidence of abnormally prolonged HV interval, then a permanent pacemaker should be considered. There is no indication for ICD placement in this setting. Beta-blockers would blunt a reactive tachycardia resulting from the patient's anemia.

67. E. There is AV dissociation. In patients presenting with wide complex tachycardia, the presence of AV dissociation is highly specific for VT. All the other listed parameters suffer from significant overlap between SVT and VT.

68. C. Procainamide, 15 mg/kg IV over 30 to 60 min. Wide complex tachycardia occurring after MI is most likely to be VT. Verapamil is contraindicated in this setting, as it might lead to hypotension and VF. DC cardioversion can be used if the patient does not respond to antiarrhythmic therapy or if he becomes hemodynamically unstable. Procainamide is the drug of choice because it treats ventricular as well as supraventricular arrhythmia. There is no role for digoxin and no need for urgent cardiac catheterization in this situation.

69. B. To admit the patient for IV antibiotics and pacemaker system extraction. This presentation is consistent with pacemaker-system infection, which occurred following the recent pulse generator replacement. Antibiotics PO or IV without extraction of the pacemaker system have limited efficacy in eradicating the infection. The patient should undergo pacemaker-system extraction, followed by IV antibiotics, until negative blood cultures are obtained. A new pacemaker system can then be implanted on the right side.

70. C. Inadequate synchronization may occur with peaked T waves, low-amplitude signal, and malfunctioning pacemakers. Cardioversion is the delivery of electric energy synchronized on the R wave. A synchronized shock should be used in AFib. A nonsynchronized shock may result in VF. Improper synchronization may occur in a situation in which more than one peaked signal exists, such as with pacemakers and peaked T waves. On the other hand, a low QRS signal may not synchronize at all. In patients with pacemakers, the pads are positioned at least 3 in. away from the pulse generator to minimize damage. MI and digoxin intake are not contraindications for DC cardioversion as long as digoxin toxicity is not suspected.

71. D. Procainamide. Procainamide can slow down conduction across the accessory pathway and potentially converts AFib. Diltiazem (Cardizem) and verapamil cause hypotension and reflex increase in sympathetic activation and may result in increased ventricular response. Adenosine is of no use in this setting. Lidocaine has little effect on the refractory period of the accessory pathway.

72. E. Amiodarone. Amiodarone may allow maintenance of sinus rhythm in patients with AFib and cardiomyopathy. In low doses, the side effects are minimized. Flecainide and disopyramide are not used in patients with cardiomyopathy because of their potential for proarrhythmia and their negative inotropic effects. Verapamil is not effective for maintenance of sinus rhythm. Sotalol might not be tolerated in patients with heart failure and has the potential for proarrhythmia in patients on diuretics prone to hypokalemia.

73. C. Digoxin can control the ventricular rate at rest in patients with AFib, but not with exercise. It is as effective as placebo for the acute conversion of AFib and does not help in maintaining NSR.

74. E. A 45-year-old man with paroxysmal AFib and no structural heart disease. The risk of stroke in patients younger than 60 years of age and with a normal heart is low and does not warrant anticoagulation. Patients with structural heart disease, such as ischemic, dilated, or hypertrophic cardiomyopathy, have a significant risk of stroke and should be anticoagulated if there are no contraindications otherwise. After AV junction ablation, AFib persists, and anticoagulation should be continued. Anticoagulation should be continued for at least 4 weeks postcardioversion, as atrial function does not normalize immediately after restoration of normal rhythm.

75. A. It may contribute to an increase in the digoxin level. Flecainide [amiodarone, propafenone (Rythmol), and verapamil] can increase digoxin level. Flecainide can regularize and slow the atrial rhythm in patients with AFib and can, therefore, lead to increased ventricular response because of improved conduction of the atrial impulses through the AV node. It is, therefore, important to use an AV nodal blocking agent in patients with AFib treated with flecainide. It is used for AFib as well as flutter. There are no definite data on its safety in patients with hypertrophic cardiomyopathy. It is effective for acute conversion as well as maintenance of NSR postconversion.

76. A. Change in the atrial refractory period as a result of the surgical manipulation. The occurrence of AFib post–cardiac surgery is believed to be related to shortening of the refractory period of atrial tissue as it recovers from surgical manipulation, cardioplegia, and, potentially, ischemia. This nonuniformity of recovery results in reentry as the mechanism of AFib.

77. B. Fatty infiltration of the right atrium is not a characteristic of arrhythmogenic RV dysplasia. Arrhythmogenic RV dysplasia refers to fatty infiltration or deposition of the myocardium. It involves predominantly the RV and may extend to involve the LV. The atrial myocardium is not involved. MRI scanning has been used for diagnosis and follow-up of this condition. Late potentials and VT arising predominantly from the RV are typical findings. Treatment with sotalol, radiofrequency ablation, or ICD placement depends on the degree of ventricular involvement and the presenting spectrum of arrhythmia.

78. C. All the other statements are true concerning the AP.

79. D. In patients with AFib of longer than 3 days' duration, anticoagulation should be used for 3 weeks before electrical or pharmacologic cardioversion and continued for at least 4 weeks after conversion, keeping a therapeutic international normalized ratio level of 2:3. TEE-guided cardioversion has recently been shown to be safe, provided anticoagulation is maintained during and for 4 weeks after cardioversion. Anticoagulation is not required before cardioversion if AFib is known to be of shorter than 48 hours' duration.

80. A. This tracing shows AVNRT. It is a narrow complex tachycardia using the slow pathway of the AV node in the antegrade direction (long AH) and the fast pathway of the AV node in the retrograde direction (short HA). It is unlikely to be orthodromic reentrant tachycardia in which the retrograde

limb of the circuit is an accessory pathway, because the QRS-A time is very short, not long enough to involve ventricular activation as part of the circuit. Because the QRS is narrow, VT is not a likely diagnosis. Idiopathic LV-VT can sometimes be narrow but has an RBBB morphology on the surface ECG.

SUGGESTED READING

Budaj A, Kokowicz P, Smielak-Korombel W, et al. Lack of effect of amiodarone on survival after extensive infarction. Polish Amiodarone Trial. *Coron Artery Dis* 1996;7: 315–319.

Cairns JA, Connolly SJ, Roberts R, et al. Randomised trial of outcome after myocardial infarction in patients with frequent or repetitive ventricular premature depolarisations: CAMIAT. Canadian Amiodarone Myocardial Infarction Arrhythmia Trial Investigators [published erratum appears in *Lancet* 1997;349(9067):1776]. *Lancet* 1997;349:675–682.

Connolly SJ, Gent M, Roberts RS, et al. Canadian Implantable Defibrillator Study (CIDS): study design and organization. CIDS Co-Investigators. *Am J Cardiol* 1993;72:103F–108F.

Connolly SJ, Sheldon R, Roberts RS, et al. The North American Vasovagal Pacemaker Study (VPS). A randomized trial of permanent cardiac pacing for the prevention of vasovagal syncope. *J Am Coll Cardiol* 1999;33:16–20.

Julian DG, Camm AJ, Frangin G, et al. Randomised trial of effect of amiodarone on mortality in patients with left-ventricular dysfunction after recent myocardial infarction: EMIAT. European Myocardial Infarct Amiodarone Trial Investigators [published erratum appears in *Lancet* 1997;349(9059):1180 and 1997;349(9067):1776]. *Lancet* 1997; 349:667–674.

Moller M. DIAMOND antiarrhythmic trials. Danish Investigations of Arrhythmia and Mortality on Dofetilide. *Lancet* 1996;348:1597–1598.

Moss AJ, Hall WJ, Cannom DS, et al. Improved survival with an implanted defibrillator in patients with coronary disease at high risk for ventricular arrhythmia. Multicenter Automatic Defibrillator Implantation Trial Investigators. *N Engl J Med* 1996;335: 1933–1940.

The Antiarrhythmics Versus Implantable Defibrillators (AVID) Investigators. A comparison of antiarrhythmic-drug therapy with implantable defibrillators in patients resuscitated from near-fatal ventricular arrhythmias. *N Engl J Med* 1997;337:1576–1583.

The Cardiac Arrhythmia Suppression Trial (CAST) Investigators. Preliminary report: effect of encainide and flecainide on mortality in a randomized trial of arrhythmia suppression after myocardial infarction. *N Engl J Med* 1989;321:406–412.

The Cardiac Arrhythmia Suppression Trial II Investigators. Effect of the antiarrhythmic agent moricizine on survival after myocardial infarction. *N Engl J Med* 1992;327:227–233.

Waldo AL, Camm AJ, de Ruyter H, et al. Survival with oral D-sotalol in patients with left ventricular dysfunction after myocardial infarction: rationale, design, and methods (the SWORD trial). *Am J Cardiol* 1995;75:1023–1027.

CHAPTER 2

Valvular Heart Disease

Maran Thamilarasan

QUESTIONS

Case 1 (Questions 1–3)

A 35-year-old woman is referred to your office for a murmur heard during a routine physical examination. She is asymptomatic. She jogs 2 to 3 miles per day without problems. She had frequent febrile illnesses as a child, but her medical history is otherwise unremarkable.

Physical Examination

BP is 120/70 mm Hg.
Heart rate is 73 bpm.
She is in no acute distress.
Her jugular venous pulse is not elevated.
Her lungs are clear.
The point of maximum impulse (PMI) is not displaced. Rate and rhythm are regular. S_1 is increased in intensity. S_2 is normal. A high-pitched diastolic sound is heard; it is heard best between the apex and left sternal border, 0.12 sec after S_2. No murmur is heard.
There is no organomegaly.
There is no edema. Distal pulses are normal. There is good capillary refill.

1. Which of the following maneuvers would be most useful in helping to confirm your diagnosis?

    A. Valsalva
    B. exercise
    C. squatting
    D. handgrip

2. After exercise, a short, decrescendo, low-pitched diastolic murmur is heard over the apex, ending by mid-diastole. A TTE is obtained. Which of the following would you not expect to find?

   A. a mitral pressure halftime of 230 msec
   B. a planimetered mitral valve area of 1.7 cm^2
   C. a maximum velocity of the tricuspid insufficiency jet of 2.1 m per sec
   D. a mean mitral gradient of 4 mm Hg

3. The TTE reveals classic rheumatic changes of the mitral valve. The mitral valve area is 1.8 cm^2 by planimetry, the pressure halftime is 110 msec, and the mean gradient is 3 mm Hg. The left atrial dimension is 3.7 cm (the planimetered area in the apical four-chamber view is 15.0 cm^2). LV and RV function are normal. Which of the following is appropriate?

   A. endocarditis prophylaxis alone
   B. endocarditis prophylaxis alone plus warfarin
   C. stress echocardiography to assess PA pressures poststress
   D. digoxin therapy

Case 2 (Questions 4–5)

The same patient is referred back to your office 5 years later for a follow-up evaluation. She denies any symptoms but is no longer exercising.

Physical Examination

She remains in sinus rhythm.
S_1 remains loud; the opening snap is still quite audible (0.10 sec after S_2). The murmur is now heard at rest and is longer.
A repeat TTE reveals a mitral valve area of 1.3 cm^2 with an estimated resting PA pressure of 35 mm Hg.
The splittability score is given as 6.
LV size and function are normal.

4. Which of the following would be the most reasonable next step in management?

   A. immediate referral for surgery
   B. immediate referral for percutaneous valvuloplasty
   C. stress TTE to assess for mitral and pulmonary pressures poststress
   D. follow-up in 5 years

5. A stress TTE is performed. The patient exercises for 6 METS. Her RV systolic pressure poststress is estimated at 70 mm Hg. Which of the following would be an appropriate next step?

   A. consideration for percutaneous valvuloplasty
   B. mitral valve replacement
   C. start a beta-blocker and return for follow-up in another 2 years
   D. start digoxin

6. A 50-year-old woman presents to you for evaluation. She reports easy fatigability as well as abdominal fullness and right-upper-quadrant pain. She also notes marked swelling in her legs. She has recently been diagnosed with asthma and is also undergoing evaluation for recurrent diarrhea.

BP is 100/60 mm Hg.

Heart rate is 96 bpm.

There is elevation in jugular venous pressure, with a large *a* wave and a prominent *v* wave.

Her lungs are clear.

There is a nondisplaced PMI. The rhythm is regular. S_1 and S_2 (including P_2) are normal. A diastolic murmur is heard along the sternal border, which increases with inspiration. A pansystolic murmur is also heard in this area.

Hepatomegaly is present, along with ascites and peripheral edema.

What is the most likely cause of this patient's signs and symptoms?

A. rheumatic heart disease
B. carcinoid
C. primary pulmonary hypertension
D. cirrhosis of the liver secondary to chronic hepatitis

7. A 60-year-old man presents to the emergency room with reports of weakness, lethargy, and severe dyspnea. One week before, his family noted that he reported chest pressure that lasted for several hours.

He appears to be experiencing respiratory distress.

BP is 80/50 mm Hg.

Heart rate is 130 bpm.

O_2 saturation is 87% on room air.

Chest examination reveals diffuse crackles.

Cardiac examination reveals a nondisplaced PMI. S_3 and S_4 are heard, as is an apical systolic murmur. No thrill is present.

An ECG reveals inferior Q waves without ST-segment elevation. He is urgently intubated and pressors are started. An IABP is placed.

A surface TTE reveals a normal-sized left atrium and a mild jet of MR.

Which test should you perform first?

A. cardiac catheterization
B. TEE
C. right-heart catheterization with an O_2 saturation run
D. administration of thrombolytic therapy

Case 3 (Questions 8–9)

A 65-year-old woman presents to your office for follow-up of a murmur she was told about several years before. She denies any symptoms but is not very active. Her past medical history is significant for hypertension and diabetes, both of which have been well controlled.

Physical Examination

She is in no acute distress.

BP is 125/75 mm Hg.

Resting heart rate is 70 bpm.

Her lungs are clear.

Cardiac examination reveals a displaced PMI. S_1 is soft. S_2 reveals an increased P_2 component. There is an RV lift. An S_3 is present. There is a grade III/VI holosystolic murmur heard at the apex radiating to the base.

She has no peripheral edema.

CXR demonstrates cardiomegaly with prominence of the central pulmonary vasculature.

8. A TTE is performed on this patient (Fig. 1).

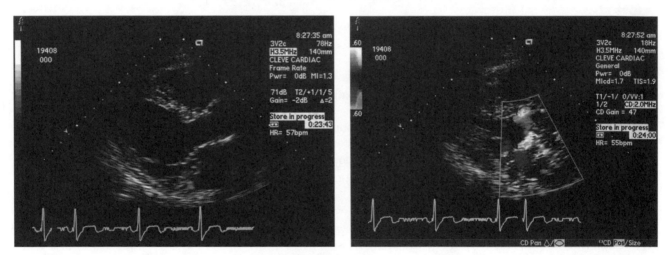

FIGURE 1

The LV systolic dimension is 4.7 cm. The EF is 45%. There is posterior leaflet prolapse. There is a very eccentric jet of MR, which is read out as 2+. Which of the following is most likely?

A. MR is unlikely to account for her presentation.

B. She likely has more severe MR than is evident on the TTE.

C. Her LV function is better than it appears on the TTE.

D. TEE is unlikely to be helpful here.

9. What should you recommend next?

A. a stress TTE to assess LV and PA pressures poststress

B. mitral valve surgery

C. starting an angiotensin-converting enzyme inhibitor (ACEI) and reassessing in 3 months

D. starting a beta-blocker

Case 4 (Questions 10–12)

A 75-year-old woman with a history of rheumatic fever presents for evaluation of significant progressive exertional dyspnea. She is no longer able to climb one flight of stairs without severe dyspnea.

Physical Examination

The patient is normotensive.

Heart rate is 70 bpm.

A malar flush is present.

Jugular venous pressure is elevated with prominent CV waves.

An RV lift is present.

Rhythm is regular.

An opening snap is barely audible, which occurs 0.07 sec after S_2. P_2 is increased. A pandiastolic rumble is heard. A high-pitched holosystolic murmur is heard at the lower sternal border that increases with inspiration.

CXR reveals an enlarged left atrium with significant calcification seen on the mitral apparatus.

A TTE is performed (Fig. 2).

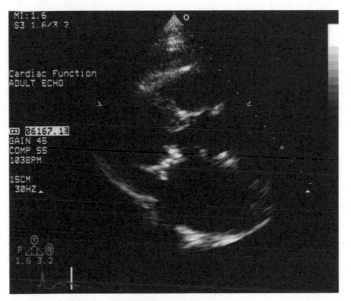

FIGURE 2

10. Which of the following would be appropriate management?

    A. mitral valve replacement
    B. mitral valve replacement with tricuspid annuloplasty
    C. percutaneous valvuloplasty
    D. digoxin and beta-blocker therapy
    E. tricuspid annuloplasty

11. If she undergoes mitral valve replacement, which valve should you recommend?

    A. bioprosthetic valve
    B. mechanical valve
    C. mitral homograft

12. The above patient refuses surgical or percutaneous intervention. Which of the following would *not* be a possible indication to initiate anticoagulation therapy with warfarin?

    A. the development of paroxysmal AFib
    B. a TIA
    C. left atrial size greater than 55 mm
    D. NSR and a left atrial size of 4.4 cm

Case 5 (Questions 13–14)

A 28-year-old man is referred to your office for a second opinion regarding his hypertension.

Physical Examination

He is in no acute distress.
BP is 160/90 mm Hg, symmetric in both arms.
Heart rate is 75 bpm.
Cardiac examination reveals a nondisplaced PMI. S_1 is normal. It is followed by a high-pitched sound widely transmitted throughout the precordium. A short II/VI systolic ejection murmur is heard. S_2 is normal.

13. What is the most important diagnostic maneuver to perform next?
    A. check plasma catecholamines
    B. check serum potassium level
    C. check lower extremity BP
    D. check plasma cortisol levels
    E. 24-hour BP recording

14. The above patient is treated appropriately and does well. Three years later, he presents to the emergency room with acute chest pain radiating to his back. He is hypotensive on presentation. An ECG reveals T-wave inversions and no ST-segment elevation. A quick bedside TTE reveals normal LV function with a pericardial effusion. What is your next step?
    A. emergency coronary angiography
    B. CT scan
    C. start IV heparin and nitrates and admit the patient to the coronary care unit
    D. start IV heparin, IIb/IIIa inhibitor, and nitrates; admit the patient to the coronary care unit
    E. none of the above

Case 6 (Questions 15–16)

A 59-year-old man presents for further evaluation of recurrent CHF.

Physical Examination

He appears in no acute distress.
BP is 100/60 mm Hg.
Carotid upstrokes are weak but not delayed.
Chest examination reveals minimal bibasilar rales.
PMI is displaced and sustained. A summation gallop is present. There is an increased P_2.
There is mild peripheral edema.
A TTE reveals a dilated LV with an EF of 25%. The aortic valve does have some calcification with restricted leaflet excursion.
Peak/mean gradients are 25/15 mm Hg.
By the continuity equation, the aortic valve area is calculated at 0.7 cm^2.

15. What should be your next step?
    A. immediate referral for aortic valve replacement (AVR)
    B. referral for cardiac transplant
    C. dobutamine TTE
    D. start an ACEI

16. With dobutamine echocardiography, the gradients across the valve increase to 50/35 mm Hg, and the calculated valve area stays at 0.7 cm^2. What should you recommend?
    A. AVR
    B. continued medical management
    C. cardiac transplant evaluation

Case 7 (Questions 17–18)

A 32-year-old man with a known bicuspid aortic valve is referred to you for management of aortic insufficiency (AI). He is completely asymptomatic, jogs 3 miles per day, and does other aerobic exercise for 30 min daily.

Physical Examination

A TTE reveals a mildly dilated LV (end-diastolic dimension of 6 cm) with an EF of 65%. There is prolapse of the conjoined aortic leaflet with 3 to 4+ insufficiency.

17. What is your recommendation?
    A. referral for surgery
    B. addition of vasodilator therapy
    C. observation for now and follow-up in 2 years
    D. cardiac catheterization

18. What should you tell him is his yearly risk of sudden death?
    A. less than 1%
    B. 2%
    C. 3% to 5%
    D. greater than 5%

Case 8 (Questions 19–20)

A 45-year-old man with rheumatic mitral stenosis (MS) presents for further evaluation. In the past 2 to 3 years, he has noted progressive dyspnea with less than moderate activity. He was started on a beta-blocker 1 year ago but remains symptomatic.

Physical Examination

A TTE reveals a mean mitral gradient of 4 mm Hg with a valve area of 1.6 cm^2.

19. What would be a reasonable next step in the evaluation and management of this patient?

    A. stress TTE
    B. referral for percutaneous intervention
    C. referral for mitral valve replacement
    D. reassurance and follow-up in 1 year

20. You decide to send this patient for percutaneous intervention. What is the most appropriate test to order at the time of or before the valvuloplasty procedure?

    A. TEE
    B. 24-hour ECG monitoring to assess for paroxysmal AFib
    C. cardiac CT to assess for aortic calcification
    D. stress nuclear perfusion study

21. Which of the following statements is *not* true about ischemic MR?

    A. Revascularization alone may sometimes reduce the MR.
    B. Surgical repair or replacement of the valve is often needed.
    C. Its prognosis is better than that of myxomatous MR.
    D. Vasodilator therapy in the setting of ischemic LV dysfunction may reduce the severity of MR.
    E. Even with initial successful valve repair, MR often recurs.

22. A 65-year-old man is referred to you for evaluation of a heart murmur. He denies any symptoms at this time.

    He is in no acute distress.
    BP is 135/75 mm Hg.
    Heart rate is 82 bpm and regular.
    Carotid upstrokes are diminished.
    The PMI is sustained and displaced. A_2 is soft. A late-peaking systolic murmur is heard at the base.
    A TTE reveals LV hypertrophy with moderate global impairment of LV function and a calculated EF of 35%.
    There is severe calcific aortic stenosis, with peak/mean gradients of 75/45 mm Hg. The aortic valve area is 0.5 cm².

    What is the role of AVR in this setting?

    A. It is absolutely indicated.
    B. It is absolutely not recommended.
    C. There are some evidence and opinions that would favor valve replacement.

23. A patient with asymptomatic aortic stenosis presents for evaluation. The aortic valve area is calculated at 0.8 cm². Mild hypertrophy is present, with preserved LV function. The patient walks for 8 METS on a treadmill, with a normal hemodynamic response and without any ectopy. Which of the following is *not* true regarding valve replacement for this patient?

    A. AVR is recommended to prevent sudden death.
    B. AVR is not recommended at this time.
    C. If he is found to have CAD that requires bypass surgery, he should undergo AVR as well.
    D. If he is found to have a dilated ascending aorta (6.4 cm), he should undergo concomitant AVR and aortic conduit.

Case 9 (Questions 24–25)

A 75-year-old man is referred to you for evaluation of aortic regurgitation (AR). He has no symptoms at this time. His past medical history is significant only for hypertension.

Physical Examination

He is in no acute distress.
BP is 170/60 mm Hg.
The arterial pulses are brisk.
A bisferiens pulse is noted in the brachial artery.
The apical impulse is displaced and hyperdynamic.
S_1 is not loud, and no opening snap is heard. A high-frequency holodiastolic murmur is heard, loudest along the right sternal border. A late diastolic apical rumble is heard as well.

24. You order a TTE. About which of the following should you be most concerned?

    A. aortic valve commissural anatomy
    B. the degree of AI
    C. aortic root dimension
    D. the mitral valve

25. The above patient returns for follow-up 6 months later. He now reports symptoms of marked exertional dyspnea. A TTE is read as 2+ central AR, with an LV end-diastolic dimension of 6.9 cm and an EF of 50%. What should you do next?

    A. cardiac catheterization with aortography
    B. start an ACEI and reassess in 6 months
    C. continue observation
    D. start a beta-blocker and reassess in 6 months

26. A 56-year-old man presents to the emergency room with the sudden onset of chest pain. He is tachypneic on presentation.

    O_2 saturation is 82% on room air.
    BP is 80/60 mm Hg.
    Heart rate is 125 bpm.
    Chest examination reveals diffuse bilateral crackles.
    Cardiac examination reveals a nondisplaced PMI. S_1 is soft. P_2 is loud. An S_3 is present. A short decrescendo diastolic murmur is heard at the upper sternal border.
    His extremities are cool.
    An ECG reveals inferior ST-segment elevation.
    He is promptly intubated, and pressors are started.
    A brief TTE is performed at the bedside. The study is difficult but reveals premature closure of the mitral valve. There is hypokinesis of the infero-posterior walls.

Which of the following should be your next course of action?

A. TEE and emergent cardiac surgical consultation

B. use of an IABP to stabilize hemodynamics, followed by emergent angiography

C. administration of thrombolytics

D. sending the patient for MRI

Case 10 (Questions 27–28)

A 77-year-old patient is admitted to the hospital for urosepsis. His medical history is significant only in that he underwent AVR 5 years earlier. A TTE 2 years earlier revealed peak/mean gradients of 24/12 mm Hg. The LVOT time velocity integral (VTI) was 19, and the aortic valve VTI was 41.

Physical Examination

He is febrile to 102 degrees.

Heart rate is 106 bpm.

Carotid upstrokes are full.

Chest examination reveals clear lung fields.

Cardiac examination reveals a hyperdynamic apical impulse, which is not displaced. S_1 and S_2 are normal. An early-peaking systolic murmur is heard at the sternal border.

A TTE reveals that peak/mean gradients are 50/30 mm Hg. LVOT VTI is 36; aortic valve VTI is 78. The aortic valve itself is not well seen.

27. What should you conclude about prosthetic aortic valve function?

    A. He has prosthetic valve stenosis.

    B. There is no evidence for dysfunction.

    C. He has severe prosthetic valve regurgitation.

    D. He likely has endocarditis in addition to prosthetic valve regurgitation.

28. The above patient remains febrile despite 1 week of antibiotic therapy. An ECG reveals a new long first-degree AV block. The patient becomes progressively dyspneic. A short regurgitant murmur is heard. What should you recommend?

    A. TEE with surgical consultation

    B. TEE

    C. a change in antibiotic regimen

Case 11 (Questions 29–30)

A 56-year-old man with MS presents for evaluation. He has class II to III symptoms.

Physical Examination

He is in no acute distress.

Jugular venous pulse mildly elevated.

Heart rate is 80 bpm and regular.

His lungs are clear.

Cardiac examination reveals a nondisplaced PMI. An opening snap is heard 0.09 msec after S_2. There is a long diastolic rumble.

There is no peripheral edema.

A TTE reveals a planimetered mitral valve area of 1.2 cm².
Mean gradient is 10 mm Hg.
Pressure halftime is 185 msec.

He undergoes percutaneous valvuloplasty. The following morning, you note that he is comfortable.

O_2 saturation is 100% on room air.
Opening snap is 0.12 msec after S_2. A shorter decrescendo diastolic rumble is heard.
A predischarge TTE report indicates a pressure halftime of 180 msec.

29. Based on the TTE, what should you do next?

    A. There was a less than optimal result from the valvuloplasty. No significant change in mitral valve area was achieved. You should send him for another procedure or surgery.
    B. There was an error in halftime measurement. You should order a repeat assessment of pressure halftime later that day.
    C. You should repeat the TTE with planimetry of the mitral valve area.

30. The TTE reveals a small left-to-right shunt at the atrial level by color. What should you recommend?

    A. observation
    B. referral for percutaneous closure
    C. referral for surgical closure
    D. indefinite anticoagulation

31. An 80-year-old man underwent successful AVR with a bioprosthetic valve 4 months ago. He presents to your office for a routine follow-up visit. He is asymptomatic. He has no clinical history of embolic events.

    He is in sinus rhythm.
    A TTE reveals a normally functioning prosthetic valve. Chamber dimensions are normal, with normal biventricular function.

    Which of the following should you recommend?

    A. antibiotic prophylaxis and office visits if he feels unwell
    B. antibiotic prophylaxis and yearly office visits
    C. warfarin therapy

32. A 67-year-old woman is referred to your office for evaluation of a heart murmur. She describes symptoms of significant and limiting exertional dyspnea.

    Normal-appearing woman.
    She is normotensive.
    Heart rate is 67 bpm and regular.
    Cardiac examination reveals a sustained but nondisplaced PMI. S_1 and S_2 are normal. An S_4 is present. A loud III/VI systolic ejection murmur is heard throughout the precordium. Carotid upstrokes are delayed and diminished.
    A TEE is performed (Fig. 3). Her serum calcium and serum lipids are normal.
    Doppler evaluation reveals a 5-m jet across the LVOT. There is moderate aortic regurgitation.

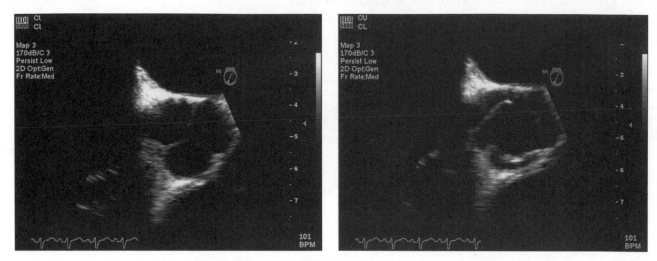

FIGURE 3

Which of the following is the most likely diagnosis?

    A. valvular aortic stenosis
    B. hypertrophic obstructive cardiomyopathy
    C. subaortic stenosis
    D. supravalvular aortic stenosis

Case 12 (Questions 33–34)

A 30-year-old woman presents to your office for a routine physical examination. She is asymptomatic.

Physical Examination

    BP is 95/65 mm Hg.
    Resting heart rate is 65 bpm.
    The physical examination is remarkable for a mild pectus deformity.
    On cardiac auscultation, a midsystolic click is heard. The click is heard earlier in systole when the patient is standing and later in systole when squatting. No murmur is heard at rest, but a soft systolic murmur becomes audible with dynamic maneuvers.

33. Which of the following is the most appropriate course of action?

    A. recommend antibiotic prophylaxis
    B. arrange for a follow-up examination in 3 years
    C. tell her she has no valve problems
    D. recommend beta-blockade
    E. recommend aspirin

34. Echocardiography demonstrates no high-risk features. What is the role of aspirin therapy in such patients, who have had no evidence of embolic events?

    A. It should be prescribed to all patients.
    B. It may play a role if a murmur is heard.
    C. There is no clear role for aspirin therapy in such patients.

35. A 50-year-old man with severe AI is referred to you for a second opinion. He is asymptomatic.

    A TTE reveals a mildly dilated LV (end-diastolic dimension, 6.2 cm; end-systolic dimension, 3.5 cm) with a normal EF.
    He has already undergone a stress TTE.
    He exercised for 14 METS.
    No symptoms or ECG changes were noted.
    The resting EF was calculated at 65%. Poststress, the EF is 60%.
    No segmental wall motion abnormalities were seen.

    What should you recommend?

    A. surgical intervention
    B. continue vasodilator therapy and reassess in 6 months
    C. cardiac catheterization
    D. stress nuclear ventriculogram

36. A 70-year-old man presents to your office with reports of exertional dyspnea.

    He is mildly hypertensive.
    Carotid upstrokes are brisk, with a secondary upstroke.
    A loud III/VI systolic murmur is heard along the sternal border radiating to the neck. S_1 and S_2 are normal. An S_4 is heard. The murmur increases in intensity with Valsalva and decreases with handgrip.

    A TTE reveals a 2-m jet across the LVOT. What should be your next step?

    A. Repeat the TTE, but have Doppler interrogation performed in other views and with a nonimaging transducer. The degree of aortic stenosis has been underestimated.
    B. Repeat the TTE with amyl nitrate.
    C. Perform TEE to better assess the valves.
    D. Perform coronary angiography.

Case 13 (Questions 37–39)

A 62-year-old man with a history of rheumatic heart disease presents to your office with reports of exertional dyspnea. No constitutional reports are present. He underwent a mitral valve replacement with a bi-leaflet tilting-disk mechanical valve 11 years before his visit.

    He is normotensive.
    Heart rate is 73 bpm.
    You note a grade II/VI holosystolic murmur at the apex.
    A TTE reveals normal LV and RV function.
    Peak mitral gradient is 30 mm Hg.
    Mean transmitral gradient is 7 mm Hg.
    Pressure halftime is 80 msec.

37. What should be your next diagnostic step?

    A. fluoroscopy of the valve
    B. TEE
    C. invasive assessment of hemodynamics
    D. drawing blood cultures

38. Which of the following would be the expected physical findings in this patient if the valve were functioning normally?

    A. prominent closing click, soft and brief diastolic rumble
    B. prominent opening and closing clicks, soft and brief diastolic rumble
    C. prominent opening click, long diastolic rumble
    D. prominent closing click, systolic murmur

39. If the patient had a ball and cage valve instead, what would you expect to hear?

    A. prominent closing click, soft and brief diastolic rumble
    B. prominent opening and closing clicks, soft and brief diastolic rumble
    C. prominent opening click, long diastolic rumble
    D. prominent closing click, systolic murmur

Case 14 (Questions 40–42)

A 65-year-old man presents to your office for evaluation of valvular heart disease. He is asymptomatic. He walks 5 miles per day without difficulty.

  A TTE reveals severe aortic stenosis, with a maximum aortic jet velocity of 4.7 m per second by Doppler echocardiography.
  LV systolic function is preserved.
  There is mild LV hypertrophy (wall thickness, 1.4 cm).
  He walks on a treadmill for 9 min with a normal hemodynamic response.

40. Continued observation is recommended. What should you tell him is his yearly risk of sudden death, provided he remains asymptomatic?

    A. less than 2%
    B. 5%
    C. 5% to 10%
    D. greater than 10%

41. What is the likelihood that he will become symptomatic within the next 3 years?

    A. 10%
    B. 10% to 25%
    C. 25% to 50%
    D. greater than 50%

42. What is the role for balloon valvuloplasty in this patient?

    A. There is no indication for it in this setting.

    B. It may result in a survival benefit, albeit with a higher procedural risk than for AVR.

    C. It would be a good choice as a bridge to surgery.

    D. It would definitely be indicated if he were to need urgent noncardiac surgery.

Case 15 (Questions 43–44)

A 52-year-old man who underwent AVR with a tilting-disk valve presents to you after a documented TIA. He presently has no symptoms. Workup at the time of his TIA included carotid Dopplers, a TTE, and TEE. These were unremarkable. The valve was well-seated and functioning normally. No thrombus was seen. Only minimal aortic atheroma was seen. No intracardiac shunt was identified. He has been on warfarin throughout and has maintained an international normalized ratio (INR) of between 2 and 3. The INR was 2.2 at the time of his TIA.

Physical Examination

He is in no acute distress.

BP is 120/80 mm Hg.

Heart rate is 68 bpm and regular.

Carotid upstrokes are full and not delayed.

A crisp valve closure sound is heard, along with a short, early-peaking systolic ejection murmur at the base. No S_3 is heard. P_2 is normal.

No peripheral edema is noted.

43. Which of the following should you recommend?

    A. Start acetylsalicylic acid, 325 mg per day.

    B. Increase warfarin to achieve an INR of 3.5 to 4.5.

    C. Increase warfarin to achieve an INR of 4.0 to 5.0.

    D. Start acetylsalicylic acid, 81 mg per day, and increase warfarin to achieve an INR of 2.5 to 3.5.

44. If his transesophageal study had revealed a small (1 to 2 mm) echodensity on the valve strut suggestive of thrombus but no obstruction to valve function, what should have been done?

    A. IV heparin therapy

    B. thrombolytic therapy

    C. reoperation

    D. IV IIb/IIIa inhibitors

Case 16 (Questions 45–46)

You are following a 50-year-old man with moderate MS who had been asymptomatic. He presents to the emergency room with reports of mild exertional dyspnea and palpitations, which have been present for the past 3 to 4 days. On arrival, he appears comfortable.

Physical Examination

O_2 saturation is 99% on room air.
Heart rate is 140 and irregular.
BP is 130/75 mm Hg.
An ECG reveals AFib.

45. Which of the following is *not* appropriate in the treatment of this patient?
    A. IV beta-blocker
    B. IV heparin
    C. immediate electrical cardioversion
    D. IV digoxin
    E. TEE-guided cardioversion after initiation of anticoagulation with IV heparin

46. The above patient spontaneously converts to sinus rhythm. Which of the following are you most likely to recommend?
    A. therapy with warfarin
    B. percutaneous valvuloplasty
    C. mitral valve replacement
    D. no change in therapy

47. A 34-year-old woman presents to your office for evaluation because she had been on treatment with anorectic agents 5 years ago. She is asymptomatic at this time. She is now at her ideal body weight.

    She is in no acute distress.
    BP is 107/68 mm Hg.
    Jugular venous pulsations appear normal.
    Her lungs are clear.
    Cardiac examination reveals a nondisplaced PMI. S_1 and S_2 are normal, with an appropriate physiologic split of S_2. P_2 is not loud. No S_3 or S_4 is heard. Auscultation is performed with the patient sitting, supine, and in the left lateral decubitus position. No murmur is heard.

    What should you most likely recommend for this patient?

    A. reassurance, with a repeat physical examination in 6 months
    B. TTE
    C. stress test

Case 17 (Questions 48–51)

A 50-year-old man presents for his first physical examination in several years. He notes that a murmur had been documented a number of years ago. He is entirely asymptomatic.

Physical Examination

BP is 120/70 mm Hg.
Heart rate is 58 bpm.
His neck veins are not distended.
Carotid upstrokes are brisk.
His lungs are clear.
Cardiac examination reveals a nondisplaced PMI. S_1 is soft. S_2 is normal (with a preserved A_2). An S_3 is heard. A III/VI holosystolic murmur is heard at the apex radiating to the base and carotids that increases with handgrip.

48. Of the four echocardiographic panels shown, which most likely represents the pathology in this particular patient (Figs. 4 through 7)?

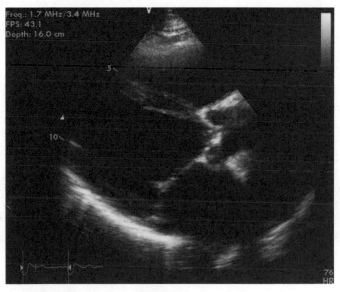

FIGURE 4

A. Figure 4
B. Figure 5
C. Figure 6
D. Figure 7

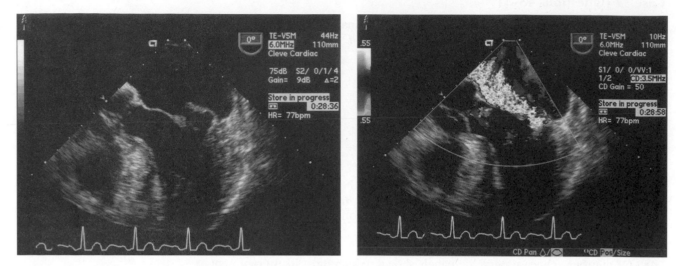

FIGURE 5

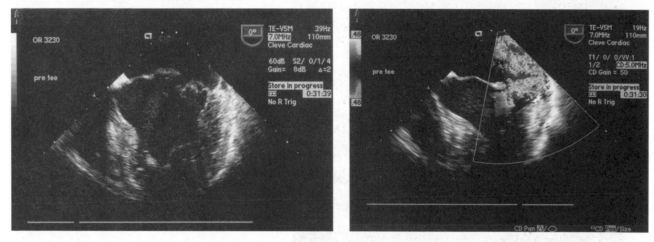

FIGURE 6

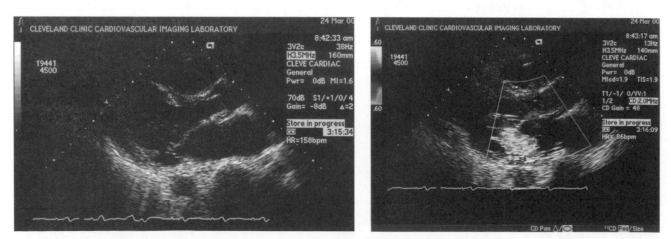

FIGURE 7

A TTE confirms your clinical suspicion. There is myxomatous mitral valve disease with posterior leaflet prolapse and severe MR. The end-systolic dimension is 3.0 cm; the end-diastolic dimension is 5.6 cm. The EF is 65%. The tricuspid regurgitation (TR) velocity is 2.9 m per second.

49. Which of the following would be most appropriate at this time?
    A. a stress TTE to assess PA pressures with stress
    B. immediate referral for mitral valve replacement
    C. the addition of an ACEI and follow-up in 2 years
    D. the addition of amiodarone to prevent AFib
    E. clinical follow-up at 2 years only

50. The above patient undergoes a stress TTE; the PA pressures do not increase significantly with stress. What are you least likely to recommend?
    A. referral for mitral valve replacement
    B. reassessment in 6 months with a TTE
    C. antibiotic prophylaxis

51. The above patient agrees to medical follow-up. He presents back to your office 2 years later with reports of dyspnea. A repeat TTE reveals an EF of 45% with an end-systolic dimension of 4.7 cm. What should you recommend?
    A. referral for mitral valve repair
    B. starting an ACEI and reassessing in 3 months
    C. mitral valve replacement
    D. starting a beta-blocker and reassessing in 3 months

Case 18 (Questions 52–53)

A 37-year-old man with a history of childhood rheumatic fever presents to establish regular cardiology follow-up. His past medical history is otherwise unremarkable. He is active and jogs 5 miles per day without any symptoms.

Physical Examination

He is in no acute distress.
BP is 150/85 mm Hg.
Heart rate is 52 bpm and regular.
His lungs are clear.
Cardiac examination reveals a nondisplaced PMI. S_1 and S_2 are normal. No opening snap is heard. There is a holosystolic murmur heard at the apex, radiating to the axilla.
He has no peripheral edema.
CXR demonstrates a calcified mitral apparatus. The cardiac silhouette and pulmonary vasculature appear within normal limits.
A TTE reveals a rheumatic-appearing mitral valve with minimal stenosis but severe regurgitation. The mitral leaflets are calcified but have good mobility. LV dimensions are normal, and the EF is 70%. RV systolic pressure is estimated at 25 mm Hg.

52. Which of the following is *not* an acceptable course of action?

    A. follow-up in 6 months with a physical examination and a TTE
    B. endocarditis prophylaxis
    C. referral for surgery
    D. initiation of an ACEI

53. The above patient does not seek follow-up for another 3 years. At this time, he reports mild dyspnea when climbing three flights of stairs. He stopped jogging 1 year ago and has gained 40 lb. What is the best course of action at this time?

    A. referral for surgery
    B. increasing ACEI
    C. starting a diuretic
    D. stress echocardiography

54. A 42-year-old man presents to you for a second opinion. He is asymptomatic, with good functional capacity, but he has been diagnosed with mitral valve prolapse with flail and severe MR. His LV EF is 70%, and the dimensions are normal. Which of the following is *not* true?

    A. There is a consensus of opinion that he needs surgery now.
    B. There are data indicating that for patients like him, there is a very high likelihood of requiring surgery in the next 10 years.
    C. There are some data indicating that he may face a risk of sudden death in the absence of intervention, approaching 1% per year.

55. A 35-year-old man presents to your office for evaluation of valvular heart disease. He reports shortness of breath with only modest amounts of exertion as well as two-pillow orthopnea. He also reports easy fatigability as well as lower extremity edema and abdominal fullness.

    He is in no acute distress.
    He is normotensive.
    Jugular venous pressure is elevated, with a prominent a wave. The v wave is not easily discerned.
    S_1 is loud. S_2 is normal. A sound is heard in diastole 0.07 msec after S_2. A diastolic rumble is heard at the apex. A diastolic murmur is also heard along the left sternal border, which increases with inspiration.
    Mild hepatomegaly is present. There is 2+ peripheral edema.

    What is your diagnosis?

    A. MS
    B. MS with tricuspid insufficiency
    C. MS and tricuspid stenosis
    D. MS and aortic stenosis

Case 19 (Questions 56–58)

An 80-year-old man presents to your office with reports of chest tightness when climbing up a flight of stairs. His past medical history is unremarkable.

Physical Examination

He is in no acute distress.
BP is 140/80 mm Hg.
Heart rate is 78 bpm and regular.
His lungs are clear.
Carotid upstrokes are diminished. The PMI is sustained but not displaced. S_4 is present. The S_2 is diminished and single. A loud late-peaking systolic murmur is heard, loudest at the second intercostal space, radiating to the neck.

56. Which of the following should be your next step?
    A. stress sestamibi
    B. stress ECG
    C. cardiac catheterization
    D. prescribe sublingual nitroglycerin as required and see how he does

57. The above patient is found to have an aortic valve area of 0.7 cm^2 with a mean gradient of 60 mm Hg. After catheterization, he develops massive upper GI bleeding. Endoscopy reveals a gastric ulcer with a bleeding vessel at its base. Cauterization is performed, which temporarily stops the bleeding. However, the bleeding recurs, and urgent partial gastrectomy is recommended. He reports chest pain during these bleeding episodes. What is the best course of action?
    A. Proceed to AVR first.
    B. Refer the patient for percutaneous balloon valvuloplasty followed by gastrectomy.
    C. Start nitroprusside and proceed with gastric surgery.
    D. Proceed with gastric surgery directly.

58. Which valve should you recommend to this 80-year-old patient with aortic stenosis?
    A. bovine pericardial valve
    B. ball-and-cage mechanical valve
    C. bi-leaflet mechanical valve
    D. aortic homograft valve

Case 20 (Questions 59–60)

A 65-year-old man with a history of well-controlled rheumatoid arthritis presents for evaluation of a heart murmur. He notes some increase in fatigue and decrease in activity level over the past 2 years but denies any specific reports of dyspnea. He leads a rather sedentary lifestyle.

Physical Examination

BP is 150/50 mm Hg.
Heart rate is 80 bpm and regular.
Carotid upstrokes are brisk, with a rapid upstroke and decline. The apical impulse is displaced and hyperdynamic. S_1 and S_2 are normal. A decrescendo, nearly holodiastolic murmur is heard along the left sternal border, loudest when the patient is sitting up.
A TTE reveals a dilated LV (end-diastolic dimension, 6.8 cm; end-systolic dimension, 3.5 cm). The EF is 55%. There is significant AR.

59. What should you most likely recommend?

   A. performing a stress test
   B. reassessing with repeat echo in 6 months
   C. starting vasodilator therapy and reassessing in 2 years
   D. referral to surgery

60. He is started on a vasodilator and returns for follow-up in 6 months. He reports no change in symptoms. A repeat echo demonstrates an end-diastolic dimension of 7.6 cm. The EF remains normal. What should you recommend now?

   A. performing a stress test
   B. surgical intervention
   C. increasing vasodilators and reassessing in 6 months
   D. performing an MRI to assess LV volumes

Case 21 (Questions 61–62)

A 42-year-old woman who underwent mitral valve replacement with a bi-leaflet tilting-disk valve for rheumatic disease presents to the emergency room with reports of severe dyspnea. Her past medical history is otherwise unremarkable.

Physical Examination

   BP is 120/60 mm Hg.
   Heart rate is 83 bpm.
   Chest examination reveals bilateral crackles, one-third up.
   Cardiac examination reveals a nondisplaced PMI. Prosthetic clicks are muffled. A long diastolic rumble is heard at the apex.

61. A TTE is ordered on the above patient. Which of the following would you expect to see?

   A. severe MR
   B. a mean gradient of 17 mm Hg
   C. a pressure halftime of 80 msec
   D. an EF of 20%

62. The above patient undergoes TEE (Fig. 8).

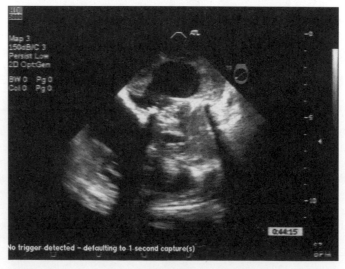

FIGURE 8

A large echodensity consistent with thrombus is seen extending from the atrial wall onto the prosthesis, causing significant restriction in leaflet mobility. What should you recommend?

A. urgent reoperation
B. thrombolytic therapy
C. IV heparin and glycoprotein IIB/IIIA inhibitor
D. an increase in warfarin dose, aiming for a higher INR

Case 22 (Questions 63–64)

A 26-year-old woman presents to your office for evaluation. She has had a murmur since childhood. She has a history of palpitations but is otherwise asymptomatic.

Physical Examination

She is in no acute distress.
Prominent *v* waves are noted in the jugular venous pulse.
Carotid upstrokes are normal.
Her chest is clear to auscultation.
Cardiac examination reveals a nondisplaced PMI. Auscultation reveals a widely split S_1 with a loud second component that sounds like a click. A holosystolic murmur is heard at the right sternal border, which increases with inspiration.
Hepatomegaly is present.
A TTE is performed (Fig. 9).

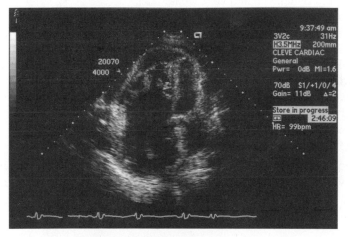

FIGURE 9

63. What is the most likely cause of her palpitations?

    A. arrhythmias secondary to an accessory pathway
    B. AV nodal reentrant tachycardia
    C. VT
    D. AFib
    E. anxiety

64. No intervention is performed for the above patient. She returns to your clinic 3 months later. She describes an episode of transient word-finding difficulty that lasted for a number of seconds. This occurred while she was recovering from a fractured tibia. A CT scan was performed, which was

negative. She is concerned that she may have a recurrence. What is the most appropriate next test for her?

A. echocardiography with saline contrast study
B. carotid Dopplers
C. 24-hour ambulatory ECG monitoring
D. cardiac catheterization with saturation run

65. In the setting of aortic stenosis with moderate insufficiency, which of the following methods would provide the most accurate estimate of aortic valve area?

A. invasive hemodynamics, using the Gorlin equation
B. Doppler echocardiography, using the continuity equation
C. pressure halftime
D. Bernoulli equation

66. Which of the following valves has the lowest incidence of endocarditis?

A. mechanical valve
B. bioprosthetic valve
C. aortic homograft valve
D. stentless mitral valve

67. A 75-year-old man is transferred to the coronary intensive care unit for refractory heart failure. He arrives intubated on mechanical ventilatory support.

BP is 95/40 mm Hg.
His extremities are cool.
Carotid upstrokes are delayed and very weak.
Coarse rales are present bilaterally.
A systolic murmur is present.
He is making 30 cc urine per hour on arrival.
A TTE reveals moderate LV dysfunction, with an EF of 30%. There is severe aortic stenosis, with a valve area of 0.6 cm^2.
Laboratory evaluation reveals BUN of 80.0 and creatinine of 2.2 (documented to be normal 6 months ago). Albumin is 2.0.

Which of the following should you *least* likely recommend?

A. percutaneous valvuloplasty
B. emergency surgery
C. IABP
D. urgent dialysis

Case 23 (Questions 68–70)

A 21-year-old man presents to your office for evaluation. He tells you that a murmur was noted a few days after his birth. He is presently asymptomatic.

Physical Examination

He is normotensive.
Heart rate is 65 bpm and regular.
Carotid upstrokes are normal.
His lungs are clear.

Cardiac examination reveals a nondisplaced PMI. An RV lift is present. A systolic thrill is present in the suprasternal notch. A high-pitched sound is heard after S_1. A crescendo-decrescendo systolic murmur is heard at the left second intercostal space. A_2 is normal.

68. Which of the following would you expect to find on echocardiography?

    A. maximum velocity across the aortic valve of 4 m per second
    B. maximum velocity across the pulmonic valve of 4 m per second
    C. a wide jet of mitral insufficiency
    D. flow reversal in the hepatic veins

69. The above patient returns 1 year later for follow-up. Which of the following is a definite indication for intervention?

    A. He tells you of an episode of syncope.
    B. He has no symptoms, but the RV to PA peak gradient is 40 to 49 mm Hg.
    C. He has no symptoms, but the RV to PA peak gradient is 30 to 39 mm Hg.
    D. He has no symptoms, but the RV to PA peak gradient is less than 30 mm Hg.

70. If intervention is recommended, what is the preferred treatment approach?

    A. percutaneous valvuloplasty
    B. Ross procedure
    C. mechanical valve
    D. bioprosthetic valve

71. What is the most common cause of TR?

    A. rheumatic tricuspid disease
    B. carcinoid
    C. congenital abnormalities
    D. pulmonary hypertension resulting from primary left-sided disease
    E. myxomatous disease of the tricuspid valve

72. Which of the following statements is true regarding treatment of tricuspid valvular disease?

    A. In patients with MS and pulmonary hypertension who develop severe tricuspid insufficiency but have normal tricuspid leaflets, placement of an annuloplasty ring is usually inadequate to treat the regurgitation.
    B. Mechanical valves are the preferred option when valve replacement becomes necessary.
    C. Bioprosthetic valves are the preferred option when valve replacement becomes necessary.

73. What is the most common organism seen in native valve endocarditis?

    A. *Streptococcus viridans*
    B. *Enterobacter faecalis*
    C. *Staphylococcus aureus*
    D. *Chlamydia pneumoniae*
    E. *Haemophilus aphrophilus, Actinobacillus actinomycetemcomitans, Cardiobacterium hominis, Eikenella corrodens,* and *Kingella kingae* organisms (HACEK)

74. A patient presents with systemic embolic events 1 month after uncompli-cated mitral valve replacement. He has been febrile for the past week. TEE demonstrates multiple echodensities on the valve ring. Which of the follow-ing are most likely to grow from blood cultures that are drawn?

    A. *S. viridans*
    B. *S. aureus*
    C. *Staphylococcus epidermidis*
    D. *E. faecalis*
    E. *Candida albicans*

75. Which of the following is not a class I indication for surgery in patients with native valve endocarditis?

    A. acute MR or AR with heart failure
    B. fungal endocarditis
    C. persistent bacteremia without other source in patients who have received 7 to 10 days of appropriate antibiotic therapy and show evidence of valve dysfunction
    D. persistent fevers with negative blood cultures

76. Which of the following are not considered high risk for development of endocarditis?

    A. presence of a prosthetic valve
    B. previous episode of endocarditis
    C. cyanotic congenital heart disease
    D. surgically repaired atrial septal defect

77. In an at-risk patient, which of the following procedures definitely requires prophylactic antibiotics?

    A. dental extraction
    B. GI endoscopy
    C. flexible bronchoscopy
    D. cardiac catheterization
    E. all of the above

78. Prophylactic regimens for GI and genitourinary procedures include all of the following except?

    A. ampicillin (2.0 g IV) and gentamicin (1.5 mg/kg IV) 30 min before the procedure for high-risk patients
    B. ampicillin (2.0 g IV) and gentamicin (1.5 mg/kg IV) 30 min before the procedure for moderate-risk patients
    C. amoxicillin (2 g PO) or ampicillin (2 g IV or IM) for moderate-risk patients
    D. vancomycin (1.0 g IV) and gentamicin (1.5 mg/kg IV) before the proce-dure for high-risk patients with a penicillin allergy

79. A 35-year-old woman is referred to your office by her internist. She desires to become pregnant. Her past medical history is significant for congenital MS, for which she underwent mitral valve replacement with a Starr-Edwards valve. Her physical examination is consistent with a nor-mally functioning mechanical prosthesis. Which of the following is not true?

A. Anticoagulation for mechanical prosthesis in pregnancy carries both maternal and fetal risk. The use of warfarin in the first trimester has been associated with an embryopathy in 4% to 10% of cases. Heparin is probably safer for the fetus but is associated with an increased risk of both thrombosis and hemorrhage in the mother.

B. If this patient chooses not to be on warfarin in the first trimester, you should recommend IV heparin to prolong the activated partial thromboplastin time to two to three times the control.

C. If this patient chooses not to be on warfarin in the first trimester, you should recommend SC heparin to prolong the activated partial thromboplastin time to two to three times the control.

D. Low-molecular-weight heparins may play a role, but as of yet there are no guidelines regarding their use in the management of patients with prosthetic valves.

80. Which of the following would have the least risk for a patient contemplating pregnancy?

    A. congenital heart disease with Eisenmenger's physiology
    B. asymptomatic aortic stenosis with a mean gradient of 60 mm Hg
    C. severe MR with functional class I
    D. severe AR in a Marfan's syndrome patient
    E. asymptomatic MS with a valve area of 1 cm^2

ANSWERS

1. B. Exercise. The most likely diagnosis is MS, based on the increased S_1 and the presence of the opening snap (high-pitched diastolic sound). The clinical history of febrile illness as a child is also suggestive. With exercise, flow is increased across the valve, and the diastolic rumble may be evident.

2. A. A mitral pressure halftime of 230 msec. The presence of the opening snap 0.12 msec after S_2 and the brief duration of the murmur suggest that the degree of stenosis is mild. A pressure halftime of 230 msec would suggest a mitral valve area of less than 1 cm^2, consistent with severe MS.

3. A. Endocarditis prophylaxis alone. The patient has mild MS with good functional capacity. No further evaluation is necessary at this time. Her left atrial size is normal, and she has no history of AFib or other embolic events. She has no indication for warfarin. Her MS is only mild, so she has no indication for consideration for percutaneous valvotomy [a class III indication according to American College of Cardiology/American Heart Association practice guidelines (ACC/AHA)]. Thus, there is no need for a stress TTE. In addition, she has good functional capacity (she jogs 2 to 3 miles per day without symptoms). There is no role for digoxin with normal biventricular function and NSR.

4. C. Stress TTE to assess for mitral and pulmonary pressures poststress. The fact that she has stopped exercising may be a clue to the onset of symptoms. An assessment of functional capacity and poststress mitral and PA pressures would be useful in the management and assessment of her true hemodynamic state. There are insufficient data for immediate referral for interven-

tion. Follow-up in a short period may not be unreasonable; however, 5 years is too long a period.

5. A. Consideration for percutaneous valvuloplasty. Her functional capacity is below average for her age. Her valve is favorable for percutaneous valvuloplasty (splittability score of 6), and she had a significant rise in PA pressures poststress. This is a class IIa indication according to ACC/AHA guidelines. A beta-blocker would not be unreasonable, but she should be followed more frequently than every 2 years. She has normal LV function and is in sinus rhythm—there is no role for digoxin in this setting. Valve replacement is considered only if the valve is deemed unsuitable for percutaneous valvuloplasty or surgical repair.

6. B. Carcinoid. The history and examination are consistent with tricuspid stenosis and regurgitation (symptoms of fatigability from decreased cardiac output, signs and symptoms of systemic venous congestion, hepatic distention and right-upper-quadrant pain, peripheral edema, and ascites; there is a diastolic murmur along the sternal border that increases with inspiration, along with a prominent a wave in the jugular venous pulse; in addition, she has a pansystolic murmur and a prominent v wave). However, no evidence of MS is noted on examination. Isolated rheumatic tricuspid stenosis is very rare. Thus, other causes for tricuspid stenosis should be considered. The second most common cause of tricuspid stenosis is the carcinoid syndrome. She also has bronchospasm and diarrhea, which go along with this diagnosis. She has a normal P_2, making primary pulmonary hypertension unlikely. Liver disease in and of itself would not produce elevation in the jugular venous pulse.

7. B. TEE. The clinical history is of a patient who had an inferior wall MI approximately 1 week earlier. He now presents in shock with acute CHF. Mechanical complication of MI is first on the differential. The presence of a ventricular gallop and an apical murmur without a thrill makes papillary muscle rupture the leading diagnosis (as opposed to a VSD). Transthoracic echocardiography may miss eccentric jets in this setting. TEE should be performed to make the diagnosis. He will certainly need cardiac catheterization (at which time a saturation run may be performed), but TEE should be done quickly at the bedside to confirm the diagnosis, so that the surgical team can be mobilized.

8. B. She likely has more severe MR than is evident on the TTE. Her examination is suggestive of severe MR. The TTE confirms LV dilation, and there is mitral leaflet pathology that could be consistent with severe MR. The eccentric nature of the jet suggests that it may have been underestimated by transthoracic imaging. A more definitive imaging procedure, such as TEE, will be helpful here.

9. B. Mitral valve surgery. The presence of mild LV dysfunction with LV dilatation is a class I indication for surgery.

10. B. Mitral valve replacement with tricuspid annuloplasty. She has severe MS (increased PA pressure, opening snap less than 0.08 msec after S_2, and a holodiastolic murmur, suggesting persistent pressure gradient) and is quite symptomatic. She does not appear to be a candidate for percutaneous intervention. A soft opening snap suggests that the valve is not

pliable. The presence of valvular calcification on CXR would likewise suggest this. The TTE confirms this, with extensive leaflet as well as subvalvular thickening and calcification. In addition, she has significant TR. She may benefit from an annuloplasty ring at the time of surgery.

11. A. Bioprosthetic valve. She is in an age group (older than 70 years) in which the risk to benefit ratio would favor a biologic valve. Durability in this age group is reasonable. She has no other clinical indications for antico-agulation (she is in sinus rhythm, and there is no history of embolic events). A homograft may prove to be a reasonable option, but there is not wide-spread availability or use as of yet.

12. D. NSR and a left atrial size of 4.4 cm are not possible indications. AFib (paroxysmal or persistent) and a prior embolic event are class I indications for anticoagulation in a patient with MS. Anticoagulation based on atrial size alone is controversial—the guidelines list a size greater than 55 mm in the setting of severe MS as a IIb indication. There is no established role for anticoagulation in the absence of the above.

13. C. Check lower extremity BP. He has a bicuspid aortic valve (an ejection sound is heard, along with a short systolic ejection murmur). There is an association between bicuspid aortic valves and coarctation of the aorta. Therefore, looking for discrepancy between upper and lower extremity BPs would be paramount.

14. B. CT scan. Patients with bicuspid aortic valves (and, in this case, aortic coarctation) have an associated aortopathy. They are, thus, at risk for aortic dissection. In this patient, a CT scan (or TEE or MRI) should be performed to look for this. Anticoagulant therapy should not be initiated until this pos-sibility is ruled out, especially with a pericardial effusion.

15. C. Dobutamine TTE. This is a patient presenting with low-gradient aortic stenosis in the setting of LV dysfunction. It is possible that the patient has severe aortic stenosis, but the gradients are now low secondary to decreased stroke volume. Alternatively, the aortic stenosis may not be truly significant, but the severity is overestimated by continuity in the set-ting of low cardiac output. In this setting, low-dose dobutamine echocar-diography may be useful. With inotropic stimulation, an improvement in stroke volume and cardiac output may help to differentiate truly severe aortic stenosis from what has been labeled pseudo aortic stenosis. If true severe aortic stenosis is not present, then valve area will increase. It would not be prudent to send such a patient for aortic valve surgery without per-forming such an evaluation. It would be necessary to exclude severe ste-nosis before proceeding with transplant evaluation. An ACEI may be beneficial, but it would be important to proceed with the workup as described above first. Afterload reduction would need to be introduced with very careful hemodynamic monitoring if true severe aortic stenosis were in fact present.

16. A. AVR. The patient has true, severe aortic stenosis. The fact that he can generate a mean gradient greater than 30 mm Hg suggests he has some con-tractile reserve.

17. B. Addition of vasodilator therapy. The patient is asymptomatic with good functional capacity. He has a normal EF with a mildly dilated LV. Surgery is a class III indication in this setting. Vasodilator therapy does seem to have some benefit in this asymptomatic population with preserved EF and LV dilatation and is a class I indication. Observation alone may not be unreasonable, but the patient requires closer follow-up than in 2 years. There is no role for cardiac catheterization at this juncture.

18. A. Less than 1%. From the available published literature, as summarized in the ACC/AHA consensus guidelines, the risk is approximately 0.2% per year in those asymptomatic patients with preserved LV function.

19. A. Stress TTE. There appears to be a discrepancy between the degree of symptoms and resting hemodynamics. Further workup is warranted. A stress TTE revealed a poststress PA pressure of 70 mm Hg and a mean transmitral gradient of 17 mm Hg. Follow-up in 1 year without further workup is inappropriate given the degree of symptoms. There is insufficient information as of yet to proceed directly with intervention.

20. A. TEE. Left atrial and appendage thrombus should be excluded before proceeding with percutaneous valvuloplasty (class IIa indication). TEE is much more sensitive in the detection of thrombus (especially in the left atrial appendage) than TTE and is indicated before the mitral valvuloplasty procedure. The other studies may be helpful in individual patients but will not usually impact the decision regarding valvuloplasty.

21. C. Generally, patients with ischemic MR, owing to concomitant coronary disease and LV dysfunction, have a worse prognosis than those with primary valvular MR. The optimal treatment for ischemic MR is a matter of debate. If MR results transiently from papillary muscle dysfunction due to ischemia, then revascularization alone may be sufficient to treat the MR. If there are regional wall motion abnormalities with annular dilatation and papillary muscle retraction, then direct intervention on the valve may be required. In those with significant impairment of LV function, vasodilator therapy to reduce afterload and favorably influence LV geometry can reduce MR severity. There is increasing data that such patients may benefit from annuloplasty rings as well.

22. C. There are some evidence and opinions that would favor valve replacement. As the patient remains asymptomatic, this is not a class I indication for surgery. However, he does have impaired LV function. By ACC/AHA guidelines, this is a class IIa indication for surgery.

23. A. There is no indication for aortic valve surgery for the prevention of sudden death in this patient population without LV dysfunction, severe hypertrophy, exercise-induced hypotension, or VT (which are class IIa or IIb indications).

24. C. Aortic root dimension. The patient clinically has severe AI. The murmur is loudest at the right sternal border, suggesting aortic root dilation as a potential cause of his AI. The presence of root dilatation (greater than or equal to 5 cm) may lead to earlier surgery and, hence, is vital to know. The diastolic rumble is most likely an Austin-Flint murmur and not concomitant MS (there is no opening snap, and S_1 is not loud).

25. A. Cardiac catheterization with aortography. Clinically, the patient has severe AR. He is symptomatic. Consistent with this, the TTE reveals a dilated LV with low normal systolic function. The degree of AR must be underestimated by this study. When there is such discrepancy, one should proceed with aortography to confirm AR severity and to assess coronaries before surgical referral. As he is symptomatic, continued observation or medical therapy is not the preferred treatment approach. Beta-blockers, by prolonging the diastolic filling period, could actually increase regurgitant volume.

26. A. TEE and emergent cardiac surgical consultation. The patient has a clinical presentation of severe acute AI (short diastolic murmur, soft S_1 from premature mitral valve closure, low output state, and pulmonary edema). In the context of chest pain, this scenario suggests aortic dissection until proven otherwise. The dissection flap likely involves the ostium of the right coronary artery, producing the inferior ST-segment elevation. Thrombolytics should not be used until dissection is ruled out. Even if there is no dissection, balloon pumps should not be used with severe AI. The augmented diastolic pressure worsens the severity of the insufficiency. MRI would also provide the diagnosis, but given the hemodynamic instability of the patient, a bedside TEE would be a safer and quicker option to arrive at the diagnosis.

27. B. There is no evidence for dysfunction. The physical examination does not suggest either stenosis or insufficiency. He appears to be in a high-output state, secondary to his febrile illness. As a result, the gradients are increased. The LVOT VTI is also increased, secondary to the increased cardiac output. The LVOT to aortic valve VTI ratio is the same in the two TTEs, which would speak against any significant obstruction.

28. A. TEE with surgical consultation. The clinical scenario, with a new first-degree AV block and acute AR, is highly suspicious for prosthetic valve abscess and even possibly partial dehiscence. A TEE should be performed, but prompt surgical consultation should also be requested. The patient is developing heart failure and is persistently febrile despite 1 week of antibiotic therapy.

29. C. You should repeat the TTE with planimetry of the mitral valve area. With acute changes in atrial and ventricular compliance (as with valvuloplasty), the halftime is unreliable. Usually, 72 hours or longer is required after the procedure before the halftime can be used with reasonable reliability. Planimetry, if performed correctly, would provide a good estimate of stenosis severity. Clinically, the patient seems to have had a good result (longer S_2-OS interval, shorter murmur).

30. A. Observation. Most of these small shunts will close over the next 6 months without any intervention. The shunt is left to right by color. He has good O_2 saturation on room air, making any significant right-to-left shunting unlikely. Anticoagulation with an atrial septal defect or patent foramen ovale may be recommended in certain settings but not indefinitely, given the good chance that the defect will close.

31. B. Antibiotic prophylaxis and yearly office visits. He clearly requires antibiotic prophylaxis with a prosthetic valve. These patients still require close follow-up with complete evaluations on a yearly basis. Some advocate a 3-month period of warfarin therapy after bioprosthetic valve placement. He is now 4 months out and has no other indications or a high-risk profile (LV dysfunction, prior embolic event, AFib)—thus, warfarin is no longer needed at this time.

32. C. Subaortic stenosis. The TEE reveals a normal-appearing aortic valve. The examination suggests a fixed obstruction with delayed and diminished carotid upstrokes. This patient has evidence of fixed obstruction of the blood leaving the heart on physical examination. The aortic valve is normal on TEE excluding significant valvar aortic stenosis. Supravalvular aortic stenosis is uncommon, is associated with congenital syndrome (Williams syndrome), or is acquired (hypercipidemia). It is unlikely in this patient, given her normal appearance and normal Ca^{2+} and lipids. Hypertrophic cardiomyopathy is associated with dynamic obstruction and a jerky carotid upstroke. The most likely diagnosis is subaortic stenosis. This is associated with fixed obstruction, and the presence of a turbulent jet hitting the aortic valve causes aortic regurgitation in many patients, as occured here.

33. A. Recommend antibiotic prophylaxis. Endocarditis prophylaxis is a class I indication in patients with the classic click-murmur complex. Although there has been some disagreement about the need for antibiotic prophylaxis in patients with an isolated systolic click and no murmur, ACC/AHA guidelines suggest a IIa indication for echocardiography in this setting and antibiotic prophylaxis for those with high-risk echocardiographic features (leaflet thickening, elongated chordae, left atrial enlargement, LV dilatation).

34. C. There is no clear role for aspirin therapy in such patients. If there is echocardiographic evidence for high-risk mitral valve prolapse (leaflet thickening, elongated chordae, left atrial enlargement, LV dilatation), aspirin therapy is considered a class IIb indication. Therapy is clearly recommended if there has been documented stroke or TIA.

35. B. Continue vasodilator therapy and reassess in 6 months. By ACC/AHA guidelines, decline in EF after stress echocardiography in and of itself is not yet an accepted indication for referral to surgical intervention. Due to the high afterload and the increase in afterload on exercise, a small to modest decline in EF (less than 10%) may still be consistent with well-compensated AI. This patient has a normal resting EF and mildly dilated LV with excellent functional capacity.

36. B. Repeat the TTE with amyl nitrate (Fig. 10). Part A shows systolic anterior motion, part B shows LVOT flow before and after amyl nitrate. The physical examination is highly suggestive of hypertrophic cardiomyopathy (brisk, bisferiens carotid pulse; normal S_2; murmur increasing with Valsalva and decreasing with handgrip). The patient may not have a significant resting tract gradient but may have a significant provocable gradient. Generally, a TEE is not needed to make the diagnosis. Invasive hemodynamics with provocation would be useful, but angiography alone would not be sufficient.

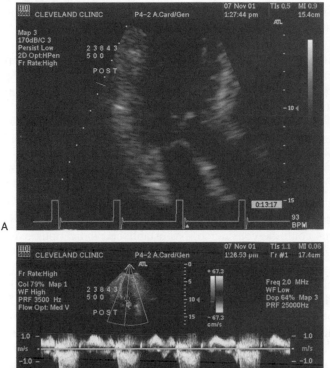

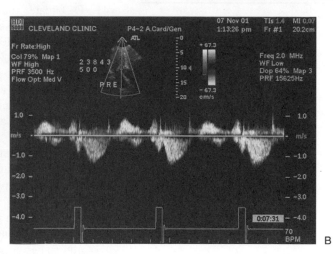

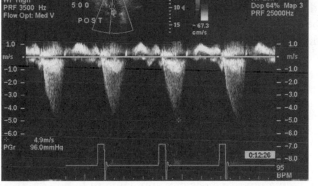

FIGURE 10

37. B. TEE. According to the examination, the patient has mitral insufficiency. The TTE is consistent with this, with an elevated peak transmitral gradient. Pressure halftime is not prolonged; thus, there does not appear be any significant stenosis (gradients elevated due to increased flow from regurgitant volume). A TEE would be most useful to confirm the diagnosis. Fluoroscopy may identify partial dehiscence but would not be helpful if there were a leak in the setting of a well-seated valve. There is no evidence for stenosis, in which fluoroscopic evaluation of leaflet motion could be diagnostic. There is no clinical evidence for endocarditis.

38. A. Prominent closing click, soft and brief diastolic rumble. The bi-leaflet mechanical valves do not typically produce a loud opening sound but do have prominent closing sounds. A brief diastolic rumble may be heard in a normally functioning prosthetic valve in the mitral position.

39. B. Prominent opening and closing clicks, soft and brief diastolic rumble. With the ball and cage valves, one would expect to hear the opening click as well.

40. A. Less than 2%. In the absence of symptoms, natural history studies would suggest a relatively low risk of sudden death.

41. D. Greater than 50%. He has a velocity across the aortic valve of greater than 4 m per second. Observational studies would suggest a high likelihood of symptom development in the next 3 years.

42. A. There is no indication for it in this setting. There is no indication for percutaneous valvuloplasty in this patient. This procedure has been advocated for such patients who may need noncardiac surgery; however, this remains a class IIb indication.

43. D. By the most recent ACC/AHA guidelines, starting acetylsalicylic acid at 81 mg per day and increasing warfarin to achieve an INR of 2.5 to 3.5 would be the preferred approach.

44. A. IV heparin therapy. Because a small clot was present, the patient would benefit from increased anticoagulant therapy. If he were to fail this, then the other alternatives could be considered. No established indications exist at this time for glycoprotein IIb/IIIa inhibitors in this clinical setting.

45. C. Immediate electrical cardioversion is not appropriate. Primary treatment includes the initiation of anticoagulation and rate control measures. This patient is not hemodynamically unstable, and, as such, immediate cardioversion is not needed. Furthermore, the clinical history suggests that he has been in AFib for longer than 24 to 48 hours. He is, thus, at increased risk for embolic events. Options include TEE-guided cardioversion with adequate anticoagulation or anticoagulation with warfarin for at least 3 weeks, followed by electrical cardioversion.

46. A. Therapy with warfarin. The role of valvuloplasty in this setting (onset of AFib) is controversial and is a class IIb indication by current guidelines.

47. A. Reassurance, with a repeat physical examination in 6 months. If a thorough physical examination reveals no signs of cardiopulmonary disease and the patient has no symptoms, then reassurance and follow-up are all that are required. Echocardiography should be performed if obesity limits the physical examination or if signs or symptoms are present. Echocardiography before invasive procedures (to assess the need for antibiotic prophylaxis) remains controversial in these patients (class IIb).

48. B. Figure 5. Figure 4 demonstrates aortic stenosis. Figure 5 is an example of predominant posterior leaflet prolapse with severe MR. Figure 6 is an example of predominant anterior leaflet prolapse with severe MR. Figure 7 is an example of a posterior leaflet that is restricted with posteriorly directed MR. The answer is B, posterior leaflet prolapse with severe MR. The presence of a soft S_1, normal carotid upstrokes, a holosystolic murmur that increases with handgrip, and an S_3 makes MR and not aortic stenosis the diagnosis. The radiation of the jet toward the base suggests an anterior jet direction, which is what would be expected with posterior leaflet prolapse. Both anterior leaflet prolapse and posterior leaflet restriction would produce a posteriorly directed jet.

49. A. A stress TTE to assess PA pressures with stress. The patient does have evidence for mild resting pulmonary hypertension. If PA pressures increased significantly with exercise (to greater than 60 mm Hg), referral for mitral valve surgery could be considered (class IIa indication by ACC/

AHA guidelines). The valve would appear amenable to repair, and replacement would not be the first choice. There are no data to suggest a beneficial role for the addition of afterload-reducing agents in the absence of systemic hypertension (again, by ACC/AHA guidelines). There is absolutely no role for the prophylactic use of amiodarone. It is reasonable to simply clinically follow the patient; however, a repeat TTE should be performed at 6 months or 1 year. Guidelines use LV dimensions and EF to guide surgical intervention, even in the absence of symptoms. As such, surveillance echocardiography is a class I indication in the setting of asymptomatic severe MR.

50. A. Referral for mitral valve replacement would be least likely recommendation. Although centers experienced in valve repair are increasingly moving to recommend surgery for asymptomatic patients with preserved LV function, it remains a class IIb indication in this setting. If surgery is recommended, valve repair and not replacement should be pursued. The patient definitely needs antibiotic prophylaxis. He also needs close follow-up.

51. A. Referral for mitral valve repair. He is now symptomatic with depressed EF and a dilated LV. This is a class I indication for surgery. Valve repair, as opposed to replacement, is the preferred surgical treatment. Medical therapy may be needed as an adjunct but is insufficient as the sole treatment.

52. C. Referral for surgery is not an acceptable course of action. This is an asymptomatic patient with preserved LV function. The presence of a rheumatic etiology with calcification makes repair significantly less likely. This is a class III indication. This patient is hypertensive, so addition of an ACEI is reasonable.

53. D. Stress echocardiography. His symptoms are equivocal and may just be related to deconditioning. A stress TTE to assess PA pressures and LV response may be useful here. There are insufficient data to refer directly to surgery at this point.

54. A. There is not a consensus of opinion that he needs surgery now. There are data from the Mayo Clinic indicating that the presence of a flail segment (ruptured chordae) implies a greater degree of MR and a higher risk. In their series, all such patients died or required surgery within a 10-year period. There was a small risk of sudden death (0.8%) in patients who were functional class I-11. However, recommendation for surgery in this setting remains controversial.

55. C. MS and tricuspid stenosis. The loud S_1, opening snap, and apical diastolic rumble are features of MS. The presence of the diastolic rumble along the sternal border that increases with inspiration, along with the prominent *a* wave in the jugular venous pulse and evidence of systemic venous congestion (hepatomegaly, peripheral edema), suggest that concomitant tricuspid stenosis is present as well.

56. C. Cardiac catheterization. According to the physical examination, the patient has severe aortic stenosis (no A_2 of S_2, late peaking murmur, and diminished carotid upstrokes). A stress test would not be appropriate in a patient with symptomatic aortic stenosis. A TTE would usually be the first

step, but proceeding directly to catheterization to measure transvalvular gradients and assess coronary anatomy would be reasonable. SL nitroglycerin could have disastrous consequences in this setting. By reducing preload, it may precipitate syncope.

57. B. Refer the patient for percutaneous balloon valvuloplasty followed by gastrectomy. He has symptomatic critical aortic stenosis. AVR, with its concomitant need for anticoagulation while on cardiopulmonary bypass, is not an attractive first option. Proceeding directly to gastric surgery would carry high risk given the ongoing symptoms. Valvuloplasty would be a reasonable bridge to lower risk from the noncardiac surgery.

58. A. Bovine pericardial valve. He is at an age at which there is substantial durability of the bioprosthetic valve. He is at increased risk for anticoagulation; thus, mechanical valves would not be the valves of first choice. According to his history, he does not appear to need anticoagulation for any other indication. Homograft is not unreasonable, but there would not appear to be any hemodynamic or durability benefits for an 80-year-old patient, and its insertion requires a more difficult operation.

59. A. Performing a stress test. The patient has significant AR with a dilated LV (although not yet at the dimensions that would be indicative of a need for surgery in the absence of symptoms: His end-systolic dimension is less than 5.5 cm, and his end-diastolic dimension is less than 7.5 cm). He leads a sedentary lifestyle, and although he has no dyspnea, he does relate some equivocal symptoms. A stress test would be useful to assess functional capacity and to objectively assess symptoms. If he were to develop symptoms at a low level of exercise, this might be an indication for surgical intervention. A vasodilator would be useful, but he would need more frequent follow-up visits given the LV dilatation.

60. B. Surgical intervention. His ventricle has dilated even further. An end-diastolic dimension of greater than 7.5 cm is a class IIa indication for surgery and is associated with an increased risk of sudden death even in the absence of symptoms.

61. B. A mean gradient of 17 mm Hg. The clinical presentation and examination are suggestive of prosthetic MS (long diastolic rumble, muffled closing click, clinical heart failure). The PMI is not displaced, so it is unlikely that she has significant LV dysfunction. There are no clinical signs of severe MR.

62. A. Urgent reoperation. She appears to have significant thrombus burden leading to valvular obstruction and has significant CHF. According to ACC/AHA guidelines, reoperation would be the preferred treatment approach in this setting. If other comorbidities were prohibitive, thrombolytic therapy could be considered.

63. A. Arrhythmias secondary to an accessory pathway. The examination is highly suggestive of Ebstein's anomaly (presence of TR, widely split S_1 with sail-like second component). The TTE confirms this. Accessory pathways are frequently associated with this condition.

64. A. Echocardiography with saline contrast study. Ebstein's anomaly is frequently associated with cardiac shunts (either patent foramen ovale or an atrial septal defect or VSD). The setting of a TIA in someone who has been immobilized (e.g., with a fracture) raises the concern of paradoxical embolism of a venous thrombus to the systemic circulation.

65. B. Doppler echocardiography, using the continuity equation. With significant insufficiency, the Gorlin formula becomes less reliable. Pressure halftime is not used to calculate aortic valve area but does give a clue to the severity of the AI.

66. C. Aortic homograft valve. Mechanical and bioprosthetic valves have a similar incidence of endocarditis, which is higher than that seen for homografts. In the setting of acute bacterial endocarditis of a prosthetic aortic valve, homografts are the valve of first choice when surgery is indicated.

67. D. The patient has severe aortic stenosis, with clinical evidence of heart failure and hypoperfusion. His low albumin suggests a chronically ill state. This is a case in which percutaneous valvuloplasty may be useful as a bridge to more definitive surgical therapy. Improved perfusion postvalvuloplasty may allow for improved overall status and a lower risk for AVR. Surgery may also be considered at this point. A balloon pump may be helpful, and some centers may opt for these approaches. Dialysis is unlikely to help in that it does not address the most likely cause of renal dysfunction: impaired renal perfusion.

68. B. Maximum velocity across the pulmonic valve of 4 m per second. The physical examination is consistent with pulmonic stenosis (presence of thrill, RV heave, ejection click, crescendo-decrescendo murmur loudest over the pulmonic area). Normal carotid upstrokes and a preserved A_2 make significant aortic stenosis unlikely. The murmur is not consistent with a regurgitant murmur.

69. A. He tells you of an episode of syncope. The presence of exertional dyspnea, angina, syncope, or near syncope are class I indications for intervention. For gradients between 30 and 49 mm Hg, there is some divergence of opinion about the role of intervention (class IIb for gradients of 30 to 39, class IIa for gradients of 40 to 49 mm Hg). There is no role for intervention in those with gradients less than 30 mm Hg who have no symptoms. A peak gradient greater than 50 mm Hg is a class I indication even in an asymptomatic patient.

70. A. Percutaneous valvuloplasty. This is the preferred treatment for young adults with pulmonic stenosis.

71. D. Pulmonary hypertension resulting from primary left-sided disease. The most common cause of tricuspid insufficiency is pulmonary hypertension that results from primary pathology on the left side of the heart. This includes aortic and mitral valvular disease as well as LV dysfunction from CAD or other cardiomyopathies.

72. C. Bioprosthetic valves are the preferred option when valve replacement is necessary. There is a greater risk of thrombosis with mechanical valves at the tricuspid position than at other valve positions; hence, bioprosthetic valves are generally preferred. In secondary TR, resulting from RV and annular dilatation from left-sided disease and pulmonary hypertension, annuloplasty is usually successful in alleviating the regurgitation.

73. A. *Streptococcus viridans. S. viridans* accounts for up to 50% of cases of native valve endocarditis. *S. aureus* is the next most common pathogen.

74. C. *Staphylococcus epidermidis.* This patient presents with early prosthetic valve endocarditis (within 2 months of surgery). This is usually acquired during the operation, and the skin species *S. epidermidis* is the most frequent pathogen encountered. Late prosthetic valve endocarditis is similar to native valve endocarditis in terms of the spectrum of pathogens involved.

75. D. Persistent fevers with negative blood cultures. According to recent ACC/AHA guidelines, this is a class III indication. All of the others listed are class I indications.

76. D. A surgically repaired atrial septal defect. This is considered to have a negligible risk by recent ACA/AHA guidelines. All of the other options listed, along with surgically constructed systemic-pulmonary shunts, are considered high-risk populations.

77. A. Dental extraction. Other procedures requiring prophylaxis include periodontal procedures, dental implants and cleaning, tonsillectomy, esophageal dilatation, sclerotherapy, cystoscopy, and urethral dilatation. For high-risk patients, recent guidelines list optional prophylactic regimens for endoscopy and flexible bronchoscopy.

78. B. Ampicillin (2.0 g IV) and gentamicin (1.5 mg/kg) 30 min before the procedure for moderate-risk patients. All of the other regimens listed are current guidelines.

79. C. This patient has a high-profile prosthesis in the mitral position. As such, in the absence of warfarin, she requires IV and not SC heparin. It is imperative that the physician discuss these issues of anticoagulation thoroughly with any patients considering pregnancy.

80. C. Severe MR with functional class I. Generally, regurgitant lesions are better tolerated than stenotic lesions, as pregnancy is associated with decreased systemic vascular resistance. Cardiac output and blood volume are increased, usually compounding stenotic lesions. Eisenmenger's and aortic stenosis with a mean gradient greater than 50 mm Hg are both associated with significant maternal and fetal risk. The AR in and of itself could likely be tolerated, but in the setting of Marfan's syndrome, the concern is for aortic root dilatation as the etiology for the AR. There is a risk of aortic dissection and rupture in these patients, particularly if the root size is greater than 4 cm. If the root is larger than 5 cm, many would advocate elective repair before conception.

SUGGESTED READING

Bonow RO, Carabello B, de Leon AC Jr, et al. ACC/AHA guidelines for the management of patients with valvular heart disease: executive summary. A report of the American College of Cardiology/American Heart Association Task Force on Practice Guidelines (Committee on Management of Patients With Valvular Heart Disease). *Circulation* 1998;98:1949–1984.

Bonow RO, Lakatos E, Maron BJ, et al. Serial long-term assessment of the natural history of asymptomatic patients with chronic AR and normal LV systolic function. *Circulation* 1991;84(4):1625–1635.

Centers for Disease Control and Prevention. Cardiac valvulopathy associated with exposure to fenfluramine and dexfenfluramine: US Department of Health and Human Services interim public health recommendations, November 1997. *JAMA* 1997;278:1729–1731.

Dajani AS, Taubert KA, Wilson W, et al. Prevention of bacterial endocarditis: recommendations by the American Heart Association. *Circulation* 1997;96:358–366.

Grigioni F, Enriquez-Sarano M, Ling LH. Sudden death in mitral regurgitation due to flail leaflet. *J Am Coll Cardiol* 1999;34(7):2078–2085.

Ling LH, Enriquez-Sarano M, Seward JB, et al. Clinical outcome of mitral regurgitation due to flail leaflet. *N Engl J Med* 1996;335(19):1417–1423.

Marso SP, Griffin BP, Topol EJ, eds. *Manual of cardiovascular medicine.* Philadelphia: Lippincott Williams & Wilkins, 2000.

Otto CM, Burwash IG, Legget ME, et al. Prospective study of asymptomatic valvular aortic stenosis. Clinical, echocardiographic, and exercise predictors of outcome. *Circulation* 1997;95(9):2262–2270.

Topol EJ, ed. *Textbook of cardiovascular medicine.* Philadelphia: Lippincott Williams & Wilkins, 2001.

CHAPTER 3

Acute Myocardial Infarction

Deepak L. Bhatt

QUESTIONS

1. A 54-year-old man comes into the emergency department reporting worsening chest pain and dyspnea on exertion. His vital signs are stable. An ECG shows T-wave inversion anterolaterally. Which of the following should be your next step?

   A. give aspirin
   B. start heparin
   C. start nitroglycerin
   D. TTE
   E. cardiac catheterization

2. The patient is given an aspirin and started on IV heparin and nitroglycerin. The patient's chest pain worsens, and he becomes hypotensive. Which of the following is an unlikely explanation for this clinical scenario?

   A. RV infarction
   B. aortic stenosis
   C. pulmonary embolus
   D. esophageal spasm
   E. vagal episode

3. Because of his hemodynamic deterioration, he is taken to the catheterization laboratory emergently. The right coronary artery (RCA) is normal. Left ventriculography is shown in systole and diastole. What is the abnormality (Fig. 1)?

NOTES

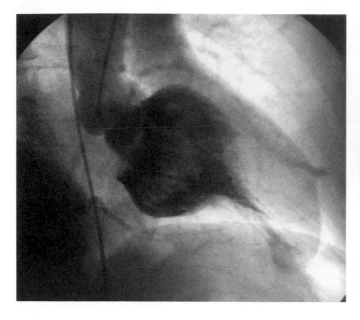

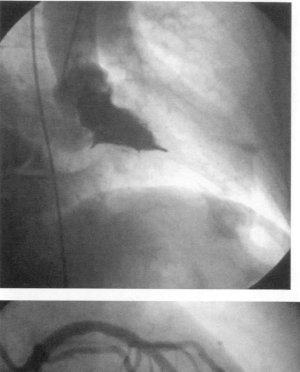

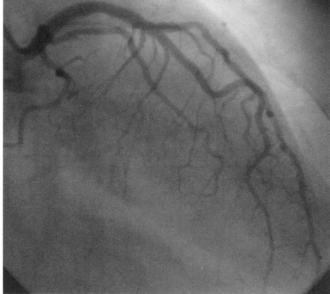

FIGURE 1 (From Bhatt DL, Heupler FA. Coronary angiography. In: Topol EJ, Prystowsky EN, Califf RM, et al., eds. *Textbook of cardiovascular medicine*, 2nd ed. Philadelphia: Lippincott Williams & Wilkins, 2002: eFigure 78.3.5E, with permission.)

    A. anomalous left anterior descending artery (LAD) with severe stenosis
    B. hypertrophic cardiomyopathy
    C. aortic stenosis
    D. LV aneurysm
    E. LV pseudoaneurysm

4. What abnormality does the arrow indicate (Fig. 2)?

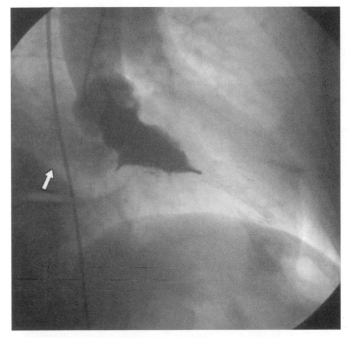

FIGURE 2 (From Bhatt DL, Heupler FA. Coronary angiography. In: Topol EJ, Prystowsky EN, Califf RM, et al., eds. *Textbook of cardiovascular medicine*, 2nd ed. Philadelphia: Lippincott Williams & Wilkins, 2002: eFigure 78.3.5F, with permission.)

A. VSD
B. aortic dissection
C. MR
D. anomalous pulmonary venous return
E. bicuspid aortic valve

5. A 64-year-old man comes into a rural emergency department reporting worsening chest pain. His vital signs are stable. The ECG is shown in Figure 3.

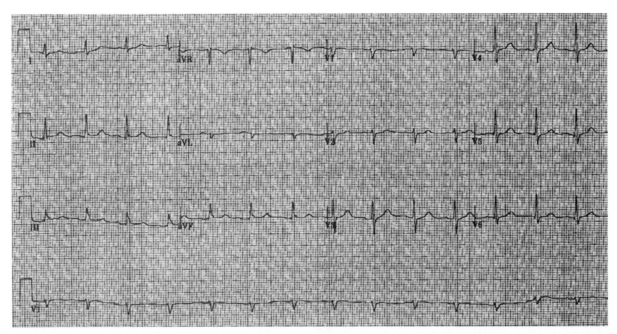

FIGURE 3

What should your next step be?

A. give aspirin
B. give aspirin, heparin, and fibrinolytics
C. give sublingual nitroglycerin and reassess
D. move to the waiting area and observe symptoms
E. discharge to home

6. The patient is given nitroglycerin with no response and a GI cocktail with partial resolution of symptoms. He is sent to the waiting area. While there, his wife sees him slump over, and he is found to be in VF. After several shocks, he is successfully defibrillated. His next ECG is shown in Figure 4.

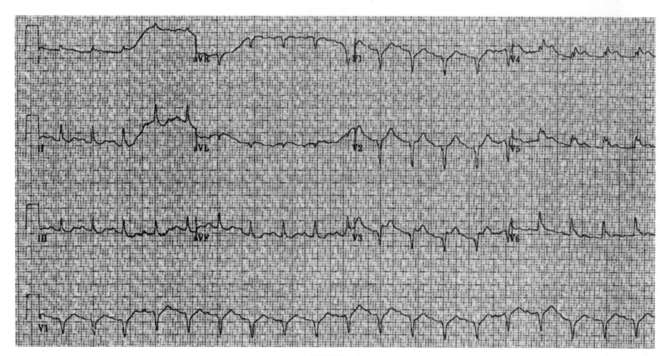

FIGURE 4

What should your next step be?

A. aspirin, heparin, and full-dose tissue plasminogen activator (t-PA)
B. aspirin, heparin, and abciximab
C. aspirin, low-molecular-weight heparin (LMWH), and abciximab
D. aspirin, LMWH, abciximab, and full-dose t-PA
E. aspirin and heparin; transfer the patient to a tertiary care center (3 hours away) for primary percutaneous coronary intervention (PCI)

7. The patient receives aspirin, heparin, and t-PA. He is transferred for catheterization. On arrival, he is sedated, intubated, and hemodynamically stable. The patient is taken to the catheterization laboratory. What do you see in Figures 5 and 6?

A. severe left main disease
B. LAD occlusion
C. diagonal occlusion
D. left circumflex artery (LCx) occlusion
E. mild LAD stenosis with thrombus

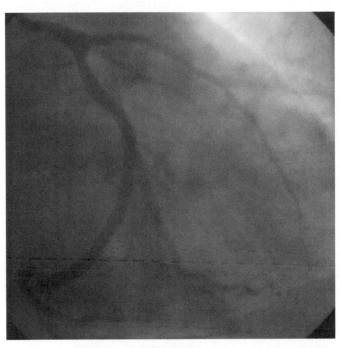

FIGURE 5

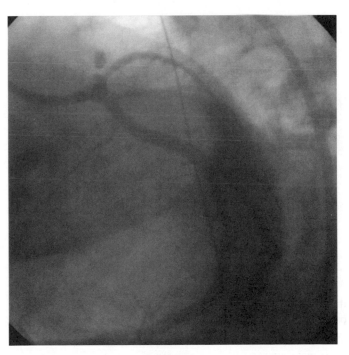

FIGURE 6

8. A 68-year-old woman comes into the emergency room with worsening chest pain at rest for the past 24 hours. The troponin level is elevated. An ECG shows 1- to 2-mm ST depression in leads II, III, and aVF. Which of the following is the *least* appropriate treatment?

   A. aspirin
   B. heparin
   C. glycoprotein (GP) IIb/IIIa inhibitors
   D. LMWH
   E. ticlopidine

9. The patient is taken to the catheterization laboratory. What is the abnormality (Fig. 7)?

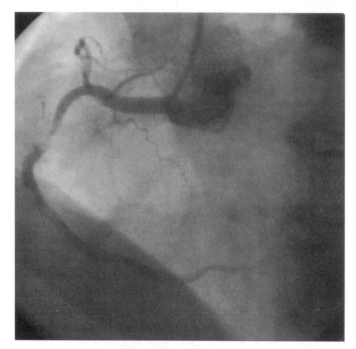

FIGURE 7

   A. spontaneous dissection
   B. coronary spasm
   C. anomalous origin of severely stenosed vessel
   D. severe stenosis with thrombus
   E. coronary aneurysm

10. During catheterization, the patient's pain continues. She has received aspirin and heparin and is on eptifibatide. What should your next step be?

   A. add tirofiban and recatheterize in 2 days
   B. emergent bypass surgery
   C. dipyridamole (Persantine) nuclear stress test
   D. IABP placement
   E. angioplasty and stenting

11. The patient has hypotension. To which of the following is this most likely due?

    A. volume depletion
    B. RV infarction
    C. pulmonary embolism
    D. aortic dissection
    E. pericarditis

12. Appropriate methods to treat RV infarction might include all of the following *except*

    A. aggressive hydration
    B. AV pacing
    C. IABP placement
    D. reperfusion
    E. diuresis

13. A 70-year-old woman comes into the emergency department reporting 3 hours of crushing chest pain. The initial ECG shows NSR with nonspecific ST-T–wave changes. Initial troponin is borderline positive. Because of the patient's severe chest pain, she is taken to the catheterization laboratory. What do the angiograms (Fig. 8) demonstrate?

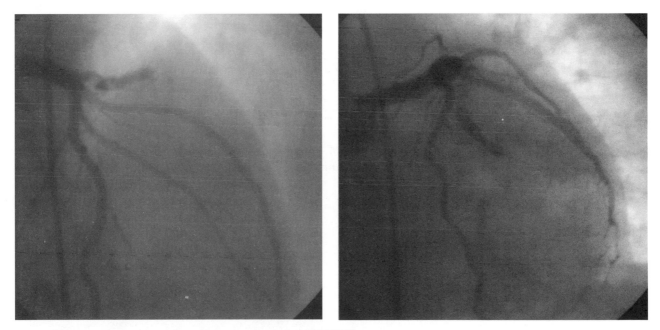

FIGURE 8

    A. severe LAD stenosis
    B. normal coronary arteries
    C. occluded LAD
    D. occluded LCx
    E. occluded RCA

14. The angiogram (Fig. 9) shows the result after PCI.

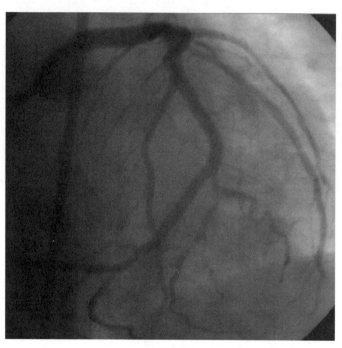

FIGURE 9

What do you see?

A. residual stenosis
B. propagation of thrombus
C. procedural dissection flap
D. patent vessel with Thrombolysis in Myocardial Infarction (TIMI)-3 flow
E. patent vessel with TIMI-1 flow

15. What physical examination findings may be present in a patient with the following findings at catheterization (Fig. 10)?

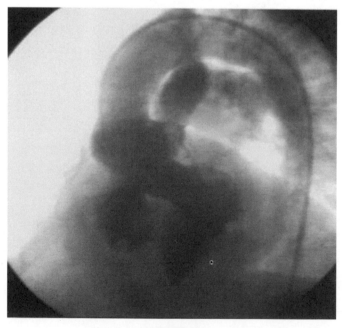

FIGURE 10

A. S_3

B. systolic and diastolic murmur

C. pericardial rub

D. crescendo-decrescendo systolic murmur

E. diastolic rumble

16. Which of the following has been shown to potentially trigger acute MI?

    A. earthquakes

    B. stress

    C. anger

    D. sexual activity

    E. all of the above

17. Which of the following is the mechanism of action of clopidogrel?

    A. thromboxane inhibition

    B. GP IIb/IIIa receptor blockade

    C. adenosine diphosphate blockade

    D. increase in cyclic adenosine monophosphate production

    E. free radical scavenger

18. In which of the following has the high-sensitivity C-reactive protein (CRP) been shown to be predictive of risk?

    A. acute MI

    B. acute coronary syndromes (ACSs)

    C. chronic stable angina

    D. peripheral vascular disease

    E. all of the above

19. Which of the following has been shown to decrease the level of the high-sensitivity CRP?

    A. unopposed estrogen

    B. amlodipine (Norvasc)

    C. simvastatin

    D. all of the above

    E. none of the above

20. Which of the following is an effective adjunct to increase the rate of smoking cessation?

    A. aldosterone

    B. bupropion

    C. buspirone

    D. cimetidine

    E. allopurinol

21. Bupropion (Zyban) is contraindicated in patients with a history of which of the following?

    A. seizures
    B. insulin-dependent diabetes mellitus
    C. severe chronic obstructive pulmonary disease (with reversible component)
    D. longer than 40-year history of tobacco use
    E. recent MI

22. Which of the following is *true* for management of acute ST segment–elevation MI?

    A. Aspirin has a much larger effect than streptokinase.
    B. Streptokinase has a much larger effect than aspirin.
    C. Streptokinase and aspirin each have a similar effect on outcome.
    D. When streptokinase and aspirin are used together, their effects are blunted.

23. Currently recommended therapies in the emergency department for acute MI include all of the following *except*

    A. aspirin
    B. t-PA
    C. clopidogrel
    D. heparin

24. Which of the following is *least* predictive of mortality in patients presenting with acute MI who are treated with fibrinolytics?

    A. location of MI (i.e., anterior vs. inferior)
    B. age
    C. heart rate
    D. BP
    E. presence or absence of diabetes
    F. Killip class

25. Which of the following have beta-blockers for acute MI been shown to do?

    A. decrease the rate of intracranial hemorrhage from fibrinolysis
    B. decrease ventricular arrhythmias
    C. improve mortality
    D. all of the above
    E. none of the above

26. In the setting of primary angioplasty for acute MI, which of the following have stents been convincingly shown to do?

    A. decrease subsequent repeat target vessel revascularization (TVR)
    B. decrease long-term mortality
    C. decrease long-term MI risk
    D. decrease the incidence of heart failure

27. Factors believed to be important in the pathogenesis of plaque rupture include which of the following?

    A. matrix metalloproteinases
    B. shear stress
    C. macrophages
    D. all of the above
    E. none of the above

28. The rate of stroke seen in the Global Utilization of Streptokinase and t-PA for Occluded Coronary Arteries (GUSTO)-III trial was approximately which of the following?

    A. 0.01%
    B. 0.1%
    C. 1%
    D. 10%

29. Which of the following is *true* about reteplase in GUSTO-III?

    A. It had a significantly higher rate of stroke than alteplase.
    B. It significantly reduced mortality compared with alteplase.
    C. It significantly reduced mortality but increased stroke compared with alteplase.
    D. It had similar rates of mortality to alteplase.

30. Which of the following statements is *not* true?

    A. Vitamin E is beneficial for acute MI patients.
    B. Fibrinolysis leads to platelet activation.
    C. Unstable angina and non–ST-elevation MI are more common causes of hospitalization in the United States than ST-elevation MI.
    D. Troponin levels are useful for risk-stratification of acute MI.

31. The Antiarrhythmics Versus Implantable Defibrillators study showed that which of the following is true for patients with acute MI who survive VF or sustained, symptomatic VT with an EF less than or equal to 40%?

    A. They benefit from an ICD more than antiarrhythmic therapy.
    B. They benefit from EP testing to decide whether an ICD is indicated.
    C. They should receive an ICD and concomitant amiodarone.
    D. All of the above are true.
    E. None of the above is true.

32. The Survival and Ventricular Enlargement study demonstrated which of the following regarding captopril among patients with MI?

    A. It decreased mortality if patients did not receive fibrinolysis.
    B. It decreased mortality in patients with symptomatic CHF.
    C. It decreased the need for subsequent CHF-related hospitalization.
    D. All of the above are true.
    E. None of the above is true.

33. With which of the following is sildenafil acetate (Viagra) most likely to interact adversely?

    A. fibrinolytic therapy
    B. primary PCI
    C. nitrates
    D. aspirin
    E. beta-blockers

34. The GUSTO-I trial showed which of the following regarding accelerated t-PA for acute MI?

    A. It reduced mortality compared with streptokinase and IV heparin.
    B. It reduced mortality compared with streptokinase and SC heparin.
    C. It increased the rate of hemorrhagic stroke compared with streptokinase.
    D. All of the above are true.
    E. None of the above is true.

35. For patients presenting with cardiogenic shock, which of the following was demonstrated in the SHOCK trial?

    A. There is a statistically significant reduction in mortality at 30 days with early revascularization.
    B. In the patients randomized to medical therapy, the rate of mortality at 30 days was almost 100%.
    C. At 6 months, mortality was reduced by over 50% in patients randomized to emergency revascularization.
    D. All of the above are true.
    E. None of the above is true.

36. Which of the following statements is *true* regarding patients who develop VF after admission for acute MI?

    A. VF in the first 48 hours is generally benign.
    B. VF in the first 48 hours is associated with a worse prognosis.
    C. Only VF developing after 48 hours affects prognosis.
    D. None of the above is true.

37. Which of the following supports the routine use of type 1 antiarrhythmics in patients with PVCs who have had an MI?

    A. the Cardiac Arrhythmia Suppression Trial (CAST) study
    B. the Basal Antiarrhythmic Study of Infarct Survival (BASIS) study
    C. the Multicenter Unsustained Tachycardia Trial (MUSTT) study
    D. all of the above
    E. none of the above

38. The MADIT-I trial showed which of the following in patients with prior MI?

    A. ICD implantation decreased mortality in patients with an EF less than or equal to 35%.
    B. ICD implantation reduced mortality in patients with an abnormal signal-averaged ECG.
    C. ICD implantation in patients with suppressible VT on EP testing had decreased mortality.
    D. ICDs decreased mortality in patients, irrespective of their baseline LV function.

39. In patients with acute MI who undergo angiography, which of the following statements is *true* regarding TIMI flow?

    A. TIMI-3 flow is associated with a higher mortality than TIMI-2 flow.
    B. TIMI-2 or -3 flow is associated with a patent artery.
    C. TIMI-2 and -3 flows are associated with similar rates of mortality.
    D. All of the above are true.
    E. None of the above is true.

40. In diabetic patients with acute MI, the rate of mortality compared with non-diabetic patients is approximately which of the following?

    A. the same
    B. twice as high
    C. five times as high
    D. ten times as high

41. Which of the following statements about acute MI is *false*?

    A. An elevated white blood cell count is associated with a greater risk of mortality.
    B. Aspirin, beta-blockers, and ACE inhibitors remain underused.
    C. Passive smoking is a risk factor for lung cancer as well as for heart disease.
    D. Patients with a history of heart failure should not receive beta-blockers.

42. For acute MI, which of the following is *true*?

    A. Large, randomized studies have found that nitrates reduce long-term mortality.
    B. ACE inhibitors have been shown to reduce mortality.
    C. Multiple randomized studies have found that heparin reduces mortality.
    D. All of the above are true.
    E. None of the above is true.

43. Which of the following is a true statement about the class III antiarrhythmic dofetilide in acute MI?

    A. It decreases the rate of death compared with placebo.
    B. It increases the rate of death compared with placebo.
    C. It is effective for the treatment of AFib and flutter.
    D. It decreases the risk of torsades de pointes.
    E. A, C, and D are true.

44. In acute MI, which of the following is *true* about IV lidocaine?

    A. When used prophylactically, it reduces mortality by more than 50%.
    B. It should not be used prophylactically.
    C. It should be administered routinely in patients with an EF of less than 35%.
    D. It should be given to all patients who receive streptokinase.

45. During acute MI, which of the following is *true* about IV magnesium?

    A. It should be routinely administered due to its significant survival benefit.
    B. It should be administered as an adjunct to primary PCI.
    C. It does not have a clear benefit in patients undergoing reperfusion therapy.
    D. It has a significant additive effect when used with fibrinolytics.

46. Warfarin is strongly indicated in patients with acute MI who have which of the following conditions?

    A. AFib
    B. symptomatic LV dysfunction
    C. asymptomatic LV dysfunction
    D. all of the above
    E. none of the above

47. Which of the following statements is *true* regarding MI due to cocaine abuse?

    A. Cocaine promotes coagulation.
    B. Cocaine accelerates atherosclerosis.
    C. Cocaine can trigger coronary spasm.
    D. Cocaine can raise BP.
    E. All of the above are true.
    F. None of the above is true.

48. A 64-year-old man presents with chest pain and is noted to have ST elevation in his inferior leads. His BP is 80/40, and his pulse is 130 bpm. The heart sounds are distant, and the neck veins are elevated. Which of the following would be the best next step?

    A. fibrinolysis
    B. coronary angiography
    C. TTE
    D. heparinization
    E. all of the above

49. A quick bedside TTE is performed and shows a large pericardial effusion. Which of the following would be the best next step?

    A. fibrinolysis
    B. IABP placement
    C. pericardiocentesis
    D. all of the above
    E. none of the above

50. Which of the following is approximately the 30-day mortality in the GUSTO-I trial in patients aged 75 years or older?

    A. 1%
    B. 5%
    C. 20%
    D. 50%
    E. 90%

51. In the GUSTO-I trial, the benefit of t-PA over streptokinase was greatest in those patients who were treated

    A. within 2 hours after MI
    B. between 2 and 4 hours after MI
    C. between 4 and 6 hours after MI
    D. over 6 hours after MI
    E. there was no time dependency observed in this trial

52. Which of the following was a finding of the GUSTO-II angioplasty study?

    A. Primary percutaneous transluminal coronary angioplasty (PTCA) reduced 30-day mortality when compared with accelerated-dose t-PA.
    B. Accelerated t-PA reduced 30-day mortality when compared with primary PTCA.
    C. Accelerated t-PA and primary PTCA produced almost identical outcomes at 30 days.
    D. Primary PTCA with abciximab was superior to accelerated-dose t-PA.

53. Two weeks after a hospitalization for an anterior wall MI, a 58-year-old man returns with reports of fever and chest pain. Laboratory studies are significant for an elevated white blood cell count. An ECG reveals ST elevation in the anterior, lateral, and inferior leads. Which of the following is the correct diagnosis?

    A. recurrent MI
    B. aneurysm formation
    C. myocardial abscess
    D. Dressler's syndrome
    E. none of the above

54. Which of the following have been used as therapy for post-MI pericarditis?

    A. aspirin
    B. nonsteroidal antiinflammatory drugs
    C. steroids
    D. colchicine
    E. all of the above
    F. none of the above

55. Which of the following is *true* regarding pericarditis in acute MI?

    A. Fibrinolysis has no effect on the incidence of pericarditis in MI.
    B. Fibrinolysis reduces the incidence of pericarditis in MI.
    C. Fibrinolysis increases the incidence of pericarditis in MI.
    D. No data have examined this issue.

56. A 78-year-old woman with an inferior wall MI is receiving t-PA. One hour later, she reports a headache and is subsequently noted to be lethargic and not able to raise her right arm or leg. Which of the following would be the best next step?

    A. getting a stat head CT
    B. getting a stat ECG; if ST elevation resolves, stopping t-PA infusion
    C. stopping t-PA
    D. giving platelets

57. Which of the following would be useful to reverse the action of t-PA?

    A. protamine
    B. hirudin
    C. cryoprecipitate
    D. epsilon aminocaproic acid
    E. B and C
    F. C and D

58. Which of the following is *true* about ventricular septal rupture?

    A. It is more common with inferior MI than with anterior MI.
    B. It is less common with transmural MI than with nontransmural MI.
    C. It is more common with a first MI.
    D. All of the above are true.
    E. None of the above is true.

59. Which of the following is *true* about acute MR in the setting of acute MI?

    A. It is more common in women than in men.
    B. It is more common in older patients than in younger patients.
    C. It is more common in patients with a prior MI.
    D. All of the above are true.
    E. None of the above is true.

60. Regarding acute MR due to MI, which of the following statements is *false*?

    A. The posteromedial papillary muscle is supplied by the posterior descending artery.
    B. The anterolateral papillary muscle is supplied by the LAD.
    C. The anterolateral papillary muscle is supplied by the LCx.
    D. Medical therapy is preferred over surgical therapy for definitive management.
    E. All of the above are true.
    F. All of the above are false.

61. Which of the following statements about the use of IABPs is *false*?

    A. They may be useful in aortic stenosis.
    B. They may be useful in aortic regurgitation.
    C. They may be useful in MR.
    D. They may be useful in ventricular septal rupture.
    E. They may be useful in RV infarction.

62. A 68-year-old man presents with an anterior wall MI. His symptoms started 3 hours before. He has a history of hypertension and smoking. His heart rate is 90 bpm, and his BP is 240/120. He has an S_3 on examination. His lungs have rales at the bases. Which of the following is true?

    A. With his BP, fibrinolysis would be safer than primary angioplasty.
    B. His risk of intracranial hemorrhage is increased with t-PA.
    C. Placement of an IABP is strongly indicated.
    D. A TEE should be the next step.
    E. None of the above is true.

63. A 72-year-old man has sustained an inferior wall MI. His BP is 200/100. Appropriate therapies may include all of the following *except*

    A. sublingual nifedipine
    B. IV metoprolol
    C. PO captopril
    D. IV nitroglycerin
    E. sublingual nitroglycerin

64. A 55-year-old man with a history of mild hypertension comes into the emergency department with severe chest pain. He reports exertional and nonexertional chest discomfort over the past several months. His internist

performed a stress thallium 2 weeks ago. This was normal at 93% maximal predicted heart rate. He is given an aspirin and three sublingual nitroglycerin tablets, with partial relief of his chest discomfort. He is given a GI cocktail, with further improvement in his chest discomfort. His troponin and cardiac enzymes are negative. He is placed in the chest pain unit for further observation. What does his initial ECG show (Fig. 11)?

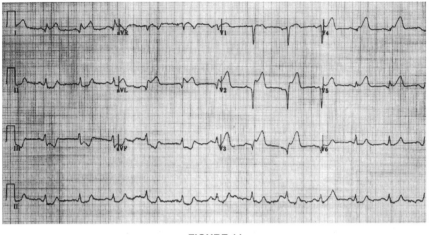

FIGURE 11

A. acute pericarditis
B. cardiac tamponade
C. ischemia
D. LV hypertrophy
E. AFib

65. The patient's second set of cardiac enzymes comes back elevated, and he is admitted to the cardiac care unit. An angiogram is performed. What is the infarct-related lesion on this angiogram (Fig. 12)?

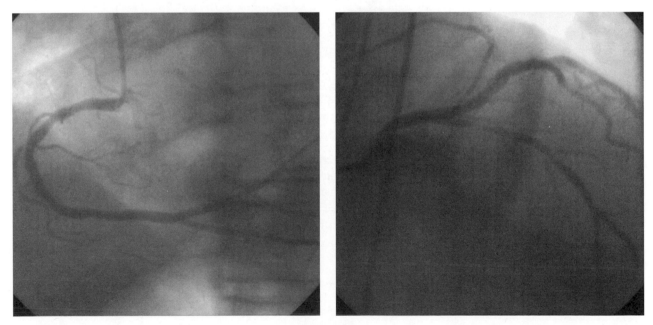

FIGURE 12

A. RCA stenosis
B. LCx stenosis
C. LAD stenosis
D. left main stenosis
E. no significant lesion

66. An 84-year-old woman presents with an acute inferior MI. She is treated conservatively with aspirin, heparin, and nitroglycerin. You are asked to evaluate her 3 days after her infarction. She has been pain free since the day of her presentation, with no angina, CHF, or arrhythmia. Which of the following would be the best next step?

A. diagnostic angiography only
B. diagnostic angiography with ad hoc PCI if the anatomy is suitable
C. symptom-limited treadmill exercise stress test before discharge
D. discharge with no further evaluation

67. This patient is taken to the catheterization suite for an angiogram. What do you see in Figure 13?

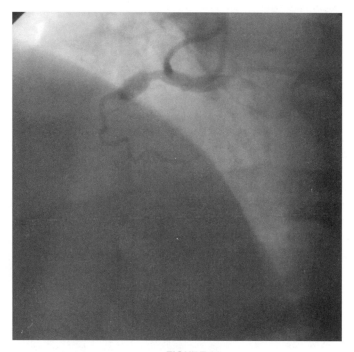

FIGURE 13

A. a severe diagonal lesion
B. a severe lateral circumflex lesion
C. collaterals to the distal LAD
D. collaterals to the RCA
E. occlusion of the RCA

68. An angioplasty is attempted, but difficulty is encountered in passing the wire through the lesion. The patient starts to get hypotensive. Which of the following is the most likely possibility to explain the hypotension?

    A. retroperitoneal bleed
    B. groin hematoma
    C. coronary perforation
    D. coronary dissection
    E. abrupt vessel occlusion

69. The patient remains hypotensive as these angiograms (Fig. 14) are performed.

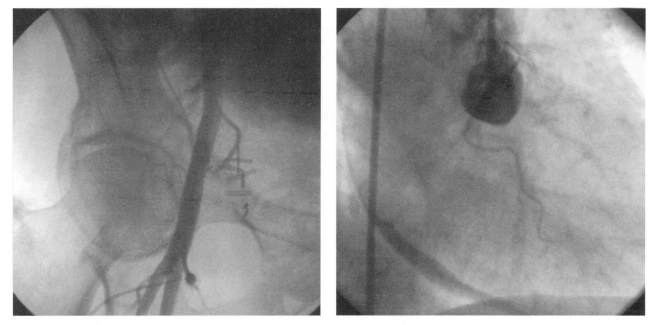

FIGURE 14

Now what do you think is the likely etiology of the hypotension?

    A. retroperitoneal bleed
    B. groin hematoma
    C. coronary perforation
    D. coronary dissection
    E. abrupt vessel occlusion

70. A 68-year-old man is brought to the emergency department reporting chest pain for the past 2 hours. The bedside troponin is positive, and the initial ECG shows ST segment depression in the anterior leads. Appropriate next steps include any of the following *except*

    A. aspirin
    B. clopidogrel
    C. tirofiban
    D. eptifibatide
    E. abciximab

71. The patient is given aspirin, heparin, nitroglycerin, metoprolol, and tirofiban, and his pain and ECG changes resolve. Which of the following would be the best next step?

    A. exercise treadmill stress test
    B. cardiac catheterization
    C. TTE
    D. positron emission tomography
    E. IABP placement

72. The cardiac catheterization is performed. The angiogram (Fig. 15) is as follows.

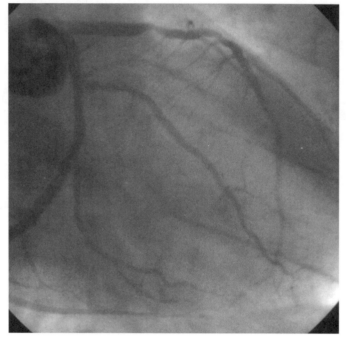

FIGURE 15

What do you see?

    A. totally occluded LAD
    B. collaterals to the LAD
    C. severe lesion in the diagonal branch
    D. severe lesion in the LCx
    E. none of the above

73. A 47-year-old woman with a history of hypertension presents to your emergency department reporting chest pain. She tells you she had a stent placed in her RCA 4 months ago. Her ECG shows ST elevation in the inferior leads. Which of the following is a possible explanation of her chest pain?

    A. stent thrombosis
    B. stent restenosis
    C. plaque rupture at a site elsewhere in her RCA
    D. all of the above
    E. none of the above

74. What does this angiogram (Fig. 16) show?

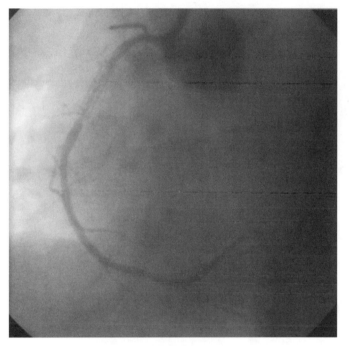

FIGURE 16

    A. severe restenosis of the RCA
    B. an intraluminal filling defect consistent with thrombus
    C. stent edge dissection
    D. extrinsic stent compression

75. A 65-year-old woman sustains a non–ST segment elevation MI from which she recovers uneventfully. She had been taking aspirin, 325 mg per day. Appropriate steps on discharge may include all of the following *except*

    A. increasing the dose of aspirin to 650 mg per day
    B. starting clopidogrel, 75 mg per day
    C. continuing aspirin at a dose of 81 mg per day
    D. continuing aspirin at a dose of 162 mg per day

76. An 83-year-old man presents to the catheterization suite with a chest pain syndrome. What does the LV angiogram show (Fig. 17)?

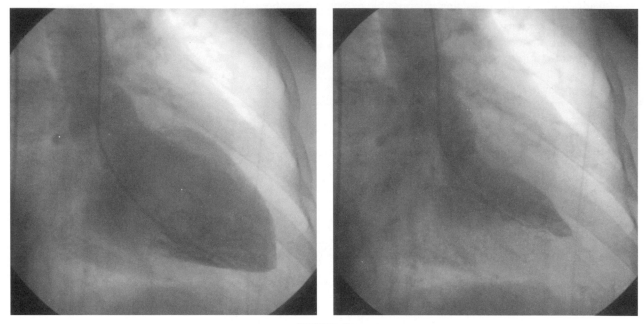

FIGURE 17

A. akinetic anterior wall
B. normal LV function
C. ventricular aneurysm
D. ventricular pseudoaneurysm
E. MR

77. Which of the following is the most likely explanation for the patient's MI (Fig. 18)?

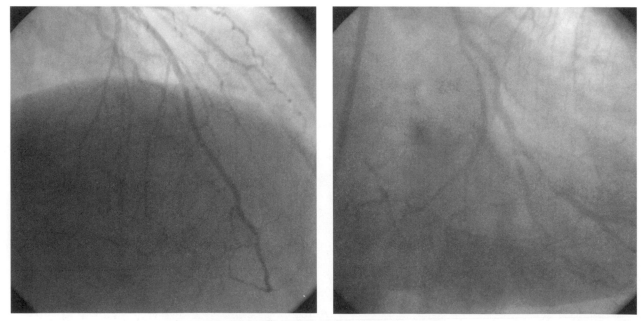

FIGURE 18

A. RCA occlusion
B. LAD occlusion
C. LCx occlusion
D. coronary dissection

78. Which of the following is *true* regarding the placement of stents during acute MI angioplasty?

A. It decreases mortality.
B. It decreases TVR.
C. It leads to large improvements in rates of TIMI-3 flow.
D. It increases the risk of arrhythmia.
E. It decreases the rate of CHF.

79. Which of the following are indicators of successful reperfusion for acute MI?

A. resolution of chest pain
B. TIMI-3 flow on angiography
C. resolution of ST segment elevation
D. all of the above
E. none of the above

80. Which of the following statements is *true* regarding the effect of gender on outcome after acute MI?

A. Female gender doubles the risk of mortality from MI.
B. Female gender triples the risk of mortality from MI.
C. There is no large difference in outcome based on gender when age and other comorbidities are considered.
D. Women have one-fourth the risk of death that men do.

81. Other than atherosclerosis, which of the following causes acute MI?

A. coronary spasm
B. spontaneous coronary dissection
C. coronary embolization
D. all of the above
E. none of the above

82. Which of the following statements is *true* regarding diabetes mellitus?

A. Diabetes raises the risk of MI the same amount as does having a history of prior MI.
B. The risk of MI due to diabetes is entirely confined to insulin-requiring diabetic patients.
C. Diabetes increases the risk of MI but does not significantly affect outcome once an MI has occurred.
D. Diabetes has minimal impact on the risk of MI once patient age is considered.

83. Which of the following statements is *not* true regarding the SHOCK trial?

A. The majority of infarctions were anterior.
B. The difference in mortality between patients randomized to emergency revascularization versus initial medical stabilization at 30 days was not statistically significant.
C. Mortality at 6 months was lower in the revascularization group than in the medical group.
D. Patients derived equal benefit from revascularization, regardless of age.

84. Which of the following measures has been demonstrated to decrease the risk of perioperative MI during vascular surgery in patients with evidence of cardiac ischemia?
    A. routine PA catheterization
    B. use of calcium channel blockers
    C. use of beta-blockers
    D. use of nitrates

ANSWERS

1. A. Give aspirin. All the answers may be appropriate, but the question asked for the next step. This sort of question is common: Several correct answers are given, but you need to pick the most important one to do first.

2. D. Esophageal spasm. If anything, nitroglycerin would be expected to improve esophageal spasm. Not all nitrate-responsive pain is cardiac in etiology. Be aware of preload-dependent states, such as aortic stenosis, dehydration, cardiac tamponade, and RV infarction, in which nitroglycerin may cause hypotension.

3. B. Hypertrophic cardiomyopathy. There is no significant disease in the LAD, just prominent septal perforators. The comment about the normal RCA, while showing you the LAD, is a trick the board examinations like to play. The real abnormality is in the ventriculography. If systolic and diastolic frames are shown, wall motion abnormalities and hypertrophic obstructive cardiomyopathy should both be considered; for coronaries, myocardial bridging should be considered.

4. C. MR. MR is often due to systolic anterior motion of the mitral valve. However, there can also be intrinsic mitral valvular abnormalities. Part of knowing the answer to questions regarding still-frame images, often of poor quality, is to know what you are looking for. The key point from this case is that you must remember that all chest pain is not due to coronary ischemia.

5. A. Give aspirin. The initial ECG is rather unremarkable, although there may be slight ST elevation noted in some of the inferior leads. A middle-aged or older patient coming in to the emergency department reporting chest pain deserves an aspirin while serial troponins, creatine kinases, and ECGs are being obtained (while the patient remains on telemetry). Early fibrinolytic therapy is important, but there is no clear-cut ST elevation or LBBB. Response to nitroglycerin, as was discussed earlier, does not necessarily indicate cardiac origin of pain.

6. A. Aspirin, heparin, and full-dose t-PA. The patient has an ST elevation MI. Anterior MI in particular is associated with increased mortality, and prompt reperfusion is indicated. Don't be confused by recent trial data—recent data will not be on the test. *Rural* is often a key word: If the time to primary PCI is longer than 90 to 120 min, fibrinolysis is probably preferred.

7. B. LAD occlusion. Always look for the LAD with its septal perforators. Although it is not uncommon to find a moderate stenosis with superimposed

thrombus after fibrinolysis, this patient has not reperfused after lytics. This rather proximal infarction is likely to be associated with significant LV dysfunction and arrhythmic risk.

8. E. Ticlopidine is the least appropriate treatment in this case. Clopidogrel in Unstable Angina to Prevent Recurrent Ischemic Events (CURE) data on clopidogrel are important but unlikely to be on the board examination (too recent). On the other hand, the LMWH and GP IIb/IIIa inhibitor data are old enough that you should know these agents have a role in ACS.

9. D. Severe stenosis with thrombus. This patient's ACS is due to a severe underlying stenosis with superimposed thrombus seen on angiography. Even when the thrombus is not angiographically apparent, ACS lesions are rich in platelet thrombus. Thus, antiplatelet agents, such as aspirin, clopidogrel, and IV GP IIb/IIIa inhibitors, are useful.

10. E. Angioplasty and stenting. Given the data from FRISC II (with LMWH) and TACTICS (Treat Angina with Aggrastat and Determine Costs of Therapy with Invasive or Conservative Strategies)–TIMI 18 (with tirofiban), an invasive approach is preferred to a conservative approach in patients presenting with ACSs. This is particularly true in patients with elevated troponin or ST depression. Even with a conservative approach, a patient with refractory ischemia on medical therapy would be a candidate for early revascularization.

11. B. RV infarction. The coronary angiogram shows an almost occluded RCA. RV infarction may complicate an RCA infarct, leading to marked hypotension.

12. E. Diuresis is not appropriate to treat RV infarction. Aggressive volume repletion is often necessary in RV infarction. Several liters of fluid may be necessary to maintain the preload. Diuresis can dramatically worsen the hypotension of RV infarction. Sequential AV pacing can be extremely useful in cases of heart block. An IABP can be used in cardiogenic shock, especially when there is concomitant LV dysfunction or ischemia. Reperfusion therapy is obviously indicated.

13. D. Occluded LCx. An LCx infarction may be electrocardiographically silent, as in this patient's case. The angiogram reveals that the LCx is occluded.

14. D. Patent vessel with TIMI-3 flow. The vessel is patent, with excellent angiographic result. It is not really possible to comment on TIMI flow on a still-frame image, but contrast dye is present distally in both the LAD and LCx, which implies that there is now TIMI-3 flow in the LCx.

15. B. Systolic and diastolic murmur. The angiograms demonstrate a VSD. Mechanical complications from an acute MI are favorite topics for board examinations.

16. E. All of the above. All of the listed factors have been shown to be potential triggers for acute MI.

17. C. Adenosine diphosphate blockade. Clopidogrel blocks the adenosine diphosphate receptor and ultimately prevents GP IIb/IIIa receptor–mediated

platelet aggregation. The board examination stresses knowledge of the basic pharmacology of the drugs used in cardiology.

18. E. All of the above. High-sensitivity CRP is a potent predictor of risk in a variety of populations with atherosclerotic disease. An elevated CRP is an independent risk factor for MI and stroke.

19. C. Simvastatin. All of the statins appear to have an effect on lowering CRP.

20. B. Bupropion. Bupropion has been shown in randomized studies to be associated with a modest increase in the rate of smoking cessation.

21. A. Seizures. Bupropion can rarely cause seizures and is generally best avoided in patients with a history of seizures. It is also contraindicated in patients with a history of bulimia and anorexia nervosa. It can be used safely in patients with recent MI.

22. C. Streptokinase and aspirin each have a similar effect on outcome. The ISIS-2 trial demonstrated that both aspirin and streptokinase had similar effects on mortality, with additive benefits.

23. C. There is currently no completed randomized clinical trial of clopidogrel for acute MI. However, the COMMIT trial (also referred to as *CCS-2*) is ongoing and is randomizing patients to clopidogrel or placebo, with patients receiving aspirin in both arms. Until the results of this trial are available to support the safety of combinations of aspirin, clopidogrel, heparin, and fibrinolysis, the use of clopidogrel in acute MI patients should be reserved for those undergoing percutaneous intervention or for secondary prevention.

24. E. Presence or absence of diabetes is least predictive of mortality. Based on the GUSTO model of mortality after acute MI, the other factors listed are major determinants of outcome. Although diabetes also increases the risk of adverse outcomes, it is not as potent as the other listed factors.

25. D. All of the above. Although much of the data regarding the benefits of beta-blockade were obtained before the fibrinolytic era, these agents appear to decrease the rate of intracranial hemorrhage in patients receiving lytics. Older data have shown their value in preventing VF.

26. A. Decrease subsequent repeat TVR. Stents have clearly been shown to decrease TVR in the setting of primary angioplasty.

27. D. All of the above. All the listed factors are believed to be important in initiating plaque rupture.

28. C. 1%. The rate of stroke in most contemporary trials of fibrinolysis is approximately 1%.

29. D. It had similar rates of mortality to alteplase. The rates of mortality and stroke were similar for reteplase and alteplase. The major advantage of reteplase was that it could be given as two boluses rather than as an infusion.

30. A. The GISSI (Gruppo Italiano Per lo Studio Della Streptokinase Nell'Infarto Miocardio)–Prevenzione trial did not find a benefit of vitamin E in acute MI. Fibrinolysis for acute MI does lead to platelet activation. Non–ST-elevation ACS is more common than ST-elevation MI. Interestingly, troponin elevation at baseline does help predict risk even in acute MI, just as it does in ACS.

31. A. They benefit from an ICD more than antiarrhythmic therapy. Patients with VF or high-risk VT who were randomized to ICD versus empiric use of a type III antiarrhythmic (predominantly amiodarone) had significantly lower rates of all-cause mortality. The strategy was not guided by EP testing.

32. C. It decreased the need for subsequent CHF-related hospitalization. In the Survival and Ventricular Enlargement trial, the ACE inhibitor captopril was demonstrated to decrease all-cause mortality in patients with *asymptomatic* LV dysfunction (EF less than or equal to 40%) after acute MI. The benefits were present even in patients receiving aspirin, fibrinolysis, or beta-blockade. There were also significant decreases in subsequent severe CHF, hospitalization for CHF, and recurrent MI.

33. C. Nitrates. Doctors need to be aware of the potential for marked hypotension when nitrates are administered to a patient who has taken sildenafil acetate recently.

34. D. All of the above are true. The GUSTO-I trial showed that accelerated t-PA reduced mortality when compared with streptokinase (either with SC heparin or IV heparin). There was an increase in the rate of hemorrhagic stroke, but this was outweighed by the reduction in overall mortality.

35. E. None of the above is true. The SHOCK trial found a significant reduction in mortality at 6 months in those patients who were randomized to emergency revascularization as opposed to initial medical therapy (50.3% vs. 63.1%; $p = .027$). This benefit was present at 30 days but was not statistically significant at that time (46.7% vs. 56.0%; $p = .11$). Despite early revascularization, the rate of mortality in patients with acute MI and cardiogenic shock is quite high, at least 50%.

36. B. VF in the first 48 hours is associated with a worse prognosis. In one study, the overall incidence of primary VF was 2.8%; in-hospital mortality nearly doubled for these patients, from 5.9% to 10.8%. In this same study, IV streptokinase did not reduce the incidence of primary VF. However, fibrinolytics do appear to reduce the incidence of secondary VF, probably by limiting infarct size. Other studies have corroborated the relationship between primary VF and worse outcome. VF after 2 days also correlates with worse outcome.

37. E. None of the above. The CAST-I and CAST-II studies found that there was no benefit, and that there was in fact detriment, in trying to suppress asymptomatic or mildly symptomatic PVCs after acute MI. The BASIS study suggested that low-dose amiodarone may be useful in some patients with complex ventricular ectopy. The MUSTT study found that EP-guided therapy with ICDs reduced the risk of sudden death in high-risk patients.

38. A. ICD implantation decreased mortality in patients with an EF less than or equal to 35%. MADIT I showed that in patients with prior MI, LV dysfunction (EF less than or equal to 35%), asymptomatic nonsustained VT, and inducible, nonsuppressible VT on EP testing, there was a reduction in all-cause mortality in patients randomized to receive an ICD instead of conventional medical therapy.

39. B. TIMI-2 or -3 flow is associated with a patent artery. TIMI flow is a powerful determinant of mortality. TIMI-3 flow is associated with a lower rate of mortality than TIMI-2 flow, which is associated with a lower mortality than TIMI-0 or -1 flow. With TIMI-2 or -3 flow, the epicardial artery is patent, but with TIMI-2, the flow is sluggish, and studies have shown that this difference in angiographic flow translates into a difference in mortality.

40. B. Twice as high. The mortality of diabetic patients is approximately 1.5 to 2.0 times higher than for nondiabetic patients after an acute MI.

41. D. An elevated white blood cell count is associated with worse outcomes, including mortality, after acute MI. Converging lines of evidence support the role of inflammation in the pathogenesis of acute MI. Despite the data supporting their use, even in patients who do not have contraindications, aspirin, fibrinolysis, beta-blockers, statins, and ACE inhibitors are all underused. Passive smoking is a risk factor for heart disease. A history of CHF is no longer considered a contraindication for beta-blockade.

42. B. ACE inhibitors have been shown to reduce mortality. Despite the widespread use of nitrates and heparin for acute MI, the evidence basis for their use is not as robust as for ACE inhibitors.

43. C. It is effective for the treatment of AFib and flutter. The Danish Investigations of Arrhythmia and Mortality on Dofetilide (DIAMOND) study enrolled patients with a recent MI and an EF less than or equal to 35% and found no significant difference in mortality between dofetilide and placebo. It was significantly more effective in restoring NSR in the 8% of patients who had atrial flutter or fibrillation at study entry. However, it was associated with an increased risk of torsades de pointes.

44. B. It should not be used prophylactically. Prophylactic IV lidocaine appears to have at best a neutral effect on mortality. Therefore, routine use of prophylactic lidocaine is no longer recommended.

45. C. It does not have a clear benefit in patients undergoing reperfusion therapy. Although there were initially some data to suggest that magnesium may be useful in acute MI, the bulk of data does not show a significant benefit, particularly in the reperfusion era. However, further studies are ongoing in an attempt to determine if particular issues of timing and dose have affected the differing results of the magnesium trials.

46. A. AFib. The role of warfarin is clear in patients with AFib to decrease the risk of stroke. There is no clearly established role for warfarin in routine MI or even in patients with LV dysfunction without LV aneurysm or thrombus.

47. E. All of the above are true. Cocaine has a number of adverse effects on the cardiovascular system.

48. C. TTE.

49. E. None of the above. Possible explanations for this patient's presentation include inferior MI with RV involvement. This could explain the inferior ST elevation and the hypotension. Other possibilities to consider include contained cardiac rupture or aortic dissection (which was the diagnosis in this case, along with compromise of the RCA ostium). When a pericardial effusion is due to aortic dissection, pericardiocentesis can precipitate hemodynamic deterioration, and unless patient death is imminent, the patient should be transferred to the operative suite for further management.

50. C. 20%. The 30-day mortality in the subgroup of patients 75 years of age or older in the streptokinase arm was 20.4% and in the t-PA arm was 19.1%. These results emphasize the high risk of death for elderly patients presenting with MI.

51. A. Within 2 hours. The benefit of t-PA over streptokinase was amplified the earlier patients were treated after the onset of their infarctions.

52. A. Primary PTCA reduced 30-day mortality when compared with accelerated-dose t-PA. The GUSTO-IIb study found that primary PTCA was superior to accelerated-dose t-PA.

53. D. Dressler's syndrome. Dressler's syndrome refers to pericarditis that occurs after MI. It can occur days to months after the MI. It is associated with chest pain, fever, and elevations of the white blood cell count and erythrocyte sedimentation rate. Cardiac or pulmonary effusions may be present. Rarely, it can lead to cardiac tamponade or constrictive pericarditis. Generally, however, it follows a more benign course.

54. E. All of the above. Aspirin, ibuprofen, and indomethacin have typically been used as first-line agents for post-MI pericarditis. Steroids or colchicine have been used in more refractory cases.

55. B. Fibrinolysis reduces the incidence of pericarditis in MI. Several studies, including GISSI 1, have examined this issue and found that fibrinolysis reduces the incidence of pericarditis in the setting of acute MI. Indeed, in the era of reperfusion therapy, the rate of both early and late pericarditis has decreased. Probably, by reducing infarct size, reperfusion decreases the incidence of pericarditis, which is more common with large MIs.

56. C. Stopping t-PA. With a strong suspicion of intracranial hemorrhage, the t-PA should be stopped, regardless of the cardiac situation. A head CT would be useful, but only after initial medical stabilization.

57. F. C and D. Protamine would be useful to reverse the action of heparin. However, to reverse the action of fibrinolytics, cryoprecipitate and epsilon aminocaproic acid would be necessary. Prompt neurosurgical consultation would also be indicated.

58. C. It is more common with a first MI. Ventricular septal rupture is more common with a first MI that is transmural. Anterior MI is a somewhat more common cause than inferior MI, although ventricular septal rupture with inferior MI generally has a worse outcome.

59. D. All of the above are true. Patients with acute MR are more likely to be older, female, and have a history of prior MI.

60. D. The posteromedial papillary muscle is supplied by the posterior descending artery, typically from the RCA. This is why inferior infarcts are more often associated with acute MR. The anterolateral papillary muscle is supplied by both the LAD and the LCx. Surgical therapy is usually warranted.

61. B. IABPs are contraindicated in the presence of moderate or severe aortic insufficiency, as the degree of regurgitation can significantly worsen.

62. B. His risk of intracranial hemorrhage is increased with t-PA. This level of hypertension greatly increases this patient's risk of intracranial hemorrhage. Control of his BP is clearly indicated. However, this will not entirely remove the associated risk of intracranial hemorrhage. If it is an option, primary angioplasty would be preferable.

63. A. Sublingual nifedipine is not an appropriate therapy. Although a few years ago sublingual nifedipine was often the treatment of choice for rapid lowering of BP, reports of MIs and strokes with this therapy, in particular associated with the practice of poking a hole in the capsule and placing it under the tongue, have led to its falling out of favor. The other listed choices are all appropriate means to lower BP.

64. C. Ischemia. The patient has clear anterior ST segment elevation (as well as ST elevation in the high lateral leads) and ST segment depression inferiorly. This is indicative of ischemia. This sort of patient should be admitted to the hospital, not observed in a chest pain center.

65. C. LAD stenosis. The patient has a lesion of his proximal LAD.

66. C. Symptom-limited treadmill exercise stress test before discharge. Of the choices listed, the treadmill exercise stress test is best, because the evidence supports a noninvasive evaluation of ischemia before discharge. Historically, this has been the submaximal exercise stress test, with a maximal stress test at a later point after discharge. Some doctors prefer to get a dipyridamole thallium scan while the patient is hospitalized to avoid the need for a subsequent imaging study.

67. E. Occlusion of the RCA. The RCA is occluded proximally.

68. C. Coronary perforation. Bleeding in the groin or retroperitoneum should always be suspected in a patient with hypotension. Coronary dissection or abrupt vessel occlusion is less likely a cause in this patient, in whom the vessel was initially occluded. The temporal relationship with wire passage and hypotension makes coronary perforation highest on the list of immediate concerns.

69. C. Coronary perforation. There is contrast-dye layering in the pericardium. The femoral artery bifurcation is unremarkable.

70. E. The GUSTO-IV trial did not find a benefit to giving abciximab as empiric therapy for non–ST segment elevation ACSs. However, abciximab is of proven benefit during PCI in ACS patients.

71. B. Cardiac catheterization. The TACTICS–TIMI-18 trial demonstrated that high-risk patients, such as those with ST segment changes or elevated troponin, benefit from an invasive evaluation and subsequent revascularization, as opposed to a conservative strategy of initial medical stabilization followed by noninvasive risk stratification.

72. E. None of the above. There is a severe lesion in the LAD itself, which is most likely the culprit.

73. D. All of the above. Stent thrombosis is more common in the first 2 weeks after stent placement, in particular if the patient is not on appropriate antiplatelet therapy, namely aspirin and clopidogrel. However, it can occur later and is a possibility in this patient with an acute MI. Restenosis is often thought of as a benign process but can present in an acute fashion. Patients with CAD in one location are at risk for plaque rupture at sites other than those with severe angiographic lesions; thus, this patient could have a lesion somewhere other than the stented segment of the RCA.

74. A. Severe restenosis of the RCA. There is severe in-stent restenosis. There is likely also thrombus present, but this is not evident angiographically.

75. A. The practice of increasing aspirin doses to this range has been out of favor in cardiology for a while and has fallen out of favor in neurology circles as well. In fact, for chronic therapy, there is no good evidence that more than 162 mg per day is of any added benefit, although the risks of gastric intolerance and bleeding appear to rise with higher aspirin doses.

76. B. Normal LV function. Make sure you get some practice looking at still frames in systole and diastole. Don't be fooled into overinterpreting random shadows that you might notice on the reproductions of the still frames.

77. A. RCA occlusion. This patient likely has an occluded or severely stenotic RCA with collaterals from the LAD. When more distal portions of vessels are shown, think of collaterals.

78. B. It decreases TVR. Stents decrease the rate of subsequent TVR compared to balloon angioplasty alone, although there is no appreciable benefit for TIMI-3 flow or mortality.

79. D. All of the above. Resolution of chest pain is a common method to indicate successful reperfusion. Resolution of ST segment elevation is a more sensitive method to detect reperfusion. TIMI-3 flow on angiography suggests epicardial reperfusion, although not necessarily reperfusion at a microvascular level.

80. C. There is no large difference in outcome based on gender when age and other comorbidities are considered. Although conclusions from various studies have differed regarding the impact of gender on outcome after acute

MI, when age and associated comorbidities, such as diabetes, are factored in, women do not appear to have a significantly worse outcome than men. However, board examinations tend to steer away from such potentially controversial areas.

81. D. All of the above. Although the predominant causes of acute MI are atherosclerotic plaque rupture and subsequent thrombosis, other rarer causes remain in the differential.

82. A. Diabetes raises the risk of MI the same amount as does having a history of prior MI. The risk of a MI is similar for diabetic patients without a history of MI and nondiabetic patients who have already had an MI.

83. D. Unlike younger patients, patients over the age of 75 did not appear to derive substantial benefit from early revascularization. Although care must be used in interpreting a subgroup from a trial, elderly patients with cardiogenic shock often have multiple comorbidities; individualized decisions should be made about the appropriateness of emergency revascularization in the elderly.

84. C. Use of beta-blockers. Use of perioperative beta-blockers appears to reduce the rate of MI and cardiac death in high-risk patients with evidence of ischemia undergoing vascular surgery.

SUGGESTED READING

Alexander JH, Granger CB, Sadowski Z, et al. Prophylactic lidocaine use in acute myocardial infarction: incidence and outcomes from two international trials. The GUSTO-I and GUSTO-IIb Investigators. *Am Heart J* 1999;137:799–805.

Anderson JL, Karagounis LA, Califf RM. Metaanalysis of five reported studies on the relation of early coronary patency grades with mortality and outcomes after acute myocardial infarction. *Am J Cardiol* 1996;78:1–8.

Antman EM, Berlin JA. Declining incidence of ventricular fibrillation in myocardial infarction. Implications for the prophylactic use of lidocaine. *Circulation* 1992;86:764–773.

Aronson D, Rayfield EJ, Chesebro JH. Mechanisms determining course and outcome of diabetic patients who have had acute myocardial infarction. *Ann Intern Med* 1997;126:296–306.

Barron HV, Cannon CP, Murphy SA, et al. Association between white blood cell count, epicardial blood flow, myocardial perfusion, and clinical outcomes in the setting of acute myocardial infarction: a Thrombolysis in Myocardial Infarction 10 substudy. *Circulation* 2000;102:2329–2334.

Barron HV, Michaels AD, Maynard C, et al. Use of angiotensin-converting enzyme inhibitors at discharge in patients with acute myocardial infarction in the United States: data from the National Registry of Myocardial Infarction 2. *J Am Coll Cardiol* 1998;32:360–367.

Barron HV, Rundle AC, Gore JM, et al. Intracranial hemorrhage rates and effect of immediate beta-blocker use in patients with acute myocardial infarction treated with tissue plasminogen activator. Participants in the National Registry of Myocardial Infarction-2. *Am J Cardiol* 2000;85:294–298.

Buxton AE, Lee KL, Fisher JD, et al. A randomized study of the prevention of sudden death in patients with coronary artery disease. Multicenter Unsustained Tachycardia Trial Investigators. *N Engl J Med* 1999;341:1882–1890.

Cannon CP, McCabe CH, Wilcox RG, et al. Association of white blood cell count with increased mortality in acute myocardial infarction and unstable angina pectoris. OPUS–TIMI-16 Investigators. *Am J Cardiol* 2001;87:636–639, A10.

Chen J, Radford MJ, Wang Y, et al. Do "America's Best Hospitals" perform better for acute myocardial infarction? *N Engl J Med* 1999;340:286–292.

de Lemos JA, Braunwald E. ST segment resolution as a tool for assessing the efficacy of reperfusion therapy. *J Am Coll Cardiol* 2001;38:1283–1294.

Ellerbeck EF, Jencks SF, Radford MJ, et al. Quality of care for Medicare patients with acute myocardial infarction. A four-state pilot study from the Cooperative Cardiovascular Project. *JAMA* 1995;273:1509–1514.

Glantz SA, Parmley WW. Passive smoking and heart disease. Epidemiology, physiology, and biochemistry. *Circulation* 1991;83:1–12.

Gottlieb SS, McCarter RJ, Vogel RA. Effect of beta-blockade on mortality among high-risk and low-risk patients after myocardial infarction. *N Engl J Med* 1998;339:489–497.

Haffner SM, Lehto S, Ronnemaa T, et al. Mortality from coronary heart disease in subjects with type 2 diabetes and in nondiabetic subjects with and without prior myocardial infarction. *N Engl J Med* 1998;339:229–234.

Hine LK, Laird N, Hewitt P, et al. Meta-analytic evidence against prophylactic use of lidocaine in acute myocardial infarction. *Arch Intern Med* 1989;149:2694–2698.

Hochman JS, Sleeper LA, Webb JG, et al. Early revascularization in acute myocardial infarction complicated by cardiogenic shock. SHOCK Investigators. Should We Emergently Revascularize Occluded Coronaries for Cardiogenic Shock. *N Engl J Med* 1999;341:625–634.

ISIS-4: a randomised factorial trial assessing early oral captopril, oral mononitrate, and intravenous magnesium sulphate in 58,050 patients with suspected acute myocardial infarction. ISIS-4 (Fourth International Study of Infarct Survival) Collaborative Group. *Lancet* 1995;345:669–685.

Kober L, Bloch Thomsen PE, Moller M, et al. Effect of dofetilide in patients with recent myocardial infarction and left-ventricular dysfunction: a randomised trial. Danish Investigations of Arrhythmia and Mortality on Dofetilide (DIAMOND) Study Group. *Lancet* 2000;356:2052–2058.

MacIntyre K, Stewart S, Capewell S, et al. Gender and survival: a population-based study of 201,114 men and women following a first acute myocardial infarction. *J Am Coll Cardiol* 2001;38:729–735.

MacMahon S, Collins R, Peto R, et al. Effects of prophylactic lidocaine in suspected acute myocardial infarction. An overview of results from the randomized, controlled trials. *JAMA* 1988;260:1910–1916.

Moss AJ, Hall WJ, Cannom DS, et al. Improved survival with an implanted defibrillator in patients with coronary disease at high risk for ventricular arrhythmia. Multicenter Automatic Defibrillator Implantation Trial Investigators. *N Engl J Med* 1996;335:1933–1940.

Mukamal KJ, Nesto RW, Cohen MC, et al. Impact of diabetes on long-term survival after acute myocardial infarction: comparability of risk with prior myocardial infarction. *Diabetes Care* 2001;24:1422–1427.

Newby KH, Thompson T, Stebbins A, et al. Sustained ventricular arrhythmias in patients receiving thrombolytic therapy: incidence and outcomes. The GUSTO Investigators. *Circulation* 1998;98:2567–2573.

Pfisterer ME, Kiowski W, Brunner H, et al. Long-term benefit of 1-year amiodarone treatment for persistent complex ventricular arrhythmias after myocardial infarction. *Circulation* 1993;87:309–311.

Poldermans D, Boersma E, Bax JJ, et al. Bisoprolol reduces cardiac death and myocardial infarction in high-risk patients as long as 2 years after successful major vascular surgery. *Eur Heart J* 2001;22:1353–1358.

Ryden L, Ariniego R, Arnman K, et al. A double-blind trial of metoprolol in acute myocardial infarction. Effects on ventricular tachyarrhythmias. *N Engl J Med* 1983;308:614–618.

Sadowski ZP, Alexander JH, Skrabucha B, et al. Multicenter randomized trial and a systematic overview of lidocaine in acute myocardial infarction. *Am Heart J* 1999;137:792–798.

NOTES

NOTES

Santoro GM, Antoniucci D, Bolognese L, et al. A randomized study of intravenous magnesium in acute myocardial infarction treated with direct coronary angioplasty. *Am Heart J* 2000;140:891–897.

Second Chinese Cardiac Study (CCS-2) Collaborative Group. Rationale, design and organization of the Second Chinese Cardiac Study (CCS-2): a randomized trial of clopidogrel plus aspirin, and of metoprolol, among patients with suspected acute myocardial infarction. *J Cardiovasc Risk* 2000;7:435–441.

The Cardiac Arrhythmia Suppression Trial (CAST) Investigators. Preliminary report: effect of encainide and flecainide on mortality in a randomized trial of arrhythmia suppression after myocardial infarction. *N Engl J Med* 1989;321:406–412.

The Cardiac Arrhythmia Suppression Trial II Investigators. Effect of the antiarrhythmic agent moricizine on survival after myocardial infarction. *N Engl J Med* 1992;327:227–233.

Volpi A, Cavalli A, Santoro E, et al. Incidence and prognosis of secondary ventricular fibrillation in acute myocardial infarction. Evidence for a protective effect of thrombolytic therapy. GISSI Investigators. *Circulation* 1990;82:1279–1288.

Volpi A, Maggioni A, Franzosi MG, et al. In-hospital prognosis of patients with acute myocardial infarction complicated by primary ventricular fibrillation. *N Engl J Med* 1987;317:257–261.

Woods KL, Fletcher S, Roffe C, et al. Intravenous magnesium sulphate in suspected acute myocardial infarction: results of the second Leicester Intravenous Magnesium Intervention Trial (LIMIT-2). *Lancet* 1992;339:1553–1558.

Woods KL, Fletcher S. Long-term outcome after intravenous magnesium sulphate in suspected acute myocardial infarction: the second Leicester Intravenous Magnesium Intervention Trial (LIMIT-2). *Lancet* 1994;343:816–819.

Ziegelstein RC, Hilbe JM, French WJ, et al. Magnesium use in the treatment of acute myocardial infarction in the United States (observations from the Second National Registry of Myocardial Infarction). *Am J Cardiol* 2001;87:7–10.

CHAPTER 4

Coronary Artery Disease

Debabrata Mukherjee

QUESTIONS
NOTES

1. A 67-year-old man presents to the emergency room with increasing frequency of angina and one episode of rest pain lasting 5 min. His medical history is significant for hypertension and hyperlipidemia. He is a 20-pack-per-year ex-smoker who quit smoking 11 years ago. His current medications include aspirin (ASA), metoprolol, ramipril, and atorvastatin.

   He is afebrile.
   Pulse is 78 bpm.
   BP is 138/76 mm Hg.
   Chest auscultation reveals an S_3 gallop.
   His presenting ECG reveals NSR and ST depression in I, aVL, V5–V6.

   You admit him to the hospital and start IV heparin, nitroglycerin (NTG), and tirofiban. Which of the following should be the next step in his management?

   A. a low-level stress test the next morning
   B. continue IV heparin, NTG, and tirofiban until completely chest-pain free for 24 hours, then discharge home
   C. coronary angiography followed by percutaneous intervention or surgical revascularization, if indicated
   D. dobutamine TTE after 48 hours

2. Which of the following is an effect of exercise training in patients who received percutaneous transluminal coronary angioplasty (PTCA) or coronary stenting?

   A. reduced restenosis
   B. lower rate of hospital readmission
   C. reduction in the volume of O_2 consumption ($\dot{V}O_2$)
   D. higher event rate related to exercise

3. Which of the following predicts future risk of coronary heart disease (CHD) in initially healthy middle-aged men?

   A. erythrocyte sedimentation rate
   B. C-reactive protein (CRP)
   C. immunoglobulin G
   D. immunoglobulin E

4. A 58-year-old man with CAD had stenting of the mid–left anterior descending coronary artery (LAD) 10 months ago. He presented with recurrent angina 4 months ago, and coronary angiography revealed diffuse in-stent restenosis. He underwent repeat percutaneous coronary intervention (PCI) with balloon angioplasty with less than 10% stenosis. He presents now with recurrent angina, and angiography reveals restenosis. Which of the following would be a reasonable next option?

   A. percutaneous transmyocardial revascularization
   B. gene therapy with vascular endothelial growth factor
   C. radiation
   D. continued medical therapy
   E. percutaneous coronary bypass

5. The HOPE (Heart Outcomes Prevention Evaluation) trial demonstrated that treatment with ramipril reduces all of the following *except*

   A. death from cardiovascular causes
   B. MI
   C. stroke
   D. hospitalization for unstable angina (UA)
   E. complications related to diabetes

6. Which one of the following types of atherosclerotic lesion (Stary type) is most likely to disrupt, thrombose, and lead to MI?

   A. I–III
   B. IV–Va
   C. Vb–Vc
   D. VI

7. The determinants of myocardial O_2 demand include all of the following *except*

   A. heart rate
   B. contractility
   C. myocardial wall tension
   D. O_2-carrying capacity of the blood

8. Which area of the myocardium is more vulnerable to ischemic damage?

   A. subepicardium
   B. midmyocardium
   C. subendocardium
   D. pericardium

9. A 73-year-old man presents to the emergency room with severe midsternal chest discomfort.

   He appears anxious and in considerable distress.
   Heart rate is 66 bpm.
   BP is 92/68 mm Hg.
   Respiratory rate is 14 breaths per minute.
   There is marked jugular venous distention evident.
   On auscultation, an S_4 gallop sound is audible, and the lung fields are clear.
   ECG reveals a 2-mm ST segment elevation in leads II, III, and aVF.

   What is the most likely diagnosis?

   A. acute pericarditis
   B. aortic dissection
   C. RV infarction
   D. inferior wall MI with RV infarction
   E. pneumonia

10. To which of the following is an S_4 in patients with acute MI (AMI) related?

    A. reduction in LV compliance
    B. rapid deceleration of transmitral flow during protodiastolic filling of the LV
    C. increased inflow into the LV
    D. reduced LV systolic function

11. With which of the following cardiac markers of necrosis is the earliest initial rise seen?

    A. troponin I
    B. troponin T
    C. myoglobin
    D. creatine kinase myocardial isoenzyme (CK-MB)
    E. low-dose heparin

12. Which of the following did the GUSTO-I (Global Utilization of Streptokinase and Tissue Plasminogen Activator for Occluded Coronary Arteries) trial demonstrate?

    A. decreased stroke risk with tissue plasminogen activator (t-PA)
    B. survival benefit of t-PA over streptokinase
    C. equivalence of t-PA and streptokinase
    D. decreased reocclusion with t-PA

13. Important predictors of mortality in the Lee statistical model derived from GUSTO include all of the following *except*

    A. systolic BP
    B. age
    C. heart rate
    D. choice of thrombolytic agent

14. High-risk exercise ECG criteria on stress testing include which of the following factors?

    A. achievement of a workload of less than 7 METS
    B. ST segment depression for longer than 2 min during the recovery period
    C. greater than or equal to 1-mm ST segment depression in stage I
    D. increase in heart rate

15. Which of the following did the 10-year follow-up of the Coronary Artery Surgery Study (CASS) demonstrate?

    A. Patients with LV dysfunction exhibit long-term benefit from an initial strategy of surgical treatment.
    B. At 10 years, there was significant improvement in cumulative survival and a difference in the percentage of patients free of death and nonfatal MI with surgery compared to medical therapy.
    C. Patients with an EF greater than or equal to 0.50 exhibited a higher proportion free of death and MI with initial surgical therapy.
    D. Patients with mild stable angina and normal LV function randomized to initial surgical treatment have improved survival compared to patients treated with medical therapy.

16. Which of the following did the Asymptomatic Cardiac Ischemia Pilot (ACIP) study demonstrate at 1 year?

    A. significant mortality benefit with revascularization compared to angina-guided medical therapy
    B. equivalent clinical outcomes with angina-guided, ischemia-guided, and revascularization strategies
    C. improved clinical outcome with angina-guided therapy compared to revascularization
    D. improved clinical outcome with ischemia-guided therapy compared to revascularization

17. Class I American College of Cardiology/American Heart Association (ACC/AHA) guidelines regarding early risk stratification for the management of patients with UA and non–ST segment elevation MI (NSTEMI) include all of the following *except*

    A. A determination of the likelihood (high, intermediate, or low) of acute ischemia caused by CAD should be made in all patients with chest discomfort.
    B. Patients who present with chest discomfort should undergo early risk stratification that focuses on anginal symptoms, physical findings, ECG findings, and biomarkers of cardiac injury.
    C. A 12-lead ECG should be obtained within 30 min in patients with ongoing chest discomfort and as rapidly as possible in patients who have a history of chest discomfort consistent with acute coronary syndrome (ACS) but whose discomfort has resolved by the time of evaluation.
    D. Biomarkers of cardiac injury should be measured in all patients who present with chest discomfort consistent with ACS. A cardiac-specific troponin is the preferred marker, and if available, it should be measured in all patients. CK-MB by mass assay is also acceptable. In patients with negative cardiac markers within 6 hours of the onset of pain, another sample should be drawn in the 6- to 12-hour time frame (e.g., at 9 hours after the onset of symptoms).

18. Class I ACC/AHA guidelines regarding immediate management of patients with UA and NSTEMI include all of the following *except*

A. The history, physical examination, 12-lead ECG, and initial cardiac marker tests should be integrated to assign patients with chest pain to one of four categories: a noncardiac diagnosis, chronic stable angina, possible ACS, and definite ACS.

B. Patients with definite or possible ACS whose initial 12-lead ECG and cardiac marker levels are normal should be observed in a facility with cardiac monitoring (e.g., chest pain unit), and a repeat ECG and cardiac marker measurement should be obtained 6 to 12 hours after the onset of symptoms.

C. If the follow-up 12-lead ECG and cardiac marker measurements are normal, a stress test (exercise or pharmacologic) to provoke ischemia may be performed in the emergency department, in a chest pain unit, or on an outpatient basis shortly after discharge. Low-risk patients with a negative stress test can be managed as outpatients.

D. Patients with definite ACS and ongoing pain, positive cardiac markers, new ST segment deviations, new deep T-wave inversions, hemodynamic abnormalities, or a positive stress test should be admitted to the hospital for further management.

E. Patients with possible ACS and negative cardiac markers who are unable to exercise or who have an abnormal resting ECG should have a coronary angiogram.

F. Patients with definite ACS and ST segment elevation should be evaluated for immediate reperfusion therapy.

19. Class I ACC/AHA guidelines regarding antiischemic therapy for patients with UA and NSTEMI include all of the following *except*

A. bed rest with continuous ECG monitoring for ischemia and arrhythmia detection in patients with ongoing rest pain

B. NTG, sublingual tablet, or spray, followed by IV administration, for immediate relief of ischemia and associated symptoms

C. supplemental O_2 for patients with cyanosis or respiratory distress; finger pulse oximetry or arterial blood gas determination to confirm adequate arterial O_2 saturation (O_2 saturation greater than 90%) and continued need for supplemental O_2 in the presence of hypoxemia

D. morphine sulfate IV when symptoms are not immediately relieved with NTG or when acute pulmonary congestion or severe agitation is present

E. a beta-blocker, with the first dose administered IV if there is ongoing chest pain, followed by PO administration, in the absence of contraindications

F. a nondihydropyridine calcium antagonist (e.g., verapamil or diltiazem), followed by PO therapy, as initial therapy

G. an ACE inhibitor when hypertension persists despite treatment with NTG and a beta-blocker in patients with LV systolic dysfunction or CHF and in ACS patients with diabetes

20. Class I ACC/AHA guidelines regarding antiplatelet and anticoagulant therapy for patients with UA and NSTEMI include all of the following *except*

A. Antiplatelet therapy should be initiated promptly. ASA is the first choice and is administered as soon as possible after presentation and continued indefinitely.
B. A thienopyridine (clopidogrel or ticlopidine) should be administered to patients who are unable to take ASA because of hypersensitivity or major GI intolerance.
C. Parenteral anticoagulation with IV unfractionated heparin (UFH) or with SC low-molecular-weight heparin (LMWH) should be added to antiplatelet therapy with ASA or a thienopyridine.
D. A platelet glycoprotein (GP) IIb/IIIa receptor antagonist should be administered in all patients.

21. Class I recommendations for revascularization with PCI and coronary artery bypass grafting (CABG) in patients with ACS include all of the following *except*

A. CABG for patients with significant left main CAD
B. CABG for patients with three-vessel disease; the survival benefit is greater in patients with abnormal LV function (EF less than 0.50)
C. CABG for patients with two-vessel disease with significant proximal LAD CAD and either abnormal LV function (EF less than 0.50) or demonstrable ischemia on noninvasive testing
D. PCI or CABG for patients with one- or two-vessel CAD without significant proximal LAD CAD
E. PCI for patients with multivessel coronary disease with suitable coronary anatomy, with normal LV function, and without diabetes
F. IV platelet GP IIb/IIIa inhibitor in UA or NSTEMI patients undergoing PCI

22. Class I recommendations regarding postdischarge care of patients with UA/non–Q-wave MI include all of the following *except*

A. Before hospital discharge, patients and designated responsible caregivers should be provided with well-understood instructions with respect to medication type, purpose, dose, frequency, and pertinent side effects.
B. Drugs required in the hospital to control ischemia should be discontinued after hospital discharge in patients who do not undergo coronary revascularization, patients with unsuccessful revascularization, or patients with recurrent symptoms after revascularization.
C. Before hospital discharge, patients should be informed about symptoms of AMI and should be instructed in how to seek help if they occur.
D. All patients should be given sublingual or spray NTG and instructed in its use.

23. Class I recommendations regarding management of patients with diabetes mellitus presenting with UA/non–Q-wave MI include all of the following *except*

A. Diabetes is an independent prognostic factor for increased risk, and this should be taken into account in the initial evaluation.
B. Medical treatment in the acute phase and decisions on whether to perform stress testing and angiography and revascularization should be geared toward more aggressive strategy in diabetic compared to nondiabetic patients.
C. Attention should be directed toward tight glucose control.
D. For patients with multivessel disease, CABG with use of the internal mammary arteries is preferred over PCI in patients who are receiving treatment for diabetes.

24. Class I indications for coronary angiography for risk stratification in patients with chronic stable angina include all of the following *except*

    A. patients with disabling [Canadian Cardiovascular Society (CCS) classes III and IV] chronic stable angina not on medical therapy
    B. patients with high-risk criteria on noninvasive testing, regardless of anginal severity
    C. patients with angina who have survived sudden cardiac death or serious ventricular arrhythmia
    D. patients with angina and symptoms and signs of CHF
    E. patients with clinical characteristics that indicate a high likelihood of severe CAD

25. Class I indications for CABG in asymptomatic patients include all of the following *except*

    A. significant left main coronary artery stenosis
    B. proximal LAD stenosis with one- or two-vessel disease
    C. three-vessel disease (survival benefit is greater in patients with abnormal LV function; e.g., with an EF less than 0.50)
    D. left main equivalent: significant (greater than or equal to 70%) stenosis of proximal LAD and proximal left circumflex coronary artery (LCx)

26. All of the following variables are associated with stent thrombosis in the modern era *except*

    A. persistent dissection
    B. total stent length
    C. deployment pressure
    D. final lumen diameter

27. Which of the following is the approximate stroke reduction (relative reduction) demonstrated by the Prospective Pravastatin Pooling (PPP) project?

    A. 10%
    B. 20%
    C. 40%
    D. 45%

28. Prognostic factors for atherosclerosis progression in saphenous vein grafts (SVGs) include all of the following *except*

    A. maximum stenosis of the graft at baseline angiography
    B. years post-SVG placement
    C. prior MI
    D. female gender
    E. high triglyceride level

29. The Atorvastatin Versus Revascularization Treatment (AVERT) trial demonstrated which of the following in patients with ischemic heart disease and stable angina pectoris?

    A. Percutaneous coronary revascularization is more effective than aggressive lipid-lowering therapy.
    B. Aggressive lipid-lowering therapy is more effective than percutaneous coronary revascularization.
    C. Aggressive lipid-lowering therapy is as effective as percutaneous coronary revascularization.

30. What was the relative risk (RR) of death in the simvastatin group in the Scandinavian Simvastatin Survival Study (4S)?
    A. 0.50
    B. 0.60
    C. 0.70
    D. 0.80
    E. 0.85

31. What was the main outcome measure of the primary prevention of acute coronary events with lovastatin in men and women with average cholesterol levels Air Force/Texas Coronary Atherosclerosis Prevention Study (AFCAPS/TexCAPS)?
    A. cardiovascular mortality
    B. first acute major coronary event defined as fatal or nonfatal MI, UA, or sudden cardiac death
    C. total mortality
    D. stroke

32. The West of Scotland Coronary Prevention Study (WOSCOPS) trial demonstrated that a fall in what percentage point in LDL is sufficient to produce the full benefit in patients taking 40-mg doses of pravastatin?
    A. 12%
    B. 24%
    C. 30%
    D. 36%

33. The Bypass Angioplasty Revascularization Investigation (BARI) randomized trial and registry both demonstrated which of the following?
    A. CABG is associated with equivalent survival to PTCA in treated diabetic patients with multivessel coronary disease suitable for either surgical or catheter-based revascularization.
    B. CABG is associated with better long-term survival than PTCA in treated diabetic patients with multivessel coronary disease suitable for either surgical or catheter-based revascularization.
    C. PTCA is associated with better long-term survival than CABG in treated diabetic patients with multivessel coronary disease suitable for either surgical or catheter-based revascularization.

34. What is the effect of cigarette smoking on the activity of ischemic heart disease?
    A. increased frequency of episodes of angina and no effect on the duration of ischemia
    B. increased frequency of episodes of angina and increased duration of ischemia
    C. increased duration of ischemia but no effect on frequency of angina
    D. no significant effect on either duration or frequency of angina

35. Which of the following did the primary end point of the Should We Emergently Revascularize Occluded Coronaries for Cardiogenic Shock (SHOCK) trial reveal?

    A. significant benefit with early revascularization compared to intensive medical therapy
    B. no significant difference with early revascularization compared to intensive medical therapy
    C. significant benefit with intensive medical therapy compared to early revascularization
    D. significant benefit with combination of thrombolysis and an IABP compared to early revascularization

36. A 76-year-old woman presents to your outpatient department with stable angina. You order a perfusion stress study, which reveals inferior and inferoseptal ischemia. Coronary angiogram reveals an 80% calcified lesion in the midportion of the right coronary artery (RCA). The LAD and the LCx have mild luminal irregularities. Based on the available literature, what percentage survival should you quote her?

    A. greater than 90% at 5 years
    B. 80% at 5 years
    C. 70% at 5 years
    D. 60% at 5 years
    E. 50% at 5 years

37. All of the following were multivariate predictors in identifying high-risk patients with left main and three-vessel CAD by adenosine–single photon emission–computed tomographic thallium imaging *except*

    A. multivessel thallium abnormality
    B. increased lung thallium uptake
    C. extent of thallium abnormality
    D. ST depression

38. Which of the following statements is *correct* regarding risk of stroke associated with abciximab among patients undergoing PCI?

    A. Abciximab in addition to ASA and heparin does not increase the risk of stroke in patients undergoing PCI.
    B. Abciximab in addition to ASA and heparin increases the risk of stroke in patients undergoing PCI.
    C. Abciximab in addition to ASA and heparin decreases the risk of stroke in patients undergoing PCI.

39. Clinical factors predictive of global and regional ventricular function after AMI as well as improvement in function between 90 min and 5 to 7 days include all of the following *except*

    A. time to treatment
    B. early infarct-related artery flow grade
    C. age
    D. body mass index

40. Factors associated with failure of medical therapy in patients with UA/non–Q-wave MI include all of the following *except*
    A. ST segment depression on the qualifying ECG
    B. history of prior angina
    C. family history of premature coronary disease (i.e., onset before 55 years of age)
    D. prior use of heparin or ASA
    E. female gender
    F. increasing age

41. Based on the Executive Summary of the Third Report of the National Cholesterol Education Program (NCEP) Expert Panel on Detection, Evaluation, and Treatment of High Blood Cholesterol in Adults (Adult Treatment Panel III), which of the following is the LDL level at which to consider drug therapy for patients with CAD?
    A. 190
    B. 160
    C. 130
    D. 100

42. What did the Thrombolysis in Myocardial Infarction (TIMI) 11B–ESSENCE metaanalysis demonstrate regarding the use of LMWH compared to UFH in patients with ACSs?
    A. Use of LMWH compared to UFH resulted in no significant difference in outcomes.
    B. Use of UFH was associated with a 20% reduction in death and serious cardiac ischemic events that appeared within the first few days of treatment, and this benefit was sustained through 43 days.
    C. Use of LMWH was associated with a 20% reduction in death and serious cardiac ischemic events that appeared within the first few days of treatment, and this benefit was sustained through 43 days.

43. What is the incidence of nonsignificant CAD in patients presenting with ACSs?
    A. 3%
    B. 6%
    C. 12%
    D. 20%
    E. 24%

44. With which of the following can bleeding due to hirudin be effectively reversed?
    A. fresh frozen plasma
    B. prothrombin complex
    C. epsilon amino caproic acid
    D. bivalirudin

45. What is the overall 30-day mortality in patients with prior bypass who present with AMI?
    A. 3%
    B. 6%
    C. 11%
    D. 16%

46. In what percentage of patients with AMI and prior CABG undergoing primary angioplasty is TIMI trial flow-grade 3 achieved?

    A. 50%
    B. 70%
    C. 90%
    D. 95%

47. A 76-year-old man presents to the emergency department with substernal chest pressure for 40 min.

    He is diaphoretic.
    Heart rate is 82 bpm.
    BP is 76/42 mm Hg.
    He has a jugular venous pressure of 12 cm of H_2O.
    On auscultation, he has an S_3 gallop and clear lung fields.
    ECG reveals ST segment elevation in leads II, III, and aVF.

    What should the diagnosis be?

    A. severe LV failure with cardiogenic shock
    B. VSD
    C. acute MR
    D. RV infarction
    E. cardiac rupture

48. In patients presenting with RV infarction, which of the following has been shown to have survival advantage?

    A. fluid loading
    B. NTG
    C. PA catheter placement
    D. primary angioplasty

49. The potential causes of a new systolic murmur after an AMI include all of the following *except*

    A. MR
    B. VSD
    C. aortic stenosis
    D. dynamic LVOT obstruction

50. In patients with CAD, what does use of PO GP IIb/IIIa inhibitors result in?

    A. significant decrease in mortality
    B. no effect on mortality
    C. significant increase in mortality
    D. mortality was not ascertained in these trials

51. What did the Clopidogrel versus Aspirin in Patients at Risk of Ischemic Events (CAPRIE) trial comparing ASA and clopidogrel show?

    A. Long-term administration of clopidogrel to patients with atherosclerotic vascular disease is as effective as ASA in reducing the combined risk of ischemic stroke, MI, and vascular death.

    B. Long-term administration of clopidogrel to patients with atherosclerotic vascular disease is more effective than ASA in reducing the combined risk of ischemic stroke, MI, and vascular death.

    C. Long-term administration of clopidogrel to patients with atherosclerotic vascular disease is less effective than ASA in reducing the combined risk of ischemic stroke, MI, and vascular death.

52. What is the clinical effect of low, fixed-dose warfarin (1 or 3 mg) combined with low-dose ASA (80 mg) in patients who have had MI?

    A. Low, fixed-dose warfarin (1 or 3 mg) combined with low-dose ASA (80 mg) in patients who have had MI does not provide clinical benefit beyond that achievable with 160-mg ASA monotherapy.

    B. Low, fixed-dose warfarin (1 or 3 mg) combined with low-dose ASA (80 mg) in patients who have had MI provides clinical benefit beyond that achievable with 160-mg ASA monotherapy.

    C. Low, fixed-dose warfarin (1 or 3 mg) combined with low-dose ASA (80 mg) in patients who have had MI has a worse clinical outcome than 160-mg ASA monotherapy.

53. What response does Figure 1 show after a ventricular premature beat in a 57-year-old woman with hypertrophic cardiomyopathy?

    A. The Brockenbrough response includes an increase in LV systolic pressure, a decrease in aortic systolic pressure, an increase in LV to aortic gradient, and diminished aortic pulse pressure.

    B. The Brockenbrough response includes an increase in LV systolic pressure, an increase in aortic systolic pressure, an increase in LV to aortic gradient, and increased aortic pulse pressure.

    C. The Brockenbrough response includes a decrease in LV systolic pressure, a decrease in aortic systolic pressure, an increase in LV to aortic gradient, and diminished aortic pulse pressure.

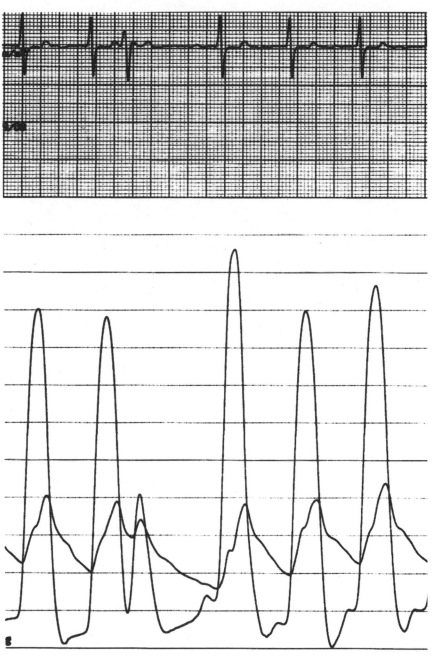

FIGURE 1

54. What does the angiogram in Figure 2 show?

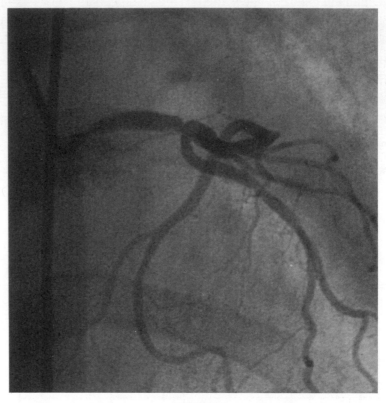

FIGURE 2

A. occluded LAD
B. occluded LCx
C. severe ostial and moderate distal left main trunk stenosis
D. normal coronary arteries

55. A 48-year-old woman presents with CHF. Based on the coronary angiogram in Figure 3, what is the etiology of her heart failure?

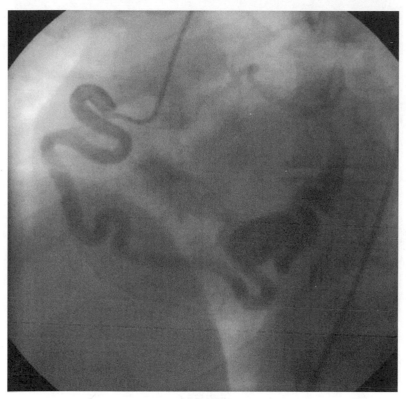

FIGURE 3

A. severe CAD
B. arteriovenous fistula
C. aortic regurgitation
D. absent RCA

56. What does the angiogram in Figure 4 show?

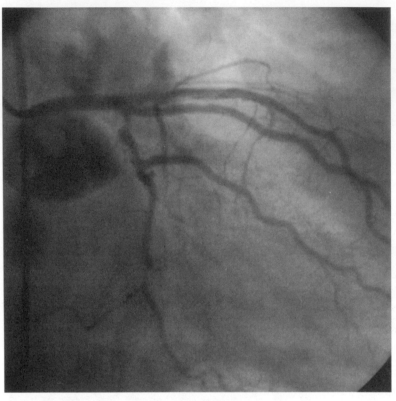

FIGURE 4

A. ostial left main trunk stenosis
B. ostial LAD artery stenosis
C. ostial LCx stenosis
D. normal coronaries

57. What does the angiogram in Figure 5 show?

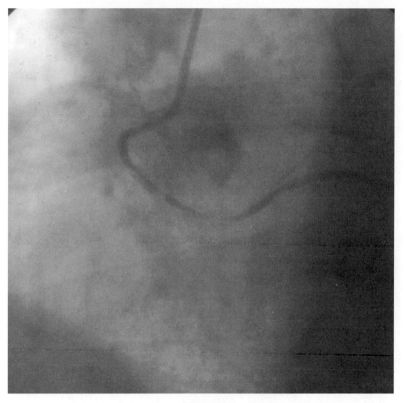

FIGURE 5

A. anomalous origin of the left main trunk
B. anomalous origin of the LAD
C. anomalous origin of the LCx
D. normal coronaries

58. What does this coronary angiogram of a 59-year-old man with acute inferior MI (Fig. 6) reveal?

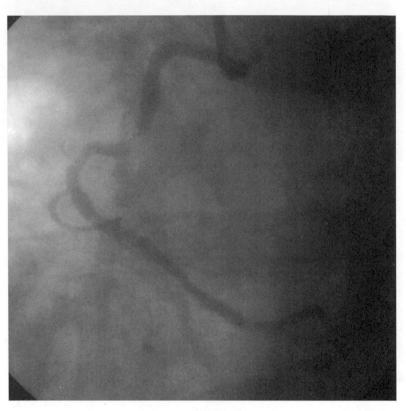

FIGURE 6

A. large angiographically visible thrombus in the mid portion of the RCA distal to a severe stenosis
B. perforation of the mid portion of the RCA
C. normal RCA
D. absent RCA

59. What does the angiogram in Figure 7 reveal?

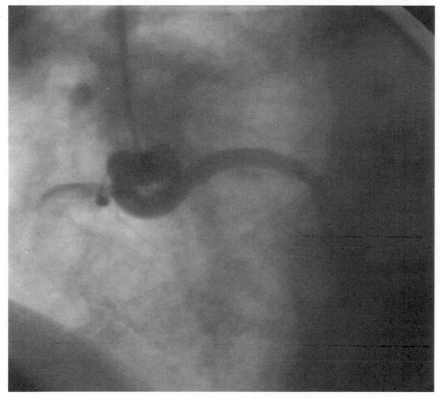

FIGURE 7

A. anomalous origin of the left main trunk
B. anomalous origin of the LAD
C. anomalous origin of the LCx
D. anomalous origin of the RCA

60. What does the angiogram in Figure 8 reveal?

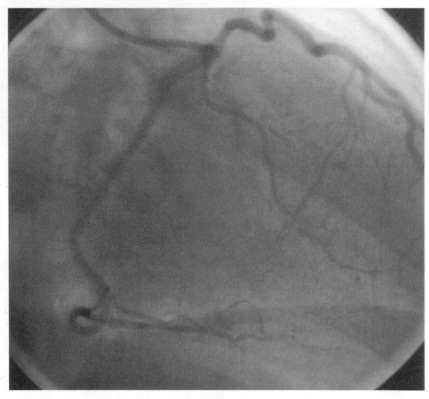

FIGURE 8

A. anomalous origin of the left main trunk
B. anomalous origin of the LAD
C. anomalous origin of the LCx
D. anomalous common origin of the LAD and the RCA

61. During coronary angioplasty of the RCA, this 72-year-old patient developed sharp chest pain with rapid development of hypotension and tachycardia. What is the most likely etiology, based on Figure 9?

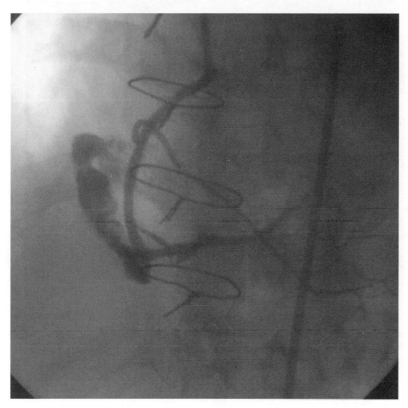

FIGURE 9

A. abrupt closure of the RCA
B. dissection of the RCA
C. perforation of the RCA
D. allergic reaction

62. What does this angiogram (Fig. 10) from a 28-year-old man with hypercholesterolemia reveal?

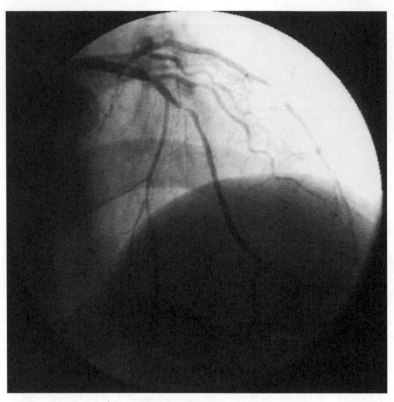

FIGURE 10

A. severe LCx stenosis
B. severe left main trunk stenosis
C. severe LAD stenosis
D. severe RCA stenosis

63. What does this angiogram (Fig. 11) from a 79-year-old woman with infero-lateral ischemia reveal?

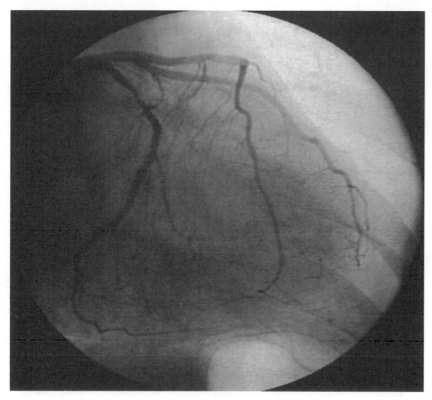

FIGURE 11

A. severe LCx stenosis
B. severe left main trunk stenosis
C. severe LAD stenosis
D. severe RCA stenosis

64. What does this angiogram (Fig. 12) from this 67-year-old man with infero-posterior ischemia reveal?

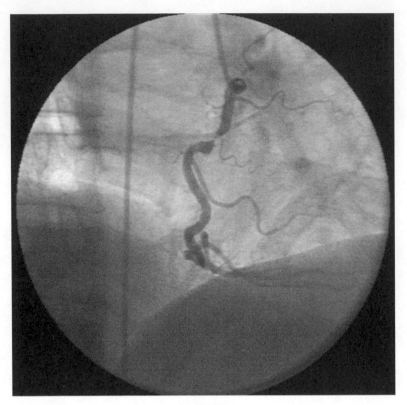

FIGURE 12

A. severe LCx stenosis
B. severe left main trunk stenosis
C. severe LAD stenosis
D. severe RCA stenosis

65. What does this angiogram (Fig. 13) from a 54-year-old man with acute lateral wall MI reveal?

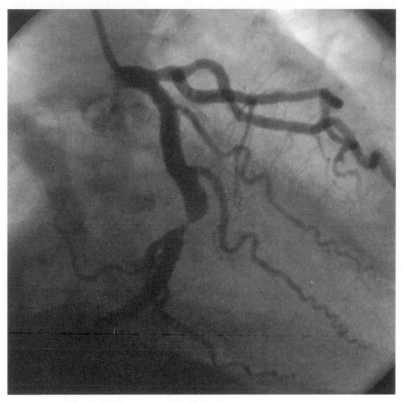

FIGURE 13

   A. severe LCx stenosis
   B. severe left main trunk stenosis
   C. severe LAD stenosis
   D. severe RCA stenosis

66. What did the Arterial Revascularization Therapies Study (ARTS) comparing bypass versus stenting in multivessel coronary disease demonstrate?

   A. At 1 year, there was no significant difference between the two groups in terms of the rates of death, stroke, or MI.
   B. At 1 year, bypass surgery had significantly better outcomes.
   C. At 1 year, coronary stenting had significantly better outcomes.
   D. The trial was aborted before 1 year.

67. What is the incidence of coronary artery aneurysms and or ectasia in patients with Kawasaki disease?

   A. 5% to 10%
   B. 10% to 15%
   C. 15% to 25%
   D. 25% to 35%
   E. approximately 40%

68. Which of the following conditions do patients with scleroderma have?

    A. increased coronary flow reserve
    B. decreased coronary flow reserve
    C. normal coronary flow reserve

69. What is the major difference in the morphology of coronary atherosclerotic lesion in patients with end-stage renal failure compared to nonuremic patients?

    A. There are significantly more fibrous plaques of coronary arteries in patients with end-stage renal failure.
    B. There are significantly more calcified plaques of coronary arteries in patients with end-stage renal failure.
    C. There are significantly more cellular plaques of coronary arteries in patients with end-stage renal failure.

70. Regarding homocysteine as a risk factor for CAD, which of the following statements is most accurate?

    A. In patients with angiographically defined CAD, homocysteine is a significant predictor of mortality in conjunction with traditional risk factors, CRP, and methylenetetrahydrofolate reductase (MTHFR) genotype.
    B. In patients with angiographically defined CAD, homocysteine is a significant predictor of mortality, independent of traditional risk factors, CRP, and MTHFR genotype.
    C. In patients with angiographically defined CAD, homocysteine is not a significant predictor of mortality, but CRP and MTHFR genotype were predictors.

ANSWERS

1. C. Coronary angiography followed by percutaneous intervention or surgical revascularization, if indicated. There is continued debate as to whether a routine, early invasive strategy is superior to a conservative strategy for the management of UA and MI without ST segment elevation. The TACTICS study enrolled 2,220 patients with UA and MI without ST segment elevation who had ECG evidence of changes in the ST segment or T wave, elevated levels of cardiac markers, a history of CAD, or all three findings. All patients were treated with ASA, heparin, and the GP IIb/IIIa inhibitor tirofiban. They were randomly assigned to an early invasive strategy, which included routine catheterization within 4 to 48 hours and revascularization as appropriate, or to a more conservative (selectively invasive) strategy, in which catheterization was performed only if the patient had objective evidence of recurrent ischemia or an abnormal stress test. The primary end point was a composite of death, nonfatal MI, and rehospitalization for an ACS at 6 months. At 6 months, the rate of the primary end point was 15.9% with use of the early invasive strategy and 19.4% with use of the conservative strategy [odds ratio (OR), 0.78; 95% confidence interval (CI), 0.62 to 0.97; $p = .025$]. The rate of death or nonfatal MI at 6 months was similarly reduced (7.3% vs. 9.5%; OR, 0.74; 95% CI, 0.54 to 1.00; $p < .05$). The authors concluded that in patients with UA and MI without ST segment elevation who were treated with the GP IIb/IIIa inhibitor tirofiban, the use of an early invasive strategy significantly reduced the incidence of major car-

diac events. These data support a policy involving broader use of the early inhibition of GP IIb/IIIa in combination with an early invasive strategy in such patients.

2. B. Lower rate of hospital readmission. Belardinelli et al. studied the effects of exercise training on functional capacity and quality of life in patients who received PTCA or coronary stenting (CS). The authors studied 118 consecutive patients with CAD (mean age, 57 ± 10 years) who underwent PTCA or CS on one (69%) or two (31%) native epicardial coronary arteries. Patients were randomized into two matched groups. Group T (n = 59) was exercised three times per week for 6 months at 60% of peak $\dot{V}o_2$. Group C (n = 59) was the control group. Only trained patients had significant improvements in peak $\dot{V}o_2$ (26%; $p <.001$) and quality of life (26.8%; $p = .001$, vs. C group). The angiographic restenosis rate was unaffected by exercise training (T group, 29%; C group, 33%; p = NS) and was not significantly different after PTCA or CS. However, residual diameter stenosis was lower in trained patients (–29.7%; $p = .045$). In patients with angiographic restenosis, thallium uptake improved only in group T (19%; $p <.001$). During the follow-up (33 ± 7 months), trained patients had a significantly lower event rate than controls [11.9% vs. 32.2%; RR, 0.71; 95% CI, 0.60 to 0.91; $p = .008$] and a lower rate of hospital readmission (18.6% vs. 46%; RR, 0.69; 95% CI, 0.55 to 0.93; $p <.001$). Moderate exercise training improved functional capacity and quality of life after PTCA or CS. During the follow-up, trained patients had fewer events and a lower hospital readmission rate than controls, despite an unchanged restenosis rate.

3. B. CRP. Inflammatory reactions in coronary plaques play an important role in the pathogenesis of acute atherothrombotic events; inflammation elsewhere is also associated with both atherogenesis generally and its thrombotic complications. Recent studies indicate that systemic markers of inflammation can identify subjects at high risk for coronary events. Koenig et al. used a sensitive immunoradiometric assay to examine the association of serum CRP with the incidence of first major CHD event in 936 men aged 45 to 64 years. The subjects, who were sampled at random from the general population, participated in the first MONICA (Monitoring Trends and Determinants in Cardiovascular Disease) Augsburg survey (1984 to 1985) and were followed for 8 years. There was a positive and statistically significant unadjusted relationship, which was linear on the log-hazards scale, between CRP values and the incidence of CHD events (n = 53). The hazard rate ratio of CHD events associated with a 1 standard deviation increase in log-CRP level was 1.67 (95% CI, 1.29 to 2.17). After adjustment for age, the hazard rate ratio was 1.60 (95% CI, 1.23 to 2.08). Adjusting further for smoking behavior, the only variable selected from a variety of potential confounders by a forward stepping process with a 5% change in the RR of CRP as the selection criterion, yielded a hazard rate ratio of 1.50 (95% CI, 1.14 to 1.97). These results confirm the prognostic relevance of CRP, a sensitive systemic marker of inflammation, to the risk of CHD in a large, randomly selected cohort of initially healthy middle-aged men. They suggest that low-grade inflammation is involved in pathogenesis of atherosclerosis, especially its thromboocclusive complications.

4. C. Radiation. A double-blind, randomized trial was undertaken to compare iridium-192 (^{192}Ir) with placebo sources in patients with previous restenosis after coronary angioplasty. Patients were randomly assigned to receive a

NOTES

0.76-mm (0.03-in.) ribbon containing sealed sources of either ^{192}Ir or placebo. All patients underwent repeat coronary angiography at 6 months. All living patients were contacted 24 months after their index study procedures. Patients were assessed with respect to the need for target-lesion revascularization or nontarget-lesion revascularization, occurrence of MI, or death. Over a 9-month period, 55 patients were enrolled; 26 were randomized to ^{192}Ir and 29 to placebo. Follow-up was obtained in 100% of living patients at a minimum of 24 months. Target-lesion revascularization was significantly lower in the ^{192}Ir group (15.4% vs. 44.8%; $p <.01$). Nontarget-lesion revascularization was similar in ^{192}Ir and placebo patients (19.2% vs. 20.7%; $p =$ NS). There were two deaths in each group. The composite end point of death, MI, or target-lesion revascularization was significantly lower in ^{192}Ir-treated versus placebo-treated patients (23.1% vs. 51.7%; $p = .03$). No patient in the ^{192}Ir group sustained a target-lesion revascularization later than 10 months. At 2-year clinical follow-up, treatment with ^{192}Ir demonstrates significant clinical benefit. Although further follow-up (including late angiography) is necessary, no clinical events have occurred to date in the ^{192}Ir group to suggest major untoward effects of vascular radiotherapy. At the intermediate follow-up time point, vascular radiotherapy continues to be a promising new treatment for restenosis. Percutaneous transmyocardial revascularization has not been shown to be effective, and gene therapy or percutaneous bypass is an investigational procedure currently indicated in no-option patients.

5. D. Hospitalization for UA. ACE inhibitors improve the outcome among patients with LV dysfunction whether or not they have heart failure. In the HOPE trial, a total of 9,297 high-risk patients (55 years of age or older) who had evidence of vascular disease or diabetes plus one other cardiovascular risk factor and who were not known to have a low EF or heart failure were randomly assigned to receive ramipril (10 mg once per day PO) or matching placebo for a mean of 5 years. The primary outcome was a composite of MI, stroke, or death from cardiovascular causes. A total of 651 patients who were assigned to receive ramipril (14.0%) reached the primary end point, as compared with 826 patients who were assigned to receive placebo (17.8%) (RR, 0.78; 95% CI, 0.70 to 0.86; $p <.001$). Treatment with ramipril reduced the rates of death from cardiovascular causes (6.1%, as compared with 8.1% in the placebo group; RR, 0.74; $p <.001$), MI (9.9% vs. 12.3%; RR, 0.80; $p <.001$), stroke (3.4% vs. 4.9%; RR, 0.68; $p <.001$), death from any cause (10.4% vs. 12.2%; RR, 0.84; $p = .005$), revascularization procedures (16.3% vs. 18.8%; RR, 0.85; $p <.001$), cardiac arrest (0.8% vs. 1.3%; RR, 0.62; $p = .02$), heart failure (9.1% vs. 11.6%; RR, 0.77; $p <.001$), and complications related to diabetes (6.4% vs. 7.6%; RR, 0.84; $p = .03$). Ramipril significantly reduced the rates of death, MI, and stroke in a broad range of high-risk patients who were not known to have a low EF or heart failure. However, treatment with ramipril had no effect on the likelihood of hospitalization for UA.

6. D. VI. MI is the most frequent cause of mortality in the United States as well as in most Western countries. Fuster et al. reviewed the processes leading to MI based on studies of vascular biology. Five phases of the progression of coronary atherosclerosis (phases 1 to 5) and eight morphologically different lesions (Stary types I, II, III, IV, Va, Vb, Vc, and VI) in the various phases were defined. The fate of plaque disruption (type VI lesion) in the genesis of the various coronary syndromes, and especially AMI, was

defined. Type VI lesion is a complicated lesion that can disrupt, thrombose, and lead to MI.

7. D. O_2-carrying capacity of the blood. The O_2-carrying capacity of the blood determines O_2 supply, not demand.

8. C. Subendocardium. The subendocardium is most susceptible to ischemic damage. Although the mechanisms of subendocardial ischemia remain to be fully defined, they are clearly associated with the transmural distribution of intramyocardial systolic pressures. Although almost all of the myocardium is perfused in diastole, a reduction of diastolic perfusion pressure or duration will result in subendocardial ischemia.

9. D. Inferior wall MI with RV infarction. The ECG is suggestive of inferior wall MI, and clinical presentation of elevated jugular venous pressure with clear lungs is suggestive of RV infarction. Tall c-v waves of tricuspid regurgitation are evident in patients with necrosis or ischemia of the RV papillary muscles.

10. A. Reduction in LV compliance. S_4 is almost universally present in patients with AMI and is related to reduction in LV compliance. Rapid deceleration of transmitral flow during protodiastolic filling of the LV and increased inflow into the LV is responsible for S_3.

11. C. Myoglobin. The earliest rise is seen with myoglobin, followed by CK-MB, troponin, and then low-dose heparin.

12. B. Survival benefit of t-PA over streptokinase. The relative efficacy of streptokinase and t-PA and the roles of IV as compared with SC heparin as adjunctive therapy in AMI were studied in GUSTO I. In 15 countries and 1,081 hospitals, 41,021 patients with evolving MI were randomly assigned to four different thrombolytic strategies, consisting of the use of streptokinase and SC heparin, streptokinase and IV heparin, accelerated t-PA and IV heparin, or a combination of streptokinase plus t-PA with IV heparin. (*Accelerated* refers to the administration of t-PA over a period of 1.5 hours—with two-thirds of the dose given in the first 30 min—rather than the conventional period of 3 hours.) The primary end point was 30-day mortality. The mortality rates in the four treatment groups were as follows: streptokinase and SC heparin, 7.2%; streptokinase and IV heparin, 7.4%; accelerated t-PA and IV heparin, 6.3%; and the combination of both thrombolytic agents with IV heparin, 7.0%. This represented a 14% reduction (95% CI, 5.9% to 21.3%) in mortality for accelerated t-PA as compared with the two streptokinase-only strategies ($p = .001$). The rates of hemorrhagic stroke were 0.49%, 0.54%, 0.72%, and 0.94% in the four groups, respectively, which represented a significant excess of hemorrhagic strokes for accelerated t-PA ($p = .03$) and for the combination strategy ($p < .001$), as compared with streptokinase only. A combined end point of death or disabling stroke was significantly lower in the accelerated t-PA group than in the streptokinase-only groups (6.9% vs. 7.8%, $p = .006$). The findings of this large-scale trial indicated that accelerated t-PA given with IV heparin provides a survival benefit over previous standard thrombolytic regimens. Reocclusion was infrequent and was similar in all four groups (range, 4.9% to 6.4%).

13. D. Choice of thrombolytic agent. Individual patients reflect a combination of clinical features that influence prognosis, and these factors must be appropriately weighted to produce an accurate assessment of risk. Using the large population of the GUSTO I trial, Lee et al. performed a comprehensive analysis of relations between baseline clinical data and 30-day mortality and developed a multivariable statistical model for risk assessment in candidates for thrombolytic therapy. For the 41,021 patients enrolled in GUSTO I, a randomized trial of four thrombolytic strategies, relations between clinical descriptors routinely collected at initial presentation and death within 30 days (which occurred in 7% of the population) were examined with both univariable and multivariable analyses. Variables studied included demographics, history and risk factors, presenting characteristics, and treatment assignment. Risk modeling was performed with logistic multiple regression and validated with bootstrapping techniques. Multivariable analysis identified age as the most significant factor influencing 30-day mortality, with rates of 1.1% in the youngest decile (younger than 45 years) and 20.5% in patients older than 75 (adjusted $\chi_2 = 717$; $p <.0001$). Other factors most significantly associated with increased mortality were lower systolic BP ($\chi_2 = 550$; $p <.0001$), higher Killip class ($\chi_2 = 350$; $p <.0001$), elevated heart rate ($\chi_2 = 275$; $p <.0001$), and anterior infarction ($\chi_2 = 143$; $p <.0001$). Together, these five characteristics contained 90% of the prognostic information in the baseline clinical data. Other significant although less important factors included previous MI, height, time to treatment, diabetes, weight, smoking status, type of thrombolytic agent, previous bypass surgery, hypertension, and prior cerebrovascular disease. Choice of the thrombolytic agent contributed less than 1% to the proportional effect of mortality.

14. C. Greater than or equal to 1-mm ST segment depression in stage I. High-risk exercise ECG variables include (a) greater than or equal to 2.0 mm ST segment depression; (b) greater than or equal to 1 mm ST segment depression in stage I; (c) ST segment depression in multiple leads; (d) ST segment depression for longer than 5 min during the recovery period; (e) achievement of a workload of less than 4 METS or a low maximal heart rate; (f) abnormal BP response; and (g) ventricular arrhythmias.

15. A. Patients with LV dysfunction exhibit long-term benefit from an initial strategy of surgical treatment. The CASS study randomized 780 patients to an initial strategy of coronary surgery or medical therapy. Of medically randomized patients, 6% had surgery within 6 months, and 40% had surgery by 10 years. At 10 years, there was no difference in cumulative survival (medical, 79% vs. surgical, 82%; NS) and no difference in the percentage free of death and nonfatal MI (medical, 69% vs. surgical, 66%; NS). Patients with an EF of less than 0.50 exhibited a better survival with initial surgery treatment (medical, 61% vs. surgical, 79%; $p = .01$). Conversely, patients with an EF greater than or equal to 0.50 exhibited a higher proportion free of death and MI with initial medical therapy (medical, 75% vs. surgical, 68%; $p = .04$), although long-term survival remained unaffected (medical, 84% vs. surgical, 83%; $p = .75$). There were no significant differences in either survival or freedom from nonfatal MI, whether stratified on the presence of heart failure, age, hypertension, or number of vessels diseased. Thus, 10-year follow-up results confirm earlier reports from CASS that patients with LV dysfunction exhibit long-term benefit from an initial strategy of surgical

treatment. Patients with mild stable angina and normal LV function randomized to initial medical treatment (with an option for later surgery if symptoms progress) have survival equivalent to those patients randomized to initial surgery.

16. A. Significant mortality benefit with revascularization compared to angina-guided medical therapy. The ACIP study assessed the ability of three treatment strategies to suppress ambulatory ECG ischemia to determine whether a large-scale trial studying the impact of these strategies on clinical outcomes was feasible. Five hundred fifty-eight patients with coronary anatomy amenable to revascularization, at least one episode of asymptomatic ischemia on the 48-hour ambulatory ECG, and ischemia on treadmill exercise testing were randomized to one of three treatment strategies: (a) medication to suppress angina (angina-guided strategy, n = 183); (b) medication to suppress both angina and ambulatory ECG ischemia (ischemia-guided strategy, n = 183); or (c) revascularization strategy (angioplasty or bypass surgery, n = 192). The revascularization group received less medication and had less ischemia on serial ambulatory ECG recordings and exercise testing than those assigned to the medical strategies. The ischemia-guided group received more medication but had suppression of ischemia similar to the angina-guided group. At 1 year, the mortality rate was 4.4% in the angina-guided group (8 of 183), 1.6% in the ischemia-guided group (3 of 183), and 0% in the revascularization group (overall, $p = .004$; angina-guided vs. revascularization, $p = .003$; other pair-wise comparisons, $p = NS$). Frequency of MI, UA, stroke, and CHF was not significantly different among the three strategies. The revascularization group had significantly fewer hospital admissions and nonprotocol revascularizations at 1 year. The incidence of death, MI, nonprotocol revascularization, or hospital admissions at 1 year was 32% with the angina-guided medical strategy, 31% with the ischemia-guided medical strategy, and 18% with the revascularization strategy ($p = .003$). After 1 year, revascularization was superior to both angina-guided and ischemia-guided medical strategies in suppressing asymptomatic ischemia and was associated with better outcome.

17. C. A 12-lead ECG should be obtained immediately (within 10 min) in patients with ongoing chest discomfort and as rapidly as possible in patients who have a history of chest discomfort consistent with ACS but whose discomfort has resolved by the time of evaluation. The remainder are all class I recommendations.

18. E. Patients with possible ACS and negative cardiac markers who are unable to exercise or who have an abnormal resting ECG should have a pharmacologic stress test instead of proceeding to coronary angiograms directly.

19. F. In patients with continuing or frequently recurring ischemia when beta-blockers are contraindicated, a nondihydropyridine calcium antagonist (e.g., verapamil or diltiazem) followed by PO therapy is indicated as initial therapy in the absence of severe LV dysfunction or other contraindications.

20. D. A platelet GP IIb/IIIa receptor antagonist should be administered, in addition to ASA and UFH, to patients with continuing ischemia or with other high-risk features and to patients in whom a PCI is planned. Eptifi-

batide and tirofiban are approved for this use. Abciximab can also be used for 12 to 24 hours in patients with UA or NSTEMI in whom a PCI is planned within the next 24 hours. The GP IIb/IIIa receptor ($\alpha_{IIb}\beta_3$ integrin) is abundant on the platelet surface. When platelets are activated, this receptor undergoes a change in configuration that increases its affinity for binding to fibrinogen and other ligands. Binding of molecules of fibrinogen to receptors on different platelets results in platelet aggregation. This mechanism is independent of the stimulus for platelet aggregation and represents the final and obligatory pathway for platelet aggregation. The platelet GP IIb/IIIa receptor antagonists act by preventing fibrinogen binding and thereby preventing platelet aggregation. The various GP IIb/IIIa antagonists, however, possess significantly different pharmacokinetic and pharmacodynamic properties. Abciximab is a Fab fragment of a humanized murine antibody that has a short plasma half-life but strong affinity for the receptor, resulting in some receptor occupancy that persists for weeks. Platelet aggregation gradually returns to normal 24 to 48 hours after the discontinuation of the drug. Abciximab is not specific for GP IIb/IIIa and inhibits the vitronectin receptor ($\alpha_v\beta_3$) on endothelial cells and the MAC-1 receptor on leukocytes as well. Eptifibatide is a cyclic heptapeptide that contains the KGD (Lys-Gly-Asp) sequence; tirofiban is a nonpeptide mimetic of the RGD (Arg-Gly-Asp) sequence of fibrinogen. Receptor occupancy with these two synthetic antagonists is in general in equilibrium with plasma levels. They have a half-life of 2 to 3 hours and are highly specific for the GP IIb/IIIa receptor, with no effect on the vitronectin receptor ($\alpha_v\beta_3$ integrin). The efficacy of GP IIb/IIIa antagonists in prevention of the complications associated with percutaneous interventions has been documented in numerous trials, many of which are composed entirely or in large part of patients with UA. Two trials with tirofiban and one trial with eptifibatide have also documented their efficacy in UA and NSTEMI patients, of whom only some underwent interventions. Abciximab has been studied primarily in PCI trials, in which its administration consistently showed a significant reduction in the rate of MI and the need for urgent revascularization. The cumulative event rates observed during the phase of medical management and at the time of PCI in the c7E3 Fab Antiplatelet Therapy in Unstable Refractory Angina (CAPTURE) (abciximab), Platelet Receptor Inhibition in Ischemic Syndrome Management in Patients Limited by Unstable Signs and Symptoms (PRISM-PLUS) (tirofiban), and Platelet Glycoprotein IIb/IIIa in Unstable Angina: Receptor Suppression Using Integrilin Therapy (PURSUIT) (eptifibatide) trials are shown in Figure 14. Each trial has shown a statistically significant reduction in the rate of death or MI during the phase of medical management; the reduction in event rates was magnified at the time of the intervention.

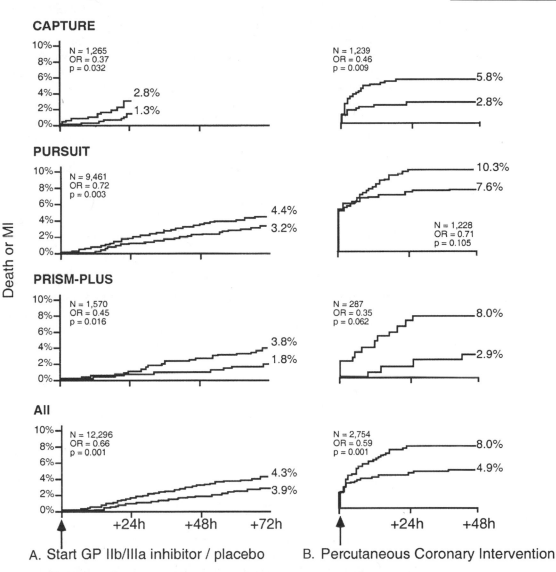

FIGURE 14 Kaplan-Meier curves showing cumulative incidence of death or MI in patients randomly assigned to platelet glycoprotein (GP) IIb/IIIa receptor antagonist (*bottom line*) or placebo. Data are derived from the CAPTURE, PURSUIT, and PRISM-PLUS trials. **A:** Events during the initial period of medical treatment until the moment of percutaneous coronary intervention (PCI) or coronary artery bypass graft. In the CAPTURE trial, abciximab was administered for 18 to 24 hours before the PCI was performed in almost all patients, as per study design; abciximab was discontinued 1 hour after the intervention. In PURSUIT, a PCI was performed in 11.2% of patients during a period of medical therapy with eptifibatide that lasted 72 hours and for 24 hours after the intervention. In PRISM-PLUS, an intervention was performed in 30.2% of patients after a 48-hour period of medical therapy with tirofiban, and the drug infusion was maintained for 12 to 24 hours after an intervention. **B:** Events occurring at the time of PCI and the next 48 hours, with the event rates reset to 0% before the intervention. Creatine kinase (CK) or CK-MB elevations exceeding two times the upper limit of normal were considered as infarction during medical management and exceeding three times the upper limit of normal for PCI-related events. OR indicates odds ratio. (Adapted from Boersma E, Akkerhuis KM, Theroux P, et al. Platelet glycoprotein IIb/IIIa receptor inhibition in non-ST-elevation acute coronary syndromes: early benefit during medical treatment only, with additional protection during percutaneous coronary intervention. *Circulation* 1999;100:2045–2048.)

21. D. PPCI or CABG is indicated in patients with a large area of viable myocardium and high-risk criteria on noninvasive testing. In general, the indications for PCI and CABG in UA or NSTEMI are similar to those in stable angina. High-risk patients with LV systolic dysfunction, two-vessel disease with severe proximal LAD involvement, severe three-vessel disease, or left main disease should be considered for CABG. Many other patients have less severe CAD that does not put them at high risk for cardiac death. However, even less severe disease can have a substantial negative affect on the quality of life. Compared with high-risk patients, low-risk patients receive negligible or very modestly increased chances of long-term survival with CABG. Therefore, in low-risk patients, quality of life and patient preferences are given more weight than are strict clinical outcomes in the selection of a treatment strategy. Low-risk patients whose symptoms do not respond well to maximal medical therapy and who experience a significant negative affect on their quality of life and functional status should be considered for revascularization.

22. B. Drugs required in the hospital to control ischemia should be continued after hospital discharge in patients who do not undergo coronary revascularization, patients with unsuccessful revascularization, or patients with recurrent symptoms after revascularization. Upward or downward titration of the doses may be required (Level of Evidence: C). The other class I recommendations include

1. Before hospital discharge, patients and/or designated responsible caregivers should be provided with well-understood instructions with respect to medication type, purpose, dose, frequency, and pertinent side effects. (Level of Evidence: C)

2. Before hospital discharge, patients should be informed about symptoms of AMI and should be instructed in how to seek help if they occur. (Level of Evidence: C)

3. All patients should be given sublingual or spray NTG and instructed in its use. (Level of Evidence: C)

4. Anginal discomfort that lasts longer than 2 or 3 min should prompt the patient to discontinue the activity or remove himself or herself from the stressful event. If pain does not subside immediately, the patient should be instructed to take NTG. If the first tablet or spray does not provide relief within 5 min, then a second and third dose, at 5-min intervals, should be taken. Pain that lasts longer than 15 to 20 min or persistent pain despite three NTG doses should prompt the patient to seek immediate medical attention by calling 9-1-1 and going to the nearest hospital emergency department, preferably by ambulance or the quickest available alternative. (Level of Evidence: C)

5. If the pattern of anginal symptoms changes (e.g., pain that is more frequent or severe, is precipitated by less effort, or now occurs at rest), the patient should contact his or her physician to determine the need for additional treatment or testing. (Level of Evidence: C)

6. ASA, 75 to 325 mg per day, in the absence of contraindications. (Level of Evidence: A)

7. Clopidogrel, 75 mg per day, in patients with a contraindication to ASA. (Level of Evidence: B)

8. Beta-blockers in the absence of contraindications. (Level of Evidence: B)

9. Lipid-lowering agents and diet in post-ACS patients, including patients who are postrevascularization with LDL cholesterol of greater than 125 mg per dL, including after revascularization. (Level of Evidence: A)

10. Lipid-lowering agents if LDL cholesterol level after diet is greater than 100 mg per dL. (Level of Evidence: C)

11. ACE inhibitors for patients with CHF, LV dysfunction (EF less than 0.40), hypertension, or diabetes. (Level of Evidence: A)

23. B. Medical treatment in the acute phase and decisions on whether to perform stress testing and angiography and revascularization should be similar in diabetic and nondiabetic patients. Diabetes occurs in approximately one-fifth of patients with UA/NSTEMI and is an independent predictor of adverse outcomes. It is associated with more extensive CAD, unstable lesions, frequent comorbidities, and less favorable long-term outcomes with coronary revascularization, especially with PTCA. The use of stents, particularly with abciximab, appears to provide more favorable results in diabetics, although more data are needed. Clinical outcome with CABG, especially using one or both internal mammary arteries, is better than that with PTCA but is still less favorable than in nondiabetics.

24. A. A class I indication for coronary angiography is when patients have disabling CCS classes III and IV chronic stable angina despite medical therapy. Patients identified as having increased risk on the basis of an assessment of clinical data and noninvasive testing are generally referred for coronary arteriography even if their symptoms are not severe. Noninvasive testing that is used appropriately is less costly than coronary angiography and has an acceptable predictive value for adverse events. This is most true when the pretest probability of severe CAD is low. When the pretest probability of severe CAD is high, direct referral for coronary angiography without noninvasive testing is probably most cost-effective because the total number of tests is reduced. Coronary angiography, the traditional gold standard for clinical assessment of coronary atherosclerosis, has limitations. It is not a reliable indicator of the functional significance of a coronary stenosis and is insensitive in detection of a thrombus (an indicator of disease activity). More important, coronary angiography is ineffective in determining which plaques have characteristics likely to lead to acute coronary events—that is, the vulnerable plaque with large lipid core, thin fibrous cap, and increased macrophages. Serial angiographic studies performed before and after acute events and early after MI suggest that plaques resulting in UA and MI commonly produced less than 50% stenosis before the acute event and were, therefore, angiographically "silent." Despite these limitations of coronary angiography, the extent and severity of coronary disease and LV dysfunction identified on angiography are the most powerful predictors of long-term patient outcome. Several prognostic indexes have been used to relate disease severity to the risk of subsequent cardiac events; the simplest and most widely used is the classification of disease into one-, two-, or three-vessel or left main CAD. In the CASS registry of medically treated patients, the 12-year survival rate of patients with normal coronary arteries was 91% compared with 74% for those with one-vessel disease, 59% for those with two-vessel disease, and 40% for those with three-vessel disease. It has been known for many years that patients with significant stenosis of the left main coronary artery have a poor prognosis when treated medically. The impact of LV dysfunction on survival was quite dramatic. In the CASS

registry, the 12-year survival rate was 73% for patients with an EF between 50% and 100%, 54% for those with an EF between 35% and 49%, and only 21% for those with an EF less than 35%.

25. B. Proximal LAD stenosis with one- or two-vessel disease. Proximal LAD stenosis with one- or two-vessel disease is a class IIa indication. Proximal LAD stenosis with one- or two-vessel disease becomes class I if there is extensive ischemia documented by noninvasive study or an LV EF less than 0.50.

26. C. Deployment pressure is not a variable associated with stent thrombosis in the modern era. There are limited studies of stent thrombosis in the modern era of second-generation stents, high-pressure deployment, and current antithrombotic regimens. Six recently completed coronary stent trials and associated nonrandomized registries that enrolled 6,186 patients (6,219 treated vessels) treated with one or more coronary stent followed by antiplatelet therapy with ASA and ticlopidine were pooled for an analysis. Within 30 days, clinical stent thrombosis developed in 53 patients (0.9%). The variables most significantly associated with the probability of stent thrombosis were persistent dissection National Heart, Lung, and Blood Institute grade B or higher after stenting (OR, 3.7; 95% CI, 1.9 to 7.7), total stent length (OR, 1.3; 95% CI, 1.2 to 1.5/10 mm), and final minimal lumen diameter within the stent (OR, 0.4; 95% CI, 0.2 to 0.7/1 mm). Stent thrombosis was documented by angiography in 45 patients (0.7%). Clinical consequences of angiographic stent thrombosis included 64.4% incidence of death or MI at the time of stent thrombosis and 8.9% 6-month mortality. Stent thrombosis occurred in less than 1% of patients undergoing stenting of native coronary artery lesions and receiving routine antiplatelet therapy with ASA plus ticlopidine. Procedure-related variables of persistent dissection, total stent length, and final lumen diameter were significantly associated with the probability of stent thrombosis.

27. B. 20%. Stroke is a leading cause of death and disability. Although clinical trials of the early lipid-lowering therapies did not demonstrate a reduction in the rates of stroke, data from recently completed statin trials strongly suggest benefit. The effect of pravastatin, 40 mg per day, on stroke events was investigated in a prospectively defined pooled analysis of three large, placebo-controlled, randomized trials that included 19,768 patients with 102,559 person-years of follow-up. In all, 598 participants had a stroke during approximately 5 years of follow-up. The two secondary prevention trials [CARE (Cholesterol And Recurrent Events) and LIPID (Long-term Intervention with Pravastatin in Ischemic Disease)] individually demonstrated reductions in nonfatal and total stroke rates. When the 13,173 patients from CARE and LIPID were combined, there was a 22% reduction in total strokes (95% CI, 7 to 35; $p = .01$) and a 25% reduction in nonfatal stroke (95% CI, 10 to 38). The beneficial effect of pravastatin on total stroke was observed across a wide range of patient characteristics. WOSCOPS (a primary prevention trial in hypercholesterolemic men) exhibited a similar, although smaller, trend for a reduction in total stroke. Among the CARE/LIPID participants, pravastatin was associated with a 23% reduction in nonhemorrhagic strokes (95% CI, 6 to 37), but there was no statistical treatment group difference in hemorrhagic or unknown type.

28. C. Prior MI is not a prognostic factor for atherosclerosis progression in SVGs. The Post-CABG trial was done to assess patients after CABG and determine prognostic factors for atherosclerosis progression. SVGs are effective in relieving angina and, in certain patient subsets, in prolonging life. However, the progression of atherosclerosis in many of these grafts limits their usefulness. The Post-CABG trial studied moderate versus aggressive lipid-lowering and low-dose warfarin versus placebo in patients with a history of coronary artery bypass surgery and found that more aggressive lipid lowering was effective in preventing progression of atherosclerosis in SVGs, but warfarin had no effect. Using variables measured at baseline, we sought the independent prognostic factors for atherosclerosis progression in SVGs, using the statistical method of generalized estimating equations with a logit-link function. Twelve independent prognostic factors for atherosclerosis progression were found. In the order of their importance, they were (a) maximum stenosis of the graft at baseline angiography, (b) years post-SVG placement, (c) the moderate LDL-cholesterol lowering strategy, (d) prior MI, (e) high triglyceride level, (f) small minimum graft diameter, (g) low HDL-C, (h) high LDL-cholesterol, (i) high mean arterial pressure, (j) low EF, (k) male gender, and (l) current smoking.

29. C. Aggressive lipid-lowering therapy is as effective as percutaneous coronary revascularization. Percutaneous coronary revascularization is widely used in improving symptoms and exercise performance in patients with ischemic heart disease and stable angina pectoris. In the AVERT study, the investigators compared percutaneous coronary revascularization with lipid-lowering treatment for reducing the incidence of ischemic events. They studied 341 patients with stable CAD, relatively normal LV function, asymptomatic or mild to moderate angina, and a serum level of LDL-cholesterol of at least 115 mg per dL (3.0 mmol/L) who were referred for percutaneous revascularization. The patients were randomly assigned either to receive medical treatment with atorvastatin at 80 mg per day (164 patients) or to undergo the recommended percutaneous revascularization procedure (angioplasty) followed by usual care, which could include lipid-lowering treatment (177 patients). The follow-up period was 18 months. Twenty-two (13%) of the patients who received aggressive lipid-lowering treatment with atorvastatin [resulting in a 46% reduction in the mean serum LDL-cholesterol level, to 77 mg per dL (2.0 mmol/L)] had ischemic events, as compared with 37 (21%) of the patients who underwent angioplasty [who had an 18% reduction in the mean serum LDL-cholesterol level, to 119 mg per dL (3.0 mmol/L)]. The incidence of ischemic events was thus 36% lower in the atorvastatin group over an 18-month period ($p = .048$, which was not statistically significant after adjustment for interim analyses). This reduction in events was due to a smaller number of angioplasty procedures, coronary-artery bypass operations, and hospitalizations for worsening angina. As compared with the patients who were treated with angioplasty and usual care, the patients who received atorvastatin had a significantly longer time to the first ischemic event ($p = .03$). In low-risk patients with stable CAD, aggressive lipid-lowering therapy is at least as effective as angioplasty and usual care in reducing the incidence of ischemic events.

30. C. 0.70. The 4S trial was designed to evaluate the effect of cholesterol lowering with simvastatin on mortality and morbidity in patients with CHD. Four thousand four hundred forty-four patients with angina pectoris or previous MI and serum cholesterol of 5.5 to 8.0 mmol per L on a lipid-lowering

diet were randomized to double-blind treatment with simvastatin or placebo. Over the 5.4-year median follow-up period, simvastatin produced mean changes in total cholesterol (TC), LDL-cholesterol, and HDL-C of –25%, –35%, and +8%, respectively, with few adverse effects. Two hundred fifty-six patients (12%) in the placebo group died, compared with 182 (8%) in the simvastatin group. The RR of death in the simvastatin group was 0.70 (95% CI, 0.58 to 0.85; p = .0003). The 6-year probabilities of survival in the placebo and simvastatin groups were 87.6% and 91.3%, respectively. There were 189 coronary deaths in the placebo group and 111 in the simvastatin group (RR, 0.58; 95% CI, 0.46 to 0.73), whereas noncardiovascular causes accounted for 49 and 46 deaths, respectively. Six hundred twenty-two patients (28%) in the placebo group and 431 (19%) in the simvastatin group had one or more major coronary events. The RR was 0.66 (95% CI, 0.59 to 0.75; p <.00001), and the respective probabilities of escaping such events were 70.5% and 79.6%. This risk was also significantly reduced in subgroups consisting of women and patients of both genders aged 60 years or older. Other benefits of treatment included a 37% reduction (p <.00001) in the risk of undergoing myocardial revascularization procedures. This study showed that long-term treatment with simvastatin is safe and improves survival in CHD patients.

31. B. First acute major coronary event defined as fatal or nonfatal MI, UA, or sudden cardiac death. The objective of this trial was to compare lovastatin with placebo for prevention of the first acute major coronary event in men and women without clinically evident atherosclerotic cardiovascular disease with average TC and LDL-cholesterol levels and below-average HDL-C levels. A randomized, double-blind, placebo-controlled trial was the design of this trial in the setting of outpatient clinics in Texas. A total of 5,608 men and 997 women with average TC and LDL-cholesterol and below-average HDL-C [as characterized by lipid percentiles for an age- and sex-matched cohort without cardiovascular disease from the National Health and Nutrition Examination Survey (NHANES) III] were studied. Mean (SD) TC level was 5.71 (0.54) mmol per L [221 (21) mg/dL] (fifty-first percentile); mean (SD) LDL-cholesterol level was 3.89 (0.43) mmol per L [150 (17) mg/dL] (sixtieth percentile); mean (SD) HDL-C level was 0.94 (0.14) mmol per L [36 (5) mg/dL] for men and 1.03 (0.14) mmol per L [40 (5) mg/dL] for women (twenty-fifth and sixteenth percentiles, respectively); and median (SD) triglyceride levels were 1.78 (0.86) mmol per L [158 (76) mg/dL] (sixty-third percentile). Lovastatin (20 to 40 mg daily) or placebo in addition to a low-saturated fat, low-cholesterol diet was studied. The main outcome measure was a first acute major coronary event defined as fatal or nonfatal MI, UA, or sudden cardiac death. After an average follow-up of 5.2 years, lovastatin reduced the incidence of first acute major coronary events (183 vs. 116 first events; RR, 0.63; 95% CI, 0.50 to 0.79; p <.001), MI (95 vs. 57 MIs; RR, 0.60; 95% CI, 0.43 to 0.83; p = .002), UA (87 vs. 60 first UA events; RR, 0.68; 95% CI, 0.49 to 0.95; p = .02), coronary revascularization procedures (157 vs. 106 procedures; RR, 0.67; 95% CI, 0.52 to 0.85; p = .001), coronary events (215 vs. 163 coronary events; RR, 0.75; 95% CI, 0.61 to 0.92; p = .006), and cardiovascular events (255 vs. 194 cardiovascular events; RR, 0.75; 95% CI, 0.62 to 0.91; p = .003). Lovastatin (20 to 40 mg daily) reduced LDL-cholesterol by 25% to 2.96 mmol per L (115 mg/dL) and increased HDL-C by 6% to 1.02 mmol per L (39 mg/dL). There were no clinically relevant differences in safety parameters between treatment groups. Lovastatin reduced the risk for the first acute major coronary event in men and women with average TC and LDL-cholesterol levels and below-average HDL-C levels.

32. B. 24%. WOSCOPS was a primary prevention trial that demonstrated the effectiveness of pravastatin (40 mg/day) in reducing morbidity and mortality from CHD in moderately hypercholesterolemic men. The authors examined the extent to which differences in LDL and other plasma lipids both at baseline and on treatment influenced CHD risk reduction. Relationships between baseline lipid concentrations and incidence of all cardiovascular events and between on-treatment lipid concentrations and risk reduction in patients taking pravastatin were examined by use of Cox regression models and by division of the cohort into quintiles. Variation in plasma lipids at baseline did not influence the RR reduction generated by pravastatin therapy. Fall in LDL level in the pravastatin-treated group did not correlate with CHD risk reduction in multivariate regression. Furthermore, maximum benefit of an approximately 45% risk reduction was observed in the middle quintile of LDL reduction (mean, 24% fall); further mean decrements in LDL (up to 39%) were not associated with a greater decrease in CHD risk. Comparison of event rates between placebo- and pravastatin-treated subjects with the same LDL-cholesterol level provided evidence for an apparent treatment effect that was independent of LDL. The investigators concluded that the treatment effect of 40 mg per day of pravastatin is proportionally the same regardless of baseline lipid phenotype. There is no CHD risk reduction unless LDL levels are reduced, but a fall in the range of 24% is sufficient to produce the full benefit in patients taking this dose of pravastatin. LDL reduction alone did not appear to account entirely for the benefits of pravastatin therapy.

33. B. CABG is associated with better long-term survival than PTCA in treated diabetic patients with multivessel coronary disease suitable for either surgical or catheter-based revascularization. Patients with treated diabetes in the randomized-trial segment of BARI who were randomized to initial revascularization with PTCA had significantly worse 5-year survival than did patients assigned to CABG. This treatment difference was not seen among diabetic patients eligible for BARI who opted to select their mode of revascularization. Among diabetics taking insulin or PO hypoglycemic drugs at entry, angiographic and clinical presentations were comparable between randomized and registry patients. The 5-year all-cause mortality rate was 34.5% in randomized diabetic patients assigned to PTCA versus 19.4% in CABG patients ($p = .0024$; RR, 1.87); corresponding cardiac mortality rates were 23.4% and 8.2%, respectively ($p = .0002$; RR, 3.10). The CABG benefit was more apparent among patients requiring insulin. In the registry, all-cause mortality was 14.4% for PTCA versus 14.9% for CABG ($p = .86$; RR, 1.10), with corresponding cardiac mortality rates of 7.5% and 6.0%, respectively ($p = .73$; RR, 1.07). These RRs in the registry increased to 1.29 and 1.41, respectively, after adjustment for all known differences between treatment groups. BARI registry results were consistent with the finding in the randomized trial that initial CABG is associated with better long-term survival than PTCA in treated diabetic patients with multivessel coronary disease suitable for either surgical or catheter-based revascularization.

34. B. Increased frequency of episodes of angina and increased duration of ischemia. Cigarette smoking has been causally linked to CHD. To investigate the effect of smoking on the activity of ischemic heart disease, 65 patients with chronic stable manifestations of coronary disease and a positive exercise tolerance test underwent continuous ambulatory monitoring to quantify the amount of ischemic ST segment depression during daily life.

Twenty-four smokers were compared with 41 nonsmokers for frequency and duration of ECG signs of ischemia during 24 hours. A total of 4,968 hours of ambulatory monitoring was analyzed. The frequency of episodes was three times greater (median) and the duration of ischemia was 12 times longer (median duration, 24 min vs. 2 min/24 hours) in smokers than in nonsmokers. This finding remained statistically significant when a number of potentially confounding factors were controlled by means of logistic regression. This study showed that patients with CAD who smoke have significantly and substantially more active myocardial ischemia during daily life than patients who do not.

35. B. No significant difference with early revascularization compared to intensive medical therapy. The leading cause of death in patients hospitalized for AMI is cardiogenic shock. The SHOCK investigators conducted a randomized trial to evaluate early revascularization in patients with cardiogenic shock. Patients with shock due to LV failure complicating MI were randomly assigned to emergency revascularization (152 patients) or initial medical stabilization (150 patients). Revascularization was accomplished by either CABG or angioplasty. Intraaortic balloon counterpulsation was performed in 86% of the patients in both groups. The primary end point was mortality from all causes at 30 days. Six-month survival was a secondary end point. The mean age of the patients was 66 years, ± 10 years; 32% were women, and 55% were transferred from other hospitals. The median time to the onset of shock was 5.6 hours after infarction, and most infarcts were anterior in location. Ninety-seven percent of the patients assigned to revascularization underwent early coronary angiography, and 87% underwent revascularization; only 2.7% of the patients assigned to medical therapy crossed over to early revascularization without clinical indication. Overall mortality at 30 days (primary end point) did not differ significantly between the revascularization and medical therapy groups (46.7% and 56.0%, respectively; difference, –9.3%; 95% CI for the difference, –20.5 to 1.9; $p = .11$). Six-month mortality was lower in the revascularization group than in the medical therapy group (50.3% vs. 63.1%, $p = .027$).

36. A. Greater than 90% at 5 years. Califf et al. analyzed the clinical outcomes in 688 patients with isolated stenosis of one major coronary artery. The survival rate among patients with disease of the RCA was higher than that among patients with LAD or LCx disease. The survival rate among patients in all three anatomic subgroups exceeded 90% at 5 years. The presence of a lesion proximal to the first septal perforator of the LAD was associated with decreased survival compared with the presence of a more distal lesion. For the entire group of one-vessel disease patients, total ischemic events (death and nonfatal infarction) occurred at similar rates regardless of the anatomic location of the lesion. LVEF was the baseline descriptor most strongly associated with survival, and the characteristics of the angina had the strongest relationship with nonfatal MI. No differences in survival or total cardiac event rates were found with surgical or nonsurgical therapy. The relief of angina was superior with surgical therapy, although the majority of nonsurgically treated patients had significant relief of angina. The survival rate of patients with one-vessel coronary disease is excellent, and the risk of nonfatal infarction is low.

37. C. Extent of thallium abnormality was not a multivariate predictor. Iskandrian et al. examined the ability of single-photon emission CT imaging with

thallium-201 during adenosine-induced coronary hyperemia to detect high-risk patients with left main or three-vessel CAD. There were 339 patients: 102 with either left main or three-vessel CAD (group one) and 237 with no CAD, one-, or two-vessel disease (group two). By means of univariate analysis, several variables were found to differ between groups one and two: (a) Q-wave MI (35% vs. 25%; $p < .05$); (b) ST segment depression (35% vs. 19%; $p < .001$); (c) age (67 ± 9 years vs. 62 ± 10 years; $p < .001$); (d) resting systolic BP (142 ± 22 mm Hg vs. 135 ± 20 mm Hg; $p < .01$); (e) abnormal thallium images (95% vs. 74%; $p < .0001$); (f) multivessel thallium abnormality (76% vs. 39%; $p < .0001$); (g) extent of thallium abnormality (24% ± 11% vs. 19% ± 13%; $p < .0001$); and (h) increased lung thallium uptake (39% vs. 15%; $p < .01$). According to stepwise discriminant analysis, only three variables were predictors of high risk: multivessel thallium abnormality ($\chi_2 = 27$), increased lung thallium uptake ($\chi_2 = 10$), and ST depression ($\chi_2 = 5$). On the basis of these variables, patients were divided into three groups with different prevalence rates for left main and three-vessel CAD: 63% in 68 patients, 30% in 137 patients, and 13% in 137 patients.

38. **A. Abciximab in addition to ASA and heparin does not increase the risk of stroke in patients undergoing PCI.** Abciximab, a potent inhibitor of the platelet GP IIb/IIIa receptor, reduces thrombotic complications in patients undergoing PCI. Because of its potent inhibition of platelet aggregation, the effect of abciximab on risk of stroke is a concern. To determine whether abciximab use among patients undergoing PCI is associated with an increased risk of stroke, Akkerhuis et al. combined analysis of data from four double-blind, placebo-controlled, randomized trials [EPIC (Evaluation of c7E3 for Prevention of Ischemic Complications), CAPTURE, EPILOG (Evaluation of PTCA to Improve Long-Term Outcome by c7E3 GP IIb/IIIa Receptor Blockade), and EPISTENT (Evaluation of Platelet IIb/IIIa Inhibitor for Stenting Trial)] conducted between November 1991 and October 1997 at a total of 257 academic and community hospitals in the United States and Europe. A total of 8,555 patients undergoing PCI with or without stent deployment for a variety of indications were randomly assigned to receive a bolus and infusion of abciximab (n = 5,476) or matching placebo (n = 3,079). Risk of hemorrhagic and nonhemorrhagic stroke within 30 days of treatment among abciximab and placebo groups was analyzed. No significant difference in stroke rate was observed between patients assigned abciximab [n = 22 (0.40%)] and those assigned placebo [n = 9 (0.29%); $p = .46$]. Excluding the EPIC abciximab bolus–only group, there were nine strokes (0.30%) among 3,023 patients who received placebo and 15 (0.32%) in 4,680 patients treated with abciximab bolus plus infusion, a difference of 0.02% (95% CI, –0.23 to 0.28). The rate of nonhemorrhagic stroke was 0.17% in patients treated with abciximab and 0.20% in patients treated with placebo (difference, –0.03%; 95% CI, –0.23 to 0.17), and the rates of hemorrhagic stroke were 0.15% and 0.10%, respectively (difference, 0.05%; 95% CI, –0.11 to 0.21). Among patients treated with abciximab, the rate of hemorrhagic stroke in patients receiving standard-dose heparin in EPIC, CAPTURE, and EPILOG was higher than in those receiving low-dose heparin in the EPILOG and EPISTENT trials (0.27% vs. 0.04%; $p = .057$). Abciximab in addition to ASA and heparin does not increase the risk of stroke in patients undergoing PCI.

39. **C. Age is not predictive.** Despite the significant survival benefit associated with successful reperfusion therapy for AMI, global indices of outcome LV

function, such as EF, have often demonstrated little or no improvement. Although these measurements are confounded by numerous clinical, physiologic, and angiographic variables, no comprehensive analysis of this issue in a large series of patients is available. Lundergan et al. used the GUSTO I database to better understand this phenomenon by determining independent predictors of LV function and their interplay with regard to outcome ventricular function and improvement in function during the initial postinfarction week. Ninety-min and 5- to 7-day posttreatment global and regional indices derived from left ventriculograms were analyzed from a population of 676 patients. These observations were combined with clinical data to describe independent determinants of ventricular function outcome. Clinical factors predictive of global and regional ventricular function as well as improvement in function between 90 min and 5 to 7 days included time to treatment, early infarct-related artery flow grade, and body mass index. These same factors contribute significantly to compensatory hyperkinesis of the noninfarct zone, which is critical to maintenance of global ventricular function during this time. The ventricular function benefits of early complete reperfusion after MI are readily demonstrable after adjustment for multiple covariables and include (a) maintenance of global ventricular function and (b) prevention or delay in ventricular dilatation.

40. E. Female gender is not associated with failure of medical therapy in patients with UA/non–Q-wave MI. Current management of patients with UA/non–Q-wave MI generally consists of intensive medical therapy, with angiography and revascularization sometimes limited to those who fail such therapy. Stone et al. analyzed the TIMI IIIB study to determine if certain baseline characteristics are predictive of patients who fail medical therapy, because such patients could then be expeditiously directed to a more invasive strategy in a cost-effective manner. The study cohort consisted of the 733 patients in the TIMI IIIB study who were randomized to conservative strategy. Patients were to be treated with bedrest, antiischemic medications, ASA, and heparin, and were to undergo risk-stratifying tests, consisting of an exercise test with ECG and thallium scintigraphy, scheduled to be performed within 3 days before, or 5 days after, hospital discharge and 24-hour Holter monitoring scheduled to begin 2 to 5 days after randomization. Baseline clinical and ECG characteristics were compared between patients who "failed" medical therapy and those who did not "fail." Failure was defined using clinical end points (death, MI, or spontaneous ischemia by 6 weeks after randomization) or a strongly positive risk-stratifying test. For each test, an ordered failure profile of results was calculated and consisted of death, MI, or rest ischemia occurring before performance of the test, a markedly abnormal test result, and no abnormality. Clinical end points occurred in 241 (33%) patients and were more likely to occur in patients who at presentation were older, had ST segment depression on the qualifying ECG, or were being treated with heparin or ASA. Characteristics independently predictive of developing a clinical event or an abnormal exercise treadmill test included (a) ST segment depression on the qualifying ECG, (b) history of prior angina, (c) family history of premature coronary disease (i.e., onset before 55 years of age), (d) prior use of heparin or ASA, and (e) increasing age. By combining these baseline risk characteristics for each outcome, the incidence of developing a clinical event ranged from 8% if none was present to 63% if all six were present, and the incidence of developing a markedly abnormal risk stratifying test ranged from 8% to 21% if none were present to approximately 90% if all six were present. Patients with these character-

istics are appropriate candidates for expeditious cardiac catheterization and consideration for revascularization, whereas patients without them may be suitable for medical management alone.

41. C. 130. For persons with CHD and CHD risk equivalents, LDL-lowering therapy greatly reduces risk for major coronary events and stroke and yields highly favorable cost-effectiveness ratios. The cut points for initiating lifestyle and drug therapies are shown in Table 1.

TABLE 1 *Guidelines for LDL Goals*

LDL Cholesterol Goals and Cut Points for Therapeutic Lifestyle Changes and Drug Therapy in Different Risk Categories

Risk Category	LDL Goal (mg/dL)	LDL Level at Which to Initiate Therapeutic Lifestyle Changes (mg/dL)	LDL Level at Which to Consider Drug Therapy (mg/dL)
CHD or CHD risk equivalents (10-yr risk >20%)	<100	≥100	(100–129; drug optional)[a]
2+ Risk factors (10-yr risk ≤20%)	<130	≥130	10-yr risk 10%–20%: ≥130 10-yr risk <10%: ≥160
0–1 Risk factor[b]	<160	≥160	≥190 (160–189: LDL-lowering drug optional)

CHD, coronary heart disease.

[a]Some authorities recommend use of LDL-lowering drugs in this category if an LDL cholesterol level of less than 100 mg/dL cannot be achieved by therapeutic lifestyle changes. Others prefer use of drugs that primarily modify triglycerides and high-density lipoprotein (e.g., nicotinic acid or fibrate). Clinical judgment also may call for deferring drug therapy in this subcategory.

[b]Almost all people with 0–1 risk factor have a 10-year risk of less than 10%; thus, 10-year risk assessment in people with 0–1 risk factor is not necessary.

Adapted from Executive summary of the Third Report of the National Cholesterol Education Program (NCEP) Expert Panel on Detection, Evaluation, and Treatment of High Blood Cholesterol in Adults (Adult Treatment Panel III). *JAMA* 2001;285:2486–2497.

If baseline LDL-cholesterol is greater than or equal to 130 mg per dL, intensive lifestyle therapy and maximal control of other risk factors should be started. Moreover, for most patients, an LDL-lowering drug will be required to achieve an LDL-cholesterol level of less than 100 mg per dL; thus, an LDL-cholesterol–lowering drug can be started simultaneously with lifestyle changes to attain the goal of therapy.

If LDL cholesterol levels are 100 to 129 mg per dL, either at baseline or on LDL-lowering therapy, several therapeutic approaches are available:

- Initiate or intensify lifestyle and/or drug therapies specifically to lower LDL.
- Emphasize weight reduction and increased physical activity in persons with the metabolic syndrome.
- Delay use or intensification of LDL-lowering therapies and institute treatment of other lipid or nonlipid risk factors; consider use of other lipid-modifying drugs (e.g., nicotinic acid or fibric acid) if the patient has elevated triglyceride or low HDL-C.

If baseline LDL-cholesterol is less than 100 mg per dL, further LDL-lowering therapy is not required. Patients should nonetheless be advised to follow the lifestyle-changes diet on their own to help keep their LDL levels optimal. Several clinical trials are currently under way to assess benefit of lowering LDL-cholesterol to well below 100 mg per dL. At present, emphasis should be placed on controlling other lipid and nonlipid risk factors and on treatment of the metabolic syndrome, if present.

42. C. Use of LMWH was associated with a 20% reduction in death and serious cardiac ischemic events that appeared within the first few days of treatment, and this benefit was sustained through 43 days. Two phase III trials of enoxaparin (LMWH) for UA/non–Q-wave MI have shown it to be superior to UFH for preventing a composite of death and cardiac ischemic events. A prospectively planned metaanalysis was performed to provide a more precise estimate of the effects of enoxaparin on multiple end points. Event rates for death, the composite end points of death or nonfatal MI, and death or nonfatal MI or urgent revascularization, and major hemorrhage were extracted from the TIMI 11B and ESSENCE databases. Treatment effects at days 2, 8, 14, and 43 were expressed as the OR (and 95% CI) for enoxaparin versus UFH. All heterogeneity tests for efficacy end points were negative, which suggests comparability of the findings in TIMI 11B and ESSENCE. Enoxaparin was associated with a 20% reduction in death and serious cardiac ischemic events that appeared within the first few days of treatment, and this benefit was sustained through 43 days. Enoxaparin's treatment benefit was not associated with an increase in major hemorrhage during the acute phase of therapy, but there was an increase in the rate of minor hemorrhage. The accumulated evidence, coupled with the simplicity of SC administration and elimination of the need for anticoagulation monitoring, indicates that enoxaparin should be considered as a replacement for UFH as the antithrombin for the acute phase of management of patients with high-risk UA/non–Q-wave MI.

43. C. 12%. A proportion of patients who present with suspected ACS are found to have insignificant CAD during coronary angiography. Of the 5,767 patients with non–ST segment elevation ACS who were enrolled in the Platelet Glycoprotein IIb/IIIa in Unstable Angina: Receptor Suppression Using Integrilin (Eptifibatide) Therapy (PURSUIT) trial and who underwent in-hospital angiography, 88% had significant CAD (any stenosis greater than 50%), 6% had mild CAD (any stenosis greater than 0% to less than or equal to 50%), and 6% had no CAD (no stenosis identified). Overall, 12% of the patients had nonsignificant CAD.

44. B. Prothrombin complex. Hirudin is a naturally occurring anticoagulant secreted by the salivary glands of the leech *Hirudo medicinalis*. It is a potent and specific anticoagulant and exerts its action by binding directly to the active catalytic site of thrombin. Unlike heparin, it does not require a cofactor (antithrombin) and does not appear to cause immune-mediated thrombocytopenia. It is also a more potent inhibitor of platelet function than heparin, probably because of a direct inhibitory effect on thrombin. Recently, recombinant hirudin has been used as an adjunct to thrombolytic agents and as an anticoagulant during PTCA. Unlike heparin, which is readily neutralized by protamine or platelet factor 4, a specific agent useful in reversing the effects of hirudin is unavailable. Irani et al. demonstrated the first clinical experience suggesting benefit from prothrombin complex concentrate in neutralizing the effect of r-hirudin. Although the specific mechanism of action remains unclear, the generation of additional thrombin probably plays a role. Also, epinephrine-induced platelet aggregation in hirudinized platelet-rich plasma is restored by addition of prothrombin complex concentrate, most probably by additional thrombin generation. Adverse effects of prothrombin complex concentrate include intravascular thrombosis, particularly in patients with liver disease and possible viral hepatitis. The concentrate is made from human plasma and is heated to 80°C for 24 hours to inactivate viruses, particularly hepatitis C virus. However,

because the product contains some activated clotting factors (II, VII, IX, and X) and has thrombogenic potential, it should be used as a last resort, especially in patients with liver disease. Clinical experience suggests that prothrombin complex concentrate in a dose of 25 to 30 U per kg can be considered for patients with life-threatening hemorrhage due to hirudin.

45. C. 11%. Patients with prior coronary bypass surgery with acute ST segment elevation MI pose an increasingly common clinical problem. Labinaz et al. assessed the characteristics and outcomes of such patients undergoing thrombolysis for AMI. They compared the characteristics and outcomes of patients in GUSTO I who had had prior bypass (n = 1,784, 4% of the population) with those without prior CABG, all of whom were randomized to receive one of four thrombolytic strategies. Patients with prior bypass were older with significantly more prior MI and angina. Overall, 30-day mortality was significantly higher in patients with prior bypass (10.7% vs. 6.7% for no prior bypass; $p <.001$); these patients also had significantly more pulmonary edema, sustained hypotension, or cardiogenic shock. Patients with prior bypass showed a 12.5% relative reduction (95% CI, 0 to 41.9) in 30-day mortality with accelerated alteplase over the streptokinase monotherapies. In the 62% of patients with prior CABG who underwent coronary angiography, the infarct-related vessel was a native coronary artery in 61.9% and a bypass graft in 38.1% of cases. The TIMI 3 flow rate was 30.5% for culprit native coronary arteries and 31.7% for culprit bypass grafts. Patients with prior bypass had more severe infarct-vessel stenoses [99% (90%, 100%) vs. 90% (80%, 99%); $p <.001$]. The 30-day mortality in patients with prior CABG was significantly higher than that for patients without prior CABG. As in the overall trial, these patients derived an incremental survival benefit from treatment with accelerated alteplase, but mortality remained high (16.7%) at 1 year. These results are at least partially explained by the higher baseline risk of these patients and by the lower rate of patency of the infarct-related artery.

46. B. 70%. Stone et al. sought to characterize the presenting characteristics of patients with previous CABG surgery and AMI and to determine the angiographic success rate and clinical outcomes of a primary PTCA strategy. Patients who have had previous CABG and AMI comprise a high-risk group with decreased reperfusion success and increased mortality after thrombolytic therapy. Little is known about the efficacy of primary PTCA in AMI. Early cardiac catheterization was performed in 1,100 patients within 12 hours of onset of AMI at 34 centers in the prospective, controlled Second Primary Angioplasty in Myocardial Infarction trial (PAMI-2), followed by primary PTCA when appropriate. Data were collected by independent study monitors, end points were adjudicated, and films were read at an independent core laboratory. Of 1,100 patients with AMI, 58 (5.3%) had undergone previous CABG. The infarct-related vessel in these patients was a bypass graft in 32 patients (55%) and a native coronary artery in 26 patients. Compared with patients without previous CABG, patients with previous CABG were older and more frequently had a previous MI and three-vessel disease. Coronary angioplasty was less likely to be performed when the infarct-related vessel was a bypass graft rather than a native coronary artery (71.9% vs. 89.8%; $p = .001$); TIMI flow grade 3 was less frequently achieved (70.2% vs. 94.3%; $p <.0001$); and in-hospital mortality was increased (9.4% vs. 2.6%; $p = .02$). As a result, mortality at 6 months was 14.3% versus 4.1% in patients with versus without previous CABG ($p = .001$). By multi-

variate analysis, independent determinants of late mortality in the entire study group were advanced age, triple-vessel disease, Killip class, and post-PTCA TIMI flow grade less than 3. Reperfusion success of a primary PTCA strategy in patients with previous CABG, although favorable with respect to historic control studies, is reduced as compared with that in patients without previous CABG.

47. D. RV infarction. The clinical triad of hypotension, clear lung fields, and elevated jugular venous pressure occurs in less than 10% of patients presenting with acute inferior MI; however, when present, they are pathognomic of RV infarction.

48. D. Primary angioplasty. To determine whether primary angioplasty improves RV function and the clinical outcome in patients with RV infarction, Bowers et al. performed TTE studies before and after angioplasty in 53 patients with acute RV infarction. *Complete reperfusion*, defined as normal flow in the main RCA and its major RV branches, was achieved in 41 patients (77%), leading to prompt and striking recovery of RV function [mean ($\pm$ SE) score for free-wall motion, 3.0 ± 0.1 at baseline and 1.4 ± 0.1 at 3 days; $p < .001$]. Twelve patients (23%) had *unsuccessful reperfusion*, defined as the failure to restore RV branch flow, with or without patency of the right main coronary artery. Unsuccessful reperfusion was associated with lack of recovery of RV function (score for free-wall motion, 3.2 ± 0.2 at baseline and 3.0 ± 0.9 at 3 days; $p = .55$), as well as persistent hypotension and low cardiac output (in 83% of the patients, vs. 12% of those with successful reperfusion; $p = .002$) and a high mortality rate (58%, vs. 2% for those with successful reperfusion; $p = .001$). In patients with RV infarction, complete reperfusion of the RCA by angioplasty results in the dramatic recovery of RV performance and an excellent clinical outcome.

49. C. Aortic stenosis is not a potential cause of a new systolic murmur after an AMI. Papillary muscle rupture leading to acute MR and ventricular septal rupture are well-recognized complications of AMI. A systolic murmur is usually audible in both these cases. Dynamic LVOT obstruction has traditionally been associated with hypertrophic obstructive cardiomyopathy. Recently, acute dynamic LVOT obstruction has been described as a complication of MI. Haley et al. described cases of three patients, all of whom presented with a systolic murmur and ECG evidence of MI. All three patients developed cardiogenic shock and were subsequently found by TTE to manifest an acute dynamic LVOT obstruction. Cardiogenic shock persisted until therapy was directed toward decreasing the degree of the dynamic LVOT obstruction. The treatment of ACSs in the presence of a dynamic LVOT obstruction differs from the traditional treatment of ACSs and includes the use of beta-blockers and alpha$_1$-agonists as well as the avoidance of therapies that aggravate the magnitude of the LVOT obstructive gradient, including nitrates, inotropic agents, and afterload reduction. The development of a systolic murmur in the setting of AMI complicated by cardiogenic shock with only a small elevation in creatine kinase suggests the presence of a dynamic LVOT obstruction as well as the classical mechanical complications of MI; namely, ventricular septal rupture and papillary muscle rupture. The presence of a dynamic LVOT obstruction is reliably detected by transthoracic TTE or by TEE if transthoracic image quality is suboptimal.

50. C. Significant increase in mortality. Numerous clinical trials have established the benefits of IV GP IIb/IIIa inhibition in the management of CAD. In con-

trast, the recent large-scale, placebo-controlled, randomized trials of the PO GP IIb/IIIa antagonists have failed to provide commensurate reductions in late composite ischemic end points despite potent inhibition of platelet aggregation. The ORs for death, MI, urgent revascularization, and major bleeding from the four large-scale, placebo-controlled, randomized trials with PO GP IIb/IIIa inhibitors were recently calculated and combined. Stratification by low-dose or high-dose therapy and the use of concurrent ASA were also undertaken. In 33,326 patients followed for longer than 30 days, a consistent and statistically significant increase in mortality was observed with PO GP IIb/IIIa therapy (OR, 1.37; 95% CI, 1.13 to 1.66; $p = .001$). This effect was evident regardless of ASA coadministration and treatment with either low-dose or high-dose therapy. Although a reduction in urgent revascularization was observed with PO GP IIb/IIIa inhibition, pooled analysis favored an increase in MI that did not demonstrate statistical significance. Chew et al. found a highly significant excess in mortality consistent across four trials with three different PO GP IIb/IIIa inhibitor agents, and this was associated with a reduction in the need for urgent revascularization and no increase in MI. These findings suggest the potential for a direct toxic effect with these agents and argue against a prothrombotic mechanism.

51. B. Long-term administration of clopidogrel to patients with atherosclerotic vascular disease is more effective as ASA in reducing the combined risk of ischemic stroke, MI, and vascular death. Many clinical trials have evaluated the benefit of long-term use of antiplatelet drugs in reducing the risk of clinical thrombotic events. ASA and ticlopidine have been shown to be effective, but both have potentially serious adverse effects. Clopidogrel, a new thienopyridine derivative similar to ticlopidine, is an inhibitor of platelet aggregation induced by adenosine diphosphate. CAPRIE was a randomized, blinded, international trial designed to assess the relative efficacy of clopidogrel (75 mg once daily) and ASA (325 mg once daily) in reducing the risk of a composite outcome cluster of ischemic stroke, MI, or vascular death; their relative safety was also assessed. The population studied comprised subgroups of patients with atherosclerotic vascular disease manifested as recent ischemic stroke, recent MI, or symptomatic peripheral arterial disease. Patients were followed for 1 to 3 years. Nineteen thousand one hundred five patients, with more than 6,300 in each of the clinical subgroups, were recruited over 3 years, with a mean follow-up of 1.91 years. There were 1,960 first events included in the outcome cluster on which an intention-to-treat analysis showed that patients treated with clopidogrel had an annual 5.32% risk of ischemic stroke, MI, or vascular death compared with 5.83% with ASA. These rates reflect a statistically significant ($p = .043$) relative-risk reduction of 8.7% in favor of clopidogrel (95% CI, 0.3 to 16.5). Corresponding on-treatment analysis yielded an RR reduction of 9.4%. There were no major differences in terms of safety. Reported adverse experiences in the clopidogrel and ASA groups judged to be severe included rash (0.26% vs. 0.10%), diarrhea (0.23% vs. 0.11%), upper GI discomfort (0.97% vs. 1.22%), intracranial hemorrhage (0.33% vs. 0.47%), and GI hemorrhage (0.52% vs. 0.72%), respectively. There were ten (0.10%) patients in the clopidogrel group with significant reductions in neutrophils (less than 1.2×10^9/L) and 16 (0.17%) in the ASA group. Long-term administration of clopidogrel to patients with atherosclerotic vascular disease is more effective than ASA in reducing the combined risk of ischemic stroke, MI, or vascular death. The overall safety profile of clopidogrel is at least as good as that of medium-dose ASA.

52. A. Low, fixed-dose warfarin (1 or 3 mg) combined with low-dose ASA (80 mg) in patients who have had MI does not provide clinical benefit beyond that achievable with 160-mg ASA monotherapy. Antiplatelet therapy with ASA and systematic anticoagulation with warfarin reduce cardiovascular morbidity and mortality after MI when given alone. In the Coumadin ASA Reinfarction Study (CARS), the investigators aimed to find out whether a combination of low-dose warfarin and low-dose ASA would give superior results to standard ASA monotherapy without excessive bleeding risk. Using a randomized double-blind study design, they randomly assigned 8,803 patients who had had MI, treatment with 160-mg ASA, 3-mg warfarin with 80-mg ASA, or 1-mg warfarin with 80-mg ASA. Patients took a single tablet daily and attended for prothrombin time measurements at weeks 1, 2, 3, 4, 6, and 12, and then every 3 months. Patients were followed up for a maximum of 33 months (median, 14 months). The primary event was first occurrence of reinfarction, nonfatal ischemic stroke, or cardiovascular death. One-year life-table estimates for the primary event were 8.6% (95% CI, 7.6 to 9.6) for 160-mg ASA, 8.4% (7.4 to 9.4) for 3-mg warfarin with 80-mg ASA, and 8.8% (7.6 to 10.0) for 1-mg warfarin with 80-mg ASA. Primary comparisons were done with all follow-up data. The RR of the primary event for the 160-mg ASA group compared with the 3-mg warfarin with 80-mg ASA group was 0.95 (0.81 to 1.12; $p = .57$). For spontaneous major hemorrhage (not procedure related), 1-year life-table estimates were 0.74% (0.43 to 1.10) in the 160-mg ASA group and 1.4% (0.94 to 1.80) in the 3-mg warfarin with 80-mg ASA group ($p = .014$ log rank on follow-up). For the 3,382 patients assigned 3-mg warfarin with 80-mg ASA, the international normalized ratio results at week 1 were (n = 2,985) median, 1.51 (interquartile range, 1.23 to 2.13); at week 4 (n = 2,701), median, 1.27 (1.13 to 1.64); and at month 6 (n = 2,145), median, 1.19 (1.08 to 1.44). Low, fixed-dose warfarin (1 mg or 3 mg) combined with low-dose ASA (80 mg) in patients who have had MI does not provide clinical benefit beyond that achievable with 160-mg ASA monotherapy.

53. A. The Brockenbrough response includes an increase in LV systolic pressure, a decrease in aortic systolic pressure, an increase in LV to aortic gradient, and diminished aortic pulse pressure.

54. C. The angiogram clearly shows severe ostial and moderate distal left main trunk stenosis.

55. B. Arteriovenous fistula. Coronary angiograms revealed large coronary arteriovenous fistula involving the RCA. The patient underwent surgical ligation of the fistula with resolution of her symptoms.

56. C. The angiogram reveals severe ostial and proximal LCx stenosis.

57. C. The coronary angiogram reveals anomalous origin of the LCx from the right sinus. A multipurpose catheter is the catheter of choice to cannulate an LCx arising from this site.

58. A. The angiogram reveals large angiographically visible thrombus in the mid portion of the RCA distal to a severe stenosis.

59. A. The angiogram reveals anomalous origin of the left main trunk from the right coronary sinus with a course anterior to the PA.

60. D. The angiogram reveals anomalous common origin of LAD and the RCA.

61. C. The angiogram clearly reveals perforation of the RCA.

62. C. Severe LAD stenosis. The coronary angiogram of the left circulation in the PA cranial view shows severe LAD stenosis after the takeoff of the first septal artery.

63. A. Severe LCx stenosis. The coronary angiogram of the left circulation in the right anterior oblique caudal view shows severe proximal LCx stenosis, explaining the lateral ischemia.

64. D. Severe RCA stenosis. The coronary angiogram in the RAO view shows severe mid-RCA stenosis, explaining the inferior ischemia.

65. A. Severe LCx stenosis. The coronary angiogram of the left circulation in the right anterior oblique caudal view shows severe mid-LCx stenosis.

66. A. At 1 year, there was no significant difference between the two groups in terms of the rates of death, stroke, or MI. The recent recognition that coronary artery stenting has improved the short- and long-term outcomes of patients treated with angioplasty has made it necessary to reevaluate the relative benefits of bypass surgery and percutaneous interventions in patients with multivessel disease. Serruys et al. studied a total of 1,205 patients who were randomly assigned to undergo stent implantation or bypass surgery when a cardiac surgeon and an interventional cardiologist agreed that the same extent of revascularization could be achieved by either technique. The primary clinical end point was freedom from major adverse cardiac and cerebrovascular events at 1 year. The costs of hospital resources used were also determined. At 1 year, there was no significant difference between the two groups in terms of the rates of death, stroke, or MI. Among patients who survived without a stroke or an MI, 16.8% of those in the stenting group underwent a second revascularization, as compared with 3.5% of those in the surgery group. The rate of event-free survival at 1 year was 73.8% among the patients who received stents and 87.8% among those who underwent bypass surgery ($p < .001$ by the log-rank test). The cost for the initial procedure was $4,212 less for patients assigned to stenting than for those assigned to bypass surgery, but this difference was reduced during follow-up because of the increased need for repeated revascularization; after 1 year, the net difference in favor of stenting was estimated to be $2,973 per patient. The authors concluded that, as measured 1 year after the procedure, coronary stenting for multivessel disease is less expensive than bypass surgery and offers the same degree of protection against death, stroke, and MI. However, stenting is associated with a greater need for repeated revascularization.

67. C. 15% to 25%. Kawasaki disease is a leading cause of acquired heart disease in children in the United States. An acute vasculitis of unknown etiology, it occurs predominantly in infancy and early childhood and more rarely in teenagers. Coronary artery aneurysms or ectasia develop in approximately 15% to 25% of children with the disease. Treatment with IV gamma globulin, 2 g per kg, in the acute phase reduces this risk three- to fivefold. Angiographic resolution occurs in approximately one-half of aneurysmal arterial segments, but these show persistent histologic and functional abnor-

malities. The remainder continues to be aneurysmal, often with development of progressive stenosis or occlusion. The worst prognosis occurs in children with so-called giant aneurysms (i.e., those with a maximum diameter greater than 8 mm), because thrombosis is promoted both by sluggish blood flow within the massively dilated vascular space and by the frequent development of stenotic lesions. Serial stress tests with myocardial imaging are mandatory in the management of patients with Kawasaki disease and significant CAD to determine the need for coronary angiography and transcatheter interventions or coronary bypass surgery. Continued long-term surveillance in patients with and without detected coronary abnormalities is necessary to determine the natural history of Kawasaki disease.

68. B. Decreased coronary flow reserve. The maximum coronary vasodilator capacity after IV dipyridamole (0.14 mg/kg/min × 4 min) was studied in seven patients with primary scleroderma myocardial disease and compared to that of seven control subjects by Nitenberg et al. Hemodynamic data and LV angiographic data were not different in the two groups. The coronary flow reserve was evaluated by the dipyridamole to basal coronary sinus blood flow ratio and the coronary resistance reserve by the dipyridamole to basal coronary resistance ratio. Coronary reserve was greatly impaired in the group with primary scleroderma myocardial disease: The dipyridamole to basal coronary sinus blood flow ratio was lower than in the control group (2.54 ± 1.37 vs. 4.01 ± 0.56, respectively; $p < .05$), and the dipyridamole to basal coronary resistance ratio was higher than in the control group (0.47 ± 0.25 vs. 0.23 ± 0.04, respectively; $p < .05$). Such a decreased coronary flow and resistance reserve in patients with primary scleroderma myocardial disease was not explained by an alteration in LV function. The authors concluded that this may be an important contributing factor in the pathogenesis of primary scleroderma myocardial disease.

69. B. There are significantly more calcified plaques of coronary arteries in patients with end-stage renal failure. An excessive rate of cardiac death is a well-known feature of renal failure. CHD is frequent, and the possibility has been raised that the natural history of the coronary plaque is different in uremic patients. Schwarz et al. assessed the morphology of coronary arteries in patients with end-stage renal failure and compared them with coronary arteries of matched nonuremic control patients. Fifty-four cases were identified at autopsy that met the inclusion criteria: cases, end-stage renal disease (n = 27); controls, nonrenal patients with CAD (n = 27). At autopsy, all three coronary arteries were prepared at corresponding sites for investigations: (a) qualitative analysis (after Stary), (b) quantitative measurements of intima and media thickness (by planimetry), (c) immunohistochemical analysis of the coronary plaques, and (d) x-ray diffraction of selected calcified plaques. Qualitative analysis of the coronary arteries showed significantly more calcified plaques of coronary arteries in patients with end-stage renal failure. Plaques of nonuremic patients were mostly fibroatheromatous. Media thickness of coronary arteries was significantly higher in uremic patients ($187 \, mm \pm 53 \, \mu m$ vs. $135 \, mm \pm 29 \, \mu m$ in controls), and intima thickness tended to be higher ($158 \, mm \pm 38 \, \mu m$ vs. $142 \, mm \pm 31 \, \mu m$), but this difference was not statistically significant. Plaque area ($4.09 \, mm \pm 1.50 \, mm^2$ vs. $4.39 \, mm \pm 0.88 \, mm^2$) was comparable in both groups. Lumen area, however, was significantly smaller in end-stage renal patients. Immunohistochemical analysis of the cellular infiltrate in coronary arteries showed no major differences in these advanced plaques of uremic and non-

uremic subjects. Coronary plaques in patients with end-stage renal failure were characterized by increased media thickness and marked calcification. In contrast to the previous opinion, the authors demonstrated that the most marked difference compared to nonuremic controls does not concern the size, but the composition of the plaque. Deposition of calcium within the plaques may contribute to the high complication rate in uremic patients.

70. B. In patients with angiographically defined CAD, homocysteine is a significant predictor of mortality, independent of traditional risk factors, CRP, and MTHFR genotype. Plasma homocysteine has been associated with CAD. Anderson et al. tested whether homocysteine also increases secondary risk, after initial CAD diagnosis, and whether it is independent of traditional risk factors, CRP, and MTHFR genotype. Blood samples were collected from 1,412 patients with severe angiographically defined CAD (stenosis greater than or equal to 70%). Plasma homocysteine was measured by fluorescence polarization immunoassay. The study cohort was evaluated for survival after a mean of 3 years ± 1 year of follow-up (minimum, 1.5 years; maximum, 5.0 years). The average age of the patients was 65 years ± 11 years, 77% were males, and 166 died during follow-up. Mortality was greater in patients with homocysteine in tertile three than in tertiles one and two [mortality, 15.7% vs. 9.6%; $p = .001$ (log-rank test); hazard ratio (HR), 1.63]. The relative hazard increased 16% for each 5-μmol per L increase in homocysteine ($p <.001$). In multivariate Cox regression analysis, controlling for univariate clinical and laboratory predictors, elevated homocysteine remained predictive of mortality (HR, 1.64; $p = .009$), together with age (HR, 1.72/10-year increment; $p <.0001$), EF (HR, 0.84/10% increment; $p = .0001$), diabetes (HR, 1.98; $p = .001$), CRP (HR, 1.42/tertile; $p = .004$), and hyperlipidemia. Homozygosity for the MTHFR variant was weakly predictive of homocysteine levels but not mortality. The authors concluded that in patients with angiographically defined CAD, homocysteine is a significant predictor of mortality, independent of traditional risk factors, CRP, and MTHFR genotype.

SUGGESTED READING

Adams JE 3rd, Abendschein DR, Jaffe AS. Biochemical markers of myocardial injury. Is MB creatine kinase the choice for the 1990s? *Circulation* 1993;88:750–763.

Akkerhuis KM, Deckers JW, Lincoff AM, et al. Risk of stroke associated with abciximab among patients undergoing percutaneous coronary intervention. *JAMA* 2001;286:78–82.

Anderson JL, Muhlestein JB, Horne BD, et al. Plasma homocysteine predicts mortality independently of traditional risk factors and C-reactive protein in patients with angiographically defined coronary artery disease. *Circulation* 2000;102:1227–1232.

Antman EM, Cohen M, Radley D, et al. Assessment of the treatment effect of enoxaparin for unstable angina/non-Q-wave myocardial infarction. TIMI 11B-ESSENCE meta-analysis. *Circulation* 1999;100:1602–1608.

Barry J, Mead K, Nabel EG, et al. Effect of smoking on the activity of ischemic heart disease. *JAMA* 1989;261:398–402.

Belardinelli R, Paolini I, Cianci G, et al. Exercise training intervention after coronary angioplasty: the ETICA trial. *J Am Coll Cardiol* 2001;37:1891–1900.

Beller GA. Current status of nuclear cardiology techniques. *Curr Probl Cardiol* 1991;16:451–535.

NOTES

Boersma E, Akkerhuis KM, Theroux P, et al. Platelet glycoprotein IIb/IIIa receptor inhibition in non-ST-elevation acute coronary syndromes: early benefit during medical treatment only, with additional protection during percutaneous coronary intervention. *Circulation* 1999;100:2045–2048.

Bowers TR, O'Neill WW, Grines C, et al. Effect of reperfusion on biventricular function and survival after right ventricular infarction. *N Engl J Med* 1998;338:933–940.

Braunwald E, Antman EM, Beasley JW, et al. ACC/AHA guidelines for the management of patients with unstable angina and non-ST-segment elevation myocardial infarction: executive summary and recommendations. A report of the American College of Cardiology/American Heart Association task force on practice guidelines (committee on the management of patients with unstable angina). *Circulation* 2000;102:1193–1209.

Byington RP, Davis BR, Plehn JF, et al. Reduction of stroke events with pravastatin: the Prospective Pravastatin Pooling (PPP) Project. *Circulation* 2001;103:387–392.

Califf RM, Tomabechi Y, Lee KL, et al. Outcome in one-vessel coronary artery disease. *Circulation* 1983;67:283–290.

Cannon CP, Weintraub WS, Demopoulos LA, et al. Comparison of early invasive and conservative strategies in patients with unstable coronary syndromes treated with the glycoprotein IIb/IIIa inhibitor tirofiban. *N Engl J Med* 2001;344:1879–1887.

CAPRIE Steering Committee. A randomised, blinded, trial of clopidogrel versus aspirin in patients at risk of ischaemic events (CAPRIE). *Lancet* 1996;348:1329–1339.

Chew DP, Bhatt DL, Sapp S, et al. Increased mortality with oral platelet glycoprotein IIb/IIIa antagonists: a meta-analysis of Phase III Multicenter Randomized Trials. *Circulation* 2001;103:201–206.

Coumadin Aspirin Reinfarction Study (CARS) Investigators. Randomised double-blind trial of fixed low-dose warfarin with aspirin after myocardial infarction. *Lancet* 1997;350:389–396.

Cutlip DE, Baim DS, Ho KK, et al. Stent thrombosis in the modern era: a pooled analysis of multicenter coronary stent clinical trials. *Circulation* 2001;103:1967–1971.

Detre KM, Guo P, Holubkov R, et al. Coronary revascularization in diabetic patients: a comparison of the randomized and observational components of the Bypass Angioplasty Revascularization Investigation (BARI). *Circulation* 1999;99:633–640.

Domanski MJ, Borkowf CB, Campeau L, et al. Prognostic factors for atherosclerosis progression in saphenous vein grafts: the postcoronary artery bypass graft (Post-CABG) trial. Post-CABG Trial Investigators. *J Am Coll Cardiol* 2000;36:1877–1883.

Downs JR, Clearfield M, Weis S, et al. Primary prevention of acute coronary events with lovastatin in men and women with average cholesterol levels: results of AFCAPS/TexCAPS. Air Force/Texas Coronary Atherosclerosis Prevention Study. *JAMA* 1998;279:1615–1622.

Eagle KA, Guyton RA, Davidoff R, et al. ACC/AHA guidelines for coronary artery bypass graft surgery: executive summary and recommendations: a report of the American College of Cardiology/American Heart Association Task Force on Practice Guidelines (Committee to revise the 1991 guidelines for coronary artery bypass graft surgery). *Circulation* 1999;100:1464–1480.

Fuster V. Lewis A. Conner Memorial Lecture. Mechanisms leading to myocardial infarction: insights from studies of vascular biology. *Circulation* 1994;90:2126–2146.

Gibbons RJ, Chatterjee K, Daley J, et al. ACC/AHA/ACP-ASIM guidelines for the management of patients with chronic stable angina: executive summary and recommendations. A Report of the American College of Cardiology/American Heart Association Task Force on Practice Guidelines (Committee on Management of Patients with Chronic Stable Angina). *Circulation* 1999;99:2829–2848.

Haley JH, Sinak LJ, Tajik AJ, et al. Dynamic left ventricular outflow tract obstruction in acute coronary syndromes: an important cause of new systolic murmur and cardiogenic shock. *Mayo Clin Proc* 1999;74:901–906.

Hochman JS, Sleeper LA, Webb JG, et al. Early revascularization in acute myocardial infarction complicated by cardiogenic shock. SHOCK Investigators. Should We Emergently Revascularize Occluded Coronaries for Cardiogenic Shock. *N Engl J Med* 1999;341:625–634.

Hoffman JI. Transmural myocardial perfusion. *Prog Cardiovasc Dis* 1987;29:429–464.

Influence of pravastatin and plasma lipids on clinical events in the West of Scotland Coronary Prevention Study (WOSCOPS). *Circulation* 1998;97:1440–1445.

Irani MS, White HJ Jr, Sexon RG. Reversal of hirudin-induced bleeding diathesis by prothrombin complex concentrate. *Am J Cardiol* 1995;75:422–423.

Iskandrian AS, Heo J, Lemlek J, et al. Identification of high-risk patients with left main and three-vessel coronary artery disease by adenosine-single photon emission computed tomographic thallium imaging. *Am Heart J* 1993;125:1130–1135.

Koenig W, Sund M, Frohlich M, et al. C-reactive protein, a sensitive marker of inflammation, predicts future risk of coronary heart disease in initially healthy middle-aged men: results from the MONICA (Monitoring Trends and Determinants in Cardiovascular Disease) Augsburg Cohort Study, 1984 to 1992. *Circulation* 1999;99:237–242.

Labinaz M, Sketch MH Jr, Ellis SG, et al. Outcome of acute ST-segment elevation myocardial infarction in patients with prior coronary artery bypass surgery receiving thrombolytic therapy. *Am Heart J* 2001;141:469–477.

Lee KL, Woodlief LH, Topol EJ, et al. Predictors of 30-day mortality in the era of reperfusion for acute myocardial infarction. Results from an international trial of 41,021 patients. GUSTO-I Investigators. *Circulation* 1995;91:1659–1668.

Lundergan CF, Ross AM, McCarthy WF, et al. Predictors of left ventricular function after acute myocardial infarction: effects of time to treatment, patency, and body mass index: the GUSTO-I angiographic experience. *Am Heart J* 2001;142:43–50.

Newburger JW, Burns JC. Kawasaki disease. *Vasc Med* 1999;4:187–202.

Nitenberg A, Foult JM, Kahan A, et al. Reduced coronary flow and resistance reserve in primary scleroderma myocardial disease. *Am Heart J* 1986;112:309–315.

Pitt B, Waters D, Brown WV, et al. Aggressive lipid-lowering therapy compared with angioplasty in stable coronary artery disease. Atorvastatin versus Revascularization Treatment Investigators. *N Engl J Med* 1999;341:70–76.

Randomised trial of cholesterol lowering in 4,444 patients with coronary heart disease: the Scandinavian Simvastatin Survival Study (4S). *Lancet* 1994;344:1383–1389.

Roe MT, Harrington RA, Prosper DM, et al. Clinical and therapeutic profile of patients presenting with acute coronary syndromes who do not have significant coronary artery disease. The Platelet Glycoprotein IIb/IIIa in Unstable Angina: Receptor Suppression Using Integrilin Therapy (PURSUIT) Trial Investigators. *Circulation* 2000;102:1101–1106.

Rogers WJ, Bourassa MG, Andrews TC, et al. Asymptomatic Cardiac Ischemia Pilot (ACIP) study: outcome at 1 year for patients with asymptomatic cardiac ischemia randomized to medical therapy or revascularization. The ACIP Investigators. *J Am Coll Cardiol* 1995;26:594–605.

Schwarz U, Buzello M, Ritz E, et al. Morphology of coronary atherosclerotic lesions in patients with end-stage renal failure. *Nephrol Dial Transplant* 2000;15:218–223.

Serruys PW, Unger F, Sousa JE, et al. Comparison of coronary-artery bypass surgery and stenting for the treatment of multivessel disease. *N Engl J Med* 2001;344:1117–1124.

Stone GW, Brodie BR, Griffin JJ, et al. Clinical and angiographic outcomes in patients with previous coronary artery bypass graft surgery treated with primary balloon angioplasty for acute myocardial infarction. Second Primary Angioplasty in Myocardial Infarction Trial (PAMI-2) Investigators. *J Am Coll Cardiol* 2000;35:605–611.

Stone PH, Thompson B, Zaret BL, et al. Factors associated with failure of medical therapy in patients with unstable angina and non-Q wave myocardial infarction. A TIMI-IIIB database study. *Eur Heart J* 1999;20:1084–1093.

Teirstein PS, Massullo V, Jani S, et al. Two-year follow-up after catheter-based radiotherapy to inhibit coronary restenosis. *Circulation* 1999;99:243–247.

The GUSTO Angiographic Investigators. The effects of tissue plasminogen activator, streptokinase, or both on coronary-artery patency, ventricular function, and survival after acute myocardial infarction. *N Engl J Med* 1993;329:1615–1622.

The GUSTO Investigators. An international randomized trial comparing four thrombolytic strategies for acute myocardial infarction. *N Engl J Med* 1993;329:673–682.

Yusuf S, Sleight P, Pogue J, et al. Effects of an angiotensin-converting-enzyme inhibitor, ramipril, on cardiovascular events in high-risk patients. The Heart Outcomes Prevention Evaluation Study Investigators. *N Engl J Med* 2000;342:145–153.

CHAPTER 5

Pharmacology

Michael A. Militello and Jodie M. Fink

QUESTIONS

Pharmacokinetics

1. P. M. is admitted to the coronary ICU with AFib and rapid ventricular rate. After controlling the ventricular rate with metoprolol, it is decided to initiate procainamide by IV infusion. P. M. weighs 80 kg. How much of a loading dose would be required to target a level of 8 μg per L? The average steady-state volume of distribution (Vd) for procainamide is 2 L per kg. The bioavailability of the IV formulation is 100%, whereas the PO form is only 83%.

   A. 1,000 mg
   B. 1,300 mg
   C. 1,500 mg
   D. 1,700 mg

2. L. M. has been receiving digoxin, 0.25 mg PO tablets q.d. Her serum drug level is 1.8 ng per mL. She is no longer able to take PO medications and needs to receive digoxin IV. By what percentage do you need to decrease the dose to maintain the current digoxin level?

   A. 10%
   B. 25%
   C. 40%
   D. 50%

3. What two pharmacokinetic parameters alter the half-life of medications?

   A. loading dose and clearance
   B. absorption and clearance
   C. Vd and clearance
   D. absorption and Vd

Pharmacodynamics

4. What is the relationship between drug concentration and pharmacologic effect known as?

    A. pharmacokinetics
    B. pharmacogenetics
    C. pharmacology
    D. pharmacodynamics

5. Each line in the graph below represents a beta-blocker in development (Fig. 1).

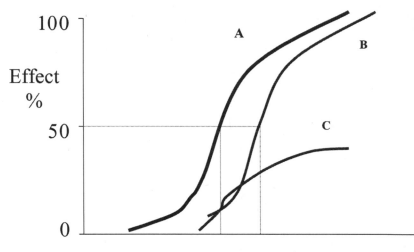

FIGURE 1 Relationship between drug concentration and effect.

Which beta-blocker is the most potent?

    A. A
    B. B
    C. C
    D. Potency cannot be determined from the above graph.

Drug Metabolism

6. F. R. is a 56-year-old man with a history of AFib treated with quinidine sulfate, extended release, for controlling his rhythm. He is also on warfarin, and you would like to start a beta-blocker to help control ventricular rate. Which of the following beta-blockers would *not* be a good choice?

    A. atenolol
    B. metoprolol
    C. nadolol
    D. bisoprolol

7. Ethanol alters the metabolism of warfarin. Two types of ethanol abuse are chronic ethanol abuse and binge ethanol drinking. How do these types of ethanol use alter warfarin metabolism? Chronic ethanol use _____ and binge ethanol drinking _____.

A. decreases warfarin metabolism, increases warfarin metabolism
B. decreases warfarin metabolism, decreases warfarin metabolism
C. increases warfarin metabolism, decreases warfarin metabolism
D. increases warfarin metabolism, increases warfarin metabolism

8. Which of the following drugs can significantly increase digoxin concentrations?

A. amiodarone
B. quinidine
C. tetracycline
D. all of the above

Angiotensin-Converting Enzyme Inhibitors

9. Which of the following ACE inhibitors are *not* prodrugs?

A. captopril, lisinopril, ramipril
B. lisinopril, enalapril, benazepril
C. captopril, lisinopril, enalaprilat
D. moexipril, captopril, lisinopril

10. ACE inhibitors have benefits on systolic dysfunction that include all of the following *except*

A. They decrease ventricular dilation and cardiac remodeling.
B. They prevent the growth effects of angiotensin II on myocytes.
C. They increase preload and decrease afterload.
D. They attenuate aldosterone-induced cardiac fibrosis.

11. Which of the following statements is *true* with regard to ACE inhibitors?

A. Mortality benefit in heart failure (HF) patients is a class effect with ACE inhibitors, and all are FDA approved for this indication.
B. ACE-inhibitor dose is negligible in CHF with regard to mortality benefit.
C. Sodium depletion is an important factor in the development of renal insufficiency associated with ACE inhibitors.
D. ACE inhibitor–associated potassium retention is related to the increase in feedback that leads to aldosterone release.

12. A patient with hypertension (HTN) has CHF, with an EF of less than 30%. Her serum creatinine is stable at 2 mg per dL, and she is currently on digoxin and furosemide. Her BP is 152/90 mm Hg. Which antihypertensive agent is indicated?

A. hydralazine
B. amlodipine
C. clonidine
D. captopril
E. verapamil

13. All of the following are contraindications to the use of ACE inhibitors *except*

A. bilateral renal artery stenosis
B. pregnancy
C. angioedema
D. cough

Angiotensin II-Receptor Blockers

14. A 25-year-old woman who delivered her first child 3 days ago has developed peripartum cardiomyopathy for which she was treated with captopril. Subsequently, she has developed angioedema and required intubation. In this patient, the next best option to treat her cardiomyopathy would be losartan, because it does not cause angioedema.

    A. true
    B. false

15. Angiotensin II-receptor blockers (ARBs) are indicated to treat which of the following disease states?

    A. HF
    B. LV dysfunction after MI
    C. HTN
    D. none of the above

16. All of the following side effects occurring with ARBs will occur with ACE inhibitors *except*

    A. cough
    B. renal dysfunction
    C. hyperkalemia
    D. hypotension

Beta-Blockers

17. The mechanisms of benefit for HF of beta-blockers include all of the following *except*

    A. increased ventricular pressure
    B. blockade of sympathetic stimulation of cell growth
    C. antiarrhythmic activity
    D. decreased programmed cell death

18. A patient with New York Heart Association class III HF was hospitalized 2 months ago for an exacerbation of his HF. The patient was discharged on lisinopril, furosemide, and digoxin. His lungs are clear, and his vitals are as follows: BP, 105/56 mm Hg; heart rate, 84 bpm; and respiration rate, 18. Which regimen is most appropriate to initiate in this patient?

    A. atenolol, 50 mg q.d.
    B. carvedilol, 3.125 mg b.i.d.
    C. carvedilol, 25 mg b.i.d.
    D. metoprolol, 50 mg b.i.d.

19. Which beta-blocker should *not* be used in patients with CHF?

    A. carvedilol
    B. metoprolol
    C. pindolol
    D. bisoprolol

20. Match the properties with the associated beta-blocking agents.

    1. pindolol   i. alpha-blockade
    2. propranolol   ii. intrinsic sympathomimetic activity (ISA)
    3. labetalol   iii. membrane-stabilizing activity
    4. bisoprolol   iv. β_1-selectivity

    A. (1) iv; (2) ii; (3) iii; (4) i
    B. (1) iii; (2) i; (3) ii; (4) iv
    C. (1) ii; (2) iii; (3) i; (4) iv
    D. (1) ii; (2) iv; (3) iii; (4) i

21. A 57-year-old man who is status post MI has a BP of 150/88 mm Hg. Which agent would be the most appropriate for treatment of his HTN?

    A. hydrochlorothiazide
    B. metoprolol
    C. clonidine
    D. losartan

Alpha$_1$-Blockers

22. All of the following medications used to treat HF have been shown to improve survival *except*

    A. captopril
    B. prazosin
    C. hydralazine and isosorbide dinitrate (ISDN)
    D. metoprolol

23. B. J. is a 56-year-old woman with long-standing HTN that is difficult to control. She is currently being treated with amlodipine, 10 mg q.d.; lisinopril, 40 mg q.d.; hydrochlorothiazide, 25 mg q.d.; and clonidine, 0.4 mg three times per day. She presented to the emergency room, and her initial BP was 200/110 mm Hg. She states she had run out of one of her medications. Which one of her medications would most likely be implicated in causing hypertensive urgency?

    A. amlodipine
    B. lisinopril
    C. hydrochlorothiazide
    D. clonidine

Calcium Channel Blockers

24. By which of the following mechanisms do diltiazem and verapamil slow ventricular rate in patients with AFib?

    A. They decrease the conduction velocity within the AV node.
    B. They decrease the refractory period of nodal tissue.
    C. They stimulate vagal tone.
    D. They prolong the refractory period of atrial tissue.

25. Short-acting dihydropyridine calcium channel blockers (CCBs) possess all of the following properties *except*

    A. They cause peripheral edema.
    B. They cause reflex tachycardia.
    C. They cause flushing.
    D. They slow ventricular response in patients with AFib.

26. Which of the following CCBs is indicated in patients presenting with a subarachnoid hemorrhage?

    A. verapamil
    B. diltiazem
    C. isradipine
    D. nimodipine

Nitroglycerin

27. All of the following are suggested mechanisms of nitrate tolerance *except*

    A. sulfhydryl-group depletion
    B. plasma volume expansion
    C. free radical depletion
    D. neurohormonal stimulation

Nitroprusside

28. A 46-year-old white man was admitted with a chief report of worsening headache and nausea and vomiting over 48 hours. The patient is status post single-lung transplant secondary to alpha$_1$-antitrypsin deficiency. His immunosuppression regimen includes cyclosporin, prednisone, and azathioprine. Due to the cyclosporin, he has HTN and renal dysfunction (baseline serum creatinine, 1.9 mg/dL). His BP is controlled with clonidine, 0.2 mg b.i.d., and mctoprolol, 25 mg b.i.d. Two months ago, he was changed to metoprolol from amlodipine due to peripheral edema. The patient was in his usual state of health until approximately 1 week ago, when he experienced diarrhea, which has since resolved. On admission, his BP was 208/110 mm Hg, and his serum creatinine was 3.8 mg per dL. What is the most appropriate regimen to control this patient's BP?

    A. change back to amlodipine, 10 mg q.d.
    B. initiate nitroprusside drip and give IV fluids
    C. add captopril to the regimen and titrate to effect
    D. give sublingual nifedipine

Hydralazine

29. A patient with CHF on lisinopril was experiencing a dry cough and hyperkalemia. What would be the most appropriate therapy to replace the ACE inhibitor?

    A. losartan
    B. metoprolol
    C. digoxin
    D. hydralazine and ISDN

Lipid-Lowering Therapy

30. A 35-year-old man, who is a smoker and has a family history of CAD (father had MI at 40 years of age), has the following lipid profile:

    Total cholesterol = 193 mg per dL
    LDL = 150 mg per dL
    HDL = 43 mg per dL
    Triglyceride (TG) = 175 mg per dL

    What, if any, medication is indicated?

    A. HMG-CoA reductase inhibitors.
    B. Bile acid sequestrants.
    C. Fibric acid derivative.
    D. No medication is indicated at this time.

31. A 55-year-old patient with HF and a past medical history of diabetes mellitus and CAD presents to the outpatient clinic for a follow-up visit. Today's lipids are as follows: total cholesterol, 249 mg per dL; TG, 561 mg per dL; HDL, 40 mg per dL; LDL, 97 mg per dL. Which agent would be most appropriate to initiate in this patient?

    A. fenofibrate
    B. atorvastatin
    C. cholestyramine
    D. no drug therapy at this time

32. Put the following regimens in order according to their LDL-lowering ability.

    atorvastatin, 10 mg per day (A)
    cholestyramine, 8 g per day (C)
    pravastatin, 20 mg per day (P)
    gemfibrozil, 600 mg b.i.d. (G)

    A. A > P > C > G
    B. P > A > G > C
    C. A > P > G > C
    D. A > C > P > G

33. A 76-year-old white man with a past medical history significant for diabetes mellitus type 2, HTN, and chronic AFib was recently diagnosed with CAD and hypercholesterolemia and was initiated on gemfibrozil, 600 mg b.i.d., and atorvastatin, 40 mg q.d. His other medications include glyburide, metoprolol, furosemide, levothyroxine, insulin, and aspirin. Two weeks later, he began to experience pain in his right calf, with pain and stiffness throughout his back, buttocks, and thigh. After another week, he was admitted to the hospital with similar heightened symptoms. On admission, his BUN was elevated, and the urinalysis showed orange, cloudy urine; protein, greater than 300; glucose, greater than 1,000; ketones, 2+; hemoglobin, 3+; red blood cell count, 6 to 10; and myoglobin, 1,367. Which of the following statements is *true*?

A. The patient is experiencing rhabdomyolysis secondary to the drug interaction of atorvastatin and glyburide.

B. Forced diuresis with urine alkalinization and discontinuation of gemfibrozil and atorvastatin are indicated for this patient.

C. Atorvastatin is contraindicated in a patient with diabetes mellitus type 2 and HTN.

D. If nicotinic acid, rather than gemfibrozil, had been used for hypercholesterolemia, this reaction would have been prevented.

34. All of the following drugs produce changes in lipid profiles *except*

A. thiazide diuretics
B. beta-blockers
C. protease inhibitors
D. ACE inhibitors

Aspirin

35. A. F. is a 52-year-old man with a history of AFib, TIAs, HTN, and rheumatic heart disease. The recommendations from the Sixth American College of Chest Physicians (ACCP) Consensus Conference on Antithrombotic Therapy suggest that this patient be initiated on _____ for antithrombotic therapy because of AFib.

A. aspirin, 81 mg q.d.
B. aspirin, 325 mg q.d.
C. warfarin, with a target-goal INR of 2.5
D. warfarin, with a target-goal INR of 3.5

36. The patient above is going to be electively cardioverted. What is the timing of PO anticoagulant therapy?

A. warfarin with a target INR of 3.5 for 4 weeks before cardioversion and continued for 6 weeks after cardioversion

B. warfarin with a target INR of 3.5 for 3 weeks before cardioversion and continued for 6 weeks after cardioversion

C. warfarin with a target INR of 2.5 for 3 weeks before cardioversion and continued for 4 weeks after cardioversion

D. warfarin with a target INR of 2.5 for 6 weeks before cardioversion and continued for 6 weeks after cardioversion

Thienopyridines

37. Which of the following side effects differentiate ticlopidine from clopidogrel?

A. diarrhea
B. rash
C. neutropenia
D. thrombotic thrombocytopenic purpura

38. By which of the following mechanisms do clopidogrel and ticlopidine exert their antiplatelet effects?

    A. cyclooxygenase inhibitor
    B. glycoprotein IIb/IIIa inhibitor
    C. adenosine diphosphate (ADP) inhibitor
    D. direct thrombin inhibitor

Glycoprotein IIb/IIIa Inhibitors

39. G. M. is a 45-year-old man presenting with a non–ST segment–elevation MI. His serum creatinine is 4.5 mg per dL, and you want to start a glycoprotein IIb/IIIa inhibitor. Which of the following agents would be the best choice?

    A. abciximab
    B. eptifibatide
    C. tirofiban
    D. All of the above agents are contraindicated in patients with renal dysfunction.

40. All of the following are considered contraindications to abciximab administration *except*

    A. readministration of abciximab
    B. thrombocytopenia with a platelet count of less than 100,000 cells per μL
    C. active internal bleeding
    D. intracranial tumor, arteriovenous malformation, or aneurysm

41. Which of the following glycoprotein IIb/IIIa inhibitors has the highest incidence of severe thrombocytopenia?

    A. tirofiban
    B. abciximab
    C. eptifibatide
    D. The incidence is not different between the different agents.

42. Which of the following glycoprotein IIb/IIIa inhibitors has the shortest half-life but the longest duration of therapy?

    A. tirofiban
    B. eptifibatide
    C. abciximab
    D. lamifiban

Heparin

43. Heparin must first bind to _____ to exert its anticoagulant activity.

    A. antithrombin
    B. thrombin
    C. factor X
    D. protein C

44. J. M. was initiated on heparin and was given a 5,000-unit bolus. Five min after the loading dose of heparin, she began to have bloody emesis, and her systolic pressure dropped to 80 mm Hg. How much protamine will she require?

    A. 25 mg
    B. 50 mg
    C. 75 mg
    D. 100 mg

45. All of the following factors increase the risk of severe allergic reactions to protamine *except*

    A. allergy to fish
    B. use of neutral protamine Hagedorn (NPH) insulin
    C. use of regular insulin
    D. vasectomized males

Low-Molecular-Weight Heparins

46. Each low-molecular-weight heparin (LMWH) has varying degrees of IIa:Xa activity. Which of the following agents has the *highest* IIa:Xa ratio?

    A. tinzaparin
    B. dalteparin
    C. enoxaparin
    D. danaparoid

47. Patients who develop heparin-induced thrombocytopenia have an *in vitro* cross reactivity with LMWH by what percent?

    A. 90% to 100%
    B. 60% to 70%
    C. 25% to 45%
    D. 5% to 10%

48. All of the following are potential advantages of LMWHs *except*

    A. There is little need for monitoring.
    B. SC bioavailability is predictable in most patients.
    C. There is convenient q.d. or b.i.d. dosing for most indications.
    D. There is no need to adjust the dose in patients with severe renal dysfunction.

Direct Thrombin Inhibitors

49. A patient with a history of heparin-associated antibodies presents with new-onset symptomatic AFib and requires anticoagulation. Other significant past medical history includes severe renal failure secondary to long-standing HTN. The patient's baseline serum creatinine is 4 mg per dL, with an estimated creatinine clearance of 10 mL per minute. Which of the following choices is the best initial therapy?

    A. lepirudin, 0.4 mg per kg bolus, then 0.15 mg per kg per hour
    B. lepirudin, 0.2 mg per kg bolus, then 0.15 mg per kg per hour
    C. argatroban, 2 µg per kg per minute
    D. enoxaparin, 1 mg per kg SC every 12 hours

50. Which of the following direct thrombin inhibitors is *not* a reversible inhibitor of thrombin?

    A. bivalirudin
    B. lepirudin
    C. argatroban
    D. melagatran

Warfarin

51. Which of the following drugs is the *least* likely to enhance the effects of warfarin?

    A. amiodarone
    B. cholestyramine
    C. metronidazole
    D. erythromycin

52. Of the following clinical conditions, all require long-term systemic anticoagulation *except*

    A. mitral valve regurgitation with a history of systemic embolism
    B. mitral valve prolapse with documented unexplained TIAs
    C. infective endocarditis with a mechanical prosthetic valve
    D. mitral annular calcification and systemic embolism not documented to be a calcific embolism

Thrombolytics

53. Which of the following is *not* a contraindication to thrombolytic therapy?

    A. acute pericarditis
    B. aortic dissection
    C. intracranial neoplasm
    D. diabetic retinopathy

54. Which of the following is *not* a risk factor for intracranial hemorrhage in patients receiving fibrinolytic therapy in the treatment of ST segment–elevation MI?

    A. HTN
    B. body weight
    C. age
    D. time to presentation

55. R. M. is a 65-year-old man presenting to the emergency department with an ST segment–elevation MI. It is decided to initiate thrombolytic therapy to induce reperfusion. The patient weighs 72 kg. What is the most effective dose of alteplase for this patient?

    A. 0.9 mg per kg, with a maximum of 90 mg
    B. 15 mg bolus; then 54 mg over 30 min; then 36 mg over 60 min
    C. 15 mg bolus; then 50 mg over 30 min; then 35 mg over 60 min
    D. 60 mg over 1 hour; then 20 mg per hour for 2 hours

Diuretics

56. J. P. is a 48-year-old woman with a history of an anterior wall MI 3 months ago. Her most recent TTE revealed an EF of 25%. She was discharged on lisinopril, 10 mg q.d.; digoxin, 0.125 mg q.d.; metoprolol succinate (Toprol XL), 100 mg q.d.; aspirin, 81 mg q.d.; simvastatin, 20 mg q.d.; and furosemide, 80 mg b.i.d. She is being seen today with a report of mild dizziness and fatigue and notes that she is making less urine over the past few days. Laboratory values are as follows: sodium, 148 mEq per L; potassium, 3.2 mmol L; chloride, 88; bicarbonate, 41; BUN, 76; SrCr, 2.8 mg per dL; glucose, 87 mg per dL. Which of the medications is most likely responsible for the above laboratory findings?

    A. lisinopril
    B. metoprolol
    C. digoxin
    D. furosemide

57. Which of the following loop diuretics is a *not* a sulfonamide and can, therefore, be given to a patient with a sulfonamide allergy?

    A. ethacrynic acid
    B. bumetanide
    C. torsemide
    D. furosemide

Thiazide

58. All of the following metabolic or electrolyte abnormalities occur with thiazide diuretics *except*

    A. hypokalemia
    B. hypocalcemia
    C. hyperuricemia
    D. hypomagnesemia

Antiarrhythmics

59. Which of the following agents is effective for converting AFib to sinus rhythm and for maintaining sinus rhythm after it is restored?

    A. digoxin
    B. amiodarone
    C. diltiazem
    D. propranolol

60. A. R. is a 65-year-old man with a history of AFib, MI, status post coronary artery bypass graft 5 years ago, HTN, deep venous thrombosis, and hypercholesterolemia, who presented to the emergency department with AFib and a rapid ventricular rate. After initiation of beta-blockers, his rate was well controlled (heart rate, 80 bpm). A. R. has been on warfarin for a deep venous thrombosis that developed after a fall. He has not been on antiarrhythmic therapy. All of the following are appropriate choices *except*

    A. amiodarone
    B. sotalol
    C. procainamide
    D. flecainide

61. M. G., a 50-year-old man, collapsed at home after shoveling his sidewalk. His son initiated cardiopulmonary resuscitation immediately, and an emergency medical service was called. When the squad arrived, it was determined that M. G. was in VF, and he was cardioverted with 200 J, 300 J, and 360 J. Epinephrine was given, and M. G. was shocked again. M. G. was still in VF. It was decided to initiate antiarrhythmic therapy. Choose the most appropriate agent from the list below.

    A. lidocaine
    B. amiodarone
    C. procainamide
    D. bretylium

62. All of the following drugs are contraindicated when coadministered with dofetilide *except*

    A. diltiazem
    B. verapamil
    C. trimethoprim
    D. ketoconazole

63. All of the following side effects may occur during amiodarone therapy *except*

    A. pulmonary toxicity
    B. hyperthyroidism
    C. peripheral neuropathy
    D. diarrhea

Inotropic Agents and Vasopressors

64. How does digoxin improve myocardial contractility?

    A. inhibition of the Na^+/K^+–adenosine triphosphatase
    B. inhibition of the breakdown of cyclic adenosine monophosphate (cAMP)
    C. increases intracellular K^+, leading to the opening of calcium channels
    D. directly stimulates calcium release from the sarcoplasmic reticulum

65. A 75-year-old man with a history of HF and AFib was initiated on amiodarone and warfarin. He has been treated for many years with captopril, furosemide, potassium, amlodipine, and digoxin. After 3 days in the hospital, the patient was sent home. One week after discharge, he developed nausea, vomiting, confusion, and symptomatic VT. His serum digoxin concentration was 3.9 ng per mL, and his serum potassium level was 5.8 mmol per L. The rhythm was treated with lidocaine, and the patient is now having episodes of nonsustained VT with a BP of 80/40 mm Hg during each episode. What should be your next course of action?

    A. discontinue the amiodarone and digoxin and observe
    B. discontinue the digoxin and administer digoxin-specific antibodies
    C. decrease the dose of digoxin
    D. discontinue digoxin and observe

66. A 34-year-old woman presented to the emergency department with a 3-day history of worsening shortness of breath and dyspnea on exertion. She stated that 2 weeks before presentation she had flu-like symptoms and thought that she had

a virus. Her vital signs on admission include (a) a heart rate of 115, (b) a respiration rate of 30, and (c) a BP of 105/50 mm Hg. An ECG obtained shows sinus tachycardia. It was decided to give the patient 250 cc of normal saline. After 10 min, her vitals were unchanged, and she was given 15 mg of metoprolol IV push over 2 min. She promptly developed symptomatic hypotension, and her heart rate dropped to 60 bpm. She was given additional fluids and developed pulmonary edema and was intubated. The patient was then transferred to the cardiac ICU, and a PA catheter was placed. Initial hemodynamics were as follows: heart rate, 75 bpm; BP, 100/50 mm Hg; cardiac index, 1.7 L per minute; pulmonary capillary wedge pressure, 24 mm Hg. Which of the following agents would be the most appropriate to increase her cardiac index?

A. dobutamine
B. dopamine
C. epinephrine
D. milrinone

67. Which of the following statements is *true*?

A. Serum levels are used to guide the selection of the dose of digoxin.
B. Because spironolactone was found to have mortality benefit in the Randomized Aldactone Evaluation Study (RALES), the addition of spironolactone should be considered for all CHF patients.
C. The benefit of long-term IV inotropic therapy may outweigh the increased mortality risk in refractory patients unable to be weaned from IV inotropic support.
D. Digoxin exhibits both symptomatic and mortality benefit in patients with CHF.

68. N. M. is a 75-year-old woman with a long-standing history of HF secondary to viral cardiomyopathy. She presents to the outpatient clinic for routine follow-up. On examination, she was short of breath and reported increasing orthopnea. She was admitted to the ICU for right-heart catheterization. Initial readings show a cardiac index of 1.8 L per minute per m², elevated pulmonary capillary wedge pressure (25 mm Hg), and high pulmonary pressures (72/45 mm Hg). Her initial BP was 105/55 mm Hg, and she had a heart rate of 105 bpm. Home medications include captopril, spironolactone, metoprolol XL, and furosemide. Which of the following inotropic agents would be most appropriate?

A. dopamine
B. dobutamine
C. milrinone
D. isoproterenol

Endocarditis

69. A 56-year-old white man who is status post coronary artery bypass graft 3 years ago is in need of a dental root canal. The patient has a history of hives due to cephalexin. What prophylactic regimen for endocarditis is indicated for this patient?

A. amoxicillin, 2 g PO 1 hour before the procedure
B. clindamycin, 600 mg PO 1 hour before the procedure
C. amoxicillin, 2 g PO 1 hour before the procedure, then 500 mg PO every 4 hours for two doses
D. azithromycin, 500 mg 1 hour before the procedure
E. No prophylaxis is recommended in this patient.

70. A 59-year-old white woman is diagnosed with enterococcal endocarditis. She has no known drug allergies. Which of the following would exhibit standard therapy?
    A. penicillin G, 5 million units IV every 4 hours for 4 to 6 weeks, plus gentamicin, 2.5 mg per kg IV every 8 hours for 4 to 6 weeks
    B. ampicillin, 2 g IV every 4 hours for 4 to 6 weeks, plus gentamicin, 1 mg per kg IV every 8 hours for 4 to 6 weeks
    C. ampicillin, 2 g IV every 4 hours for 4 to 6 weeks, plus gentamicin, 1 mg per kg IV every 8 hours for 3 to 5 days
    D. vancomycin, 30 mg per kg per 24 hours in two equally divided doses for 4 to 6 weeks

ANSWERS

1. B. 1,300 mg. To determine the loading dose of a one-compartment drug, three items are needed: (a) the drug's Vd (L/kg), (b) the desired steady-state concentration [Cpss (mg/L)], and (c) the patient's weight. Loading dose = Vd × Cpss. Kilograms and liters cancel, and you are left with the loading dose in milligrams.

2. C. 40%. The bioavailability of digoxin tablets is 75%. Therefore, when converting from PO to IV administration (bioavailability of 100%), there is a 25% increase in bioavailability. Without altering the dose of digoxin, this patient would most likely have an increase in digoxin level to approximately 2.4 ng per mL. This could lead to potential digoxin toxicity.

3. C. Half-life is a function of both clearance (Cl) and Vd. The elimination-rate constant (k_{el}) is determined by two independent factors: Cl and Vd. $k_{el} = Cl/Vd$. Half-life is determined by the equation $0.693/k_{el}$. Therefore, as the apparent Vd and Cl change, the half-life of a drug may change.

4. D. Pharmacodynamics. *Pharmacodynamics* has been defined as the study of the biologic effects resulting from the interaction between drugs and biologic systems. Pharmacokinetic principles consider drug distribution, metabolism, clearance, and bioavailability, whereas pharmacodynamic principles take this one step further and relate these factors to pharmacologic response. Pharmacogenetics is the study of heredity on variations in drug response among individuals and populations. Pharmacogenetic studies have established that genetics play an important role in the dose-concentration-response relationships of medications, whereas pharmacology is simply the study of drugs.

5. A. Drug A is the most potent agent. This is based on the fact that at any given concentration of this agent, the effect is greater than that of the other drugs at similar concentrations. Drug B has the same maximal effect; however, it occurs at a higher concentration. Drug C is similar to drug B; however, it is less efficacious, because its maximal effect occurs at a concentration that is 50% lower than that of drug B.

6. B. Metoprolol is not a good choice. Metoprolol is eliminated through the cytochrome–P450 2D6 enzyme system. Quinidine is a potent inhibitor of

this enzyme and may lead to a decreased elimination of metoprolol, leading to an enhanced pharmacologic response of metoprolol. Agents that are not eliminated through this system may cause fewer side effects.

7. C. Increases warfarin metabolism, decreases warfarin metabolism. Chronic ethanol consumption can lead to increased hepatic metabolism of many medications that are cleared through the liver. Increased hepatic metabolism is related to enhanced enzyme function. Therefore, chronic ethanol users typically need higher than usual doses of warfarin to achieve therapeutic INRs. Acute ingestion of large amounts of ethanol at a time may inhibit warfarin metabolism. This may lead to elevated INRs and increase the risk of hemorrhagic complications. Moderate ingestion of ethanol does not seem to affect the metabolism of warfarin.

8. D. All of the above. Amiodarone and quinidine are well known to increase the levels of digoxin. Pharmacokinetic interactions include increased bio-availability and decreased clearance of digoxin. Approximately 10% of patients taking digoxin have significant metabolism of digoxin in the GI tract by *Eubacterium lentum*. This bacterium is killed by tetracyclines and erythromycin, and a small subset of patients will have increased bioavailability of digoxin and, hence, elevated serum drug concentrations.

9. C. All ACE inhibitors, except for captopril, lisinopril, and enalaprilat, are prodrugs that require hepatic activation for pharmacologic activity.

10. C. Because angiotensin II can alter cardiac structure by hemodynamically and nonhemodynamically mediated mechanisms, ACE inhibitors are beneficial in HF. A hemodynamic benefit, however, is reduction in both preload and afterload.

11. C. Sodium depletion is an important factor in the development of renal insufficiency associated with ACE inhibitors. Numerous studies, including the Studies of Left Ventricular Dysfunction (SOLVD) treatment trial, Veterans' Administration Heart Failure Trial (V-HeFT) II, and Cooperative North Scandinavian Enalapril Survival Study (CONSENSUS), have shown ACE inhibitors to reduce mortality in patients with ischemic and nonischemic cardiomyopathy and mild to moderate HF. ACE inhibitors are considered to be associated with a class benefit; however, not all ACE inhibitors carry the FDA indication for HF. The ACE inhibitors that are approved for the treatment of HF include captopril, enalapril, lisinopril, quinapril, fosinopril, and ramipril.

In 1998, the Assessment of Treatment with Lisinopril and Survival (ATLAS) trial showed that high doses of lisinopril were superior to low doses in decreasing risk of death or hospitalization. Therefore, an effort to use target doses used in clinical trials is important (e.g., captopril, 50 mg t.i.d.; enalapril, 10 mg b.i.d.; lisinopril, 20 mg q.d.). Patients with hyponatremia, dehydration, and severe HF are most dependent on the maintenance of renal perfusion by angiotensin II–mediated vasoconstriction of the efferent arteriole. Prevention of hyponatremia by decreasing diuretics can reduce such risk. Potassium retention of ACE inhibitors is caused by a reduction in the feedback of angiotensin II to stimulate aldosterone release. Caution is necessary when initiating a potassium supplement in a patient on ACE-inhibitor therapy.

12. D. Captopril. Because the patient is not already receiving ACE-inhibitor therapy, an ACE inhibitor is indicated in patients with HF and a reduced EF (less than 35% to 45%) to decrease morbidity and mortality, as shown in the SOLVD, V-HeFT, and CONSENSUS trials. The patient has no contraindications to such therapy. If the patient's renal function were changing, thereby making an ACE inhibitor inappropriate, then hydralazine plus a nitrate would be indicated, because V-HeFT I showed mortality benefit compared to placebo and an alpha-blocker. Calcium channel antagonists should not be used in the treatment of HF due to their ability to worsen HF and increase mortality. However, if a CCB is necessary for an indication aside from HF (HTN or angina), amlodipine may be used in patients with HF, because in the Prospective Randomized Amlodipine Survival Evaluation (PRAISE) trial, it had no significant effect on mortality.

13. D. Cough is a common side effect of ACE inhibitors. It is not a contraindication to initiate patients on ACE inhibitors if they have preexisting cough. ACE inhibitor–associated cough is difficult at times to differentiate from cough associated with HF. Also, cough is not life threatening and is considered an annoyance. In many patients, the cough is such a nuisance that cessation of therapy will be required. Patients with bilateral renal artery stenosis are at high risk of developing acute renal failure with the use of ACE inhibitors. ACE inhibitors preferentially dilate the efferent arteriole in the nephron and in the presence of decreased afferent arterial pressures lead to a decrease in glomerular filtration. This can lead to acute renal failure and is typically reversible if the ACE inhibitor is discontinued early. In the second and third trimesters of pregnancy, ACE inhibitors can lead to oligohydramnios, fetal calvarial hypoplasia, fetal pulmonary hypoplasia, fetal growth retardation, and fetal death. Therefore, these agents should be used with extreme caution in women of childbearing potential. Finally, angioedema is a rare but potentially fatal adverse event that can occur with ACE inhibitors. Angioedema typically occurs within the first few doses; however, it may develop after years of therapy. ACE inhibitors are considered contraindicated in patients with a prior history of angioedema.

14. B. False. The risk of angioedema to the losartan is too great in this patient. There have been several case reports that identify patients experiencing angioedema to an ARB after experiencing ACE inhibitor–induced angioedema. In this patient, it would be prudent to avoid such treatments and treat with the combination of hydralazine and ISDN.

15. C. HTN. Currently, ARBs are only indicated for the treatment of HTN. Ongoing trials are evaluating the use of ARBs in patients post-MI and in patients with HF. Currently, there are little data to support the use of ARBs over ACE inhibitors in the primary treatment of HF; in combination with beta-blockers, there may be a trend toward worsened outcomes.

16. A. ARBs have a very similar side-effect profile to ACE inhibitors. They are both contraindicated in patients with bilateral renal artery stenosis, and both can cause hyperkalemia and hypotension. Cough is a major difference with these two agents. ARBs do not increase the levels of bradykinin, whereas ACE inhibitors will decrease the breakdown of bradykinins, thus leading to accumulation and, thus, to cough.

17. A. Increased ventricular pressure is not a mechanism of benefit. Beta-blockers interfere with neurohormonal actions of the sympathetic nervous system. Sympathetic activity causes an increase in ventricular volume, thereby increasing ventricular pressure as a result of peripheral vasoconstriction. Norepinephrine and sympathetic activity can lead to arrhythmias, cardiac hypertrophy, and apoptosis (programmed cell death). By administering beta-blockers, these activities are inhibited, thereby causing positive effects in patients with HF, as exhibited in several clinical trials, including Cardiac Insufficiency Bisoprolol Study (CIBIS) I, CIBIS II, Metoprolol CR/XL Controlled Release Randomized Intervention Trial in Heart Failure (MERIT-HF), and others.

18. B. Carvedilol, 3.125 mg b.i.d. All patients with stable, class II or III HF should be initiated on a beta-blocker, unless a contraindication (bronchospastic disease, symptomatic bradycardia, or advanced heart block) or intolerance is exhibited. Initiation of beta-blocker therapy is recommended in stable patients with mild to moderate HF and a low EF (less than 35% to 40%). The mortality benefit of beta-blocker use was seen when added to a preexisting regimen of an ACE inhibitor and diuretic, with or without digoxin. It should be noted that beta-blockers must be initiated at very low doses and only gradually increased if low doses have been well tolerated.

19. C. Pindolol exhibits ISA and should, therefore, not be used on patients with HF. Beta-blockers with ISA are partial beta agonists and can maintain normal sympathetic tone. This activity prevents the benefits seen with the reduced heart rate, cardiac output, and peripheral blood flow caused by other beta-blockers. Such agents include pindolol, penbutolol, carteolol, and acebutolol.

20. C. (1) ii; (2) iii; (3) i; (4) iv. Agents exhibiting alpha-blockade include labetalol and carvedilol. Agents with ISA are pindolol, penbutolol, carteolol, and acebutolol. Agents with membrane-stabilizing activity are propranolol, labetalol, and acebutolol. Beta$_1$-selective agents include bisoprolol, betaxolol, atenolol, acebutolol, and metoprolol.

21. B. Metoprolol. The American College of Cardiology and the American Heart Association recommend the use of beta-blockers in patients after surviving an MI to decrease mortality, sudden death, and reinfarction. Therefore, if this patient is not already on a beta-blocker, one would be indicated, not only for his HTN but also for secondary prevention.

22. B. Prazosin has not been shown to improve survival. Multiple trials have shown that ACE inhibitors, beta-blockers, and the combination of hydralazine and ISDN improve survival in patients who have HF. In the V-HeFT-I trial, prazosin was compared to placebo and the combination of hydralazine and ISDN; in those patients who received prazosin, there was no significant difference in mortality when compared to placebo.

23. D. Clonidine. Abrupt withdrawal of an alpha$_2$ agonist is the most likely cause of severe rebound HTN. Typically, this is seen within 24 to 48 hours of discontinuation of clonidine and typically occurs in patients taking large doses for longer than 3 months. The best treatment for this is to restart clonidine. Beta-blockers could make the situation worse due to causing unopposed alpha$_1$ stimulation.

24. A. Diltiazem and verapamil decrease conduction velocity within the AV node and increase RP of nodal tissue. This then causes slowing of ventricular rate.

25. D. Dihydropyridines are more selective for vascular smooth-muscle calcium channels than for myocardial calcium channels. Dihydropyridine CCBs do not slow AV-nodal conduction. Unlike verapamil and diltiazem, dihydropyridine CCBs cause a reflex tachycardia and do not increase AV-nodal RP. Pedal edema is one of the most common side effects of dihydropyridine-type CCBs and is associated with short half-life, short-acting agents. Because of their ability to produce such profound vasodilation, these agents can produce flushing as well.

26. D. Nimodipine. Nimodipine is the only agent indicated for patients with subarachnoid hemorrhage. Nimodipine decreases the influx of extracellular calcium, thus preventing vasospasm.

27. C. Free radical depletion is not a suggested mechanism. Long-term administration of nitroglycerin without a nitrate-free interval may lead to nitrate tolerance. Although the exact mechanism of this effect is not fully understood, there are a number of hypotheses, including volume expansion, sulfhydryl-group depletion, reflex vasoconstriction, and free radical production. The mechanism for volume depletion causing tolerance is unknown. Additionally, there is a lack of evidence suggesting that the depletion of sulfhydryl groups, which are necessary for intracellular biotransformation of nitrates to nitric oxide, is responsible for tolerance. A neurohormonal hypothesis associates the administration of nitrates with a reflexive release of vasoconstrictor hormones that decrease the vasodilating effects of nitrates; however, this has not been consistently observed. Finally, free radical production, specifically superoxide anion, leads to nitrate tolerance in animal trials and has been reversed with the administration of antioxidants.

28. B. Initiate nitroprusside drip and give IV fluids. Hypertensive emergencies are defined by the presence of end-organ damage in the face of high BP. This patient was dehydrated from the diarrhea and had uncontrolled BP due to the medication change that occurred. Use of nitroprusside would be most appropriate in this patient due to the emergent situation of the renal insufficiency and possible cerebrovascular involvement exhibited by the headache. Typically, parenteral antihypertensive agents are initiated for hypertensive emergencies. In addition, it is necessary to correct the underlying cause of the hypertensive episode, if it can be identified; therefore, rehydration in this patient is prudent. Nitroprusside is the drug of choice because it has a quick onset of action yet is easily titratable. Sublingual nifedipine is no longer advocated due to the precipitous drop in BP and the subsequent adverse effects.

29. D. Hydralazine and ISDN. In the V-HeFT-I trial, the combination of hydralazine and ISDN exhibited a mortality benefit compared to placebo and prazosin in patients with classes II and III HF. In the V-HeFT-II trial, the same combination was inferior to the mortality benefit of enalapril in patients with HF. Therefore, it is recommended that the combination of hydralazine and ISDN only be used in patients intolerant of or unable to take ACE inhibitors.

Losartan, an ARB, would be another alternative to ACE-inhibitor therapy for use in HF patients. The Evaluation of Losartan in the Elderly (ELITE) and ELITE-II trials have shown similar benefit with respect to cardiac remodeling, but no mortality benefit over ACE-inhibitor therapy was identified. In this case, because the patient has hyperkalemia, an ARB would not be appropriate, because both ACE inhibitors and ARBs can cause potassium retention. A potential benefit of ARB therapy is the potential for less cough and angioedema.

30. D. No medication is indicated at this time. Because this patient is a smoker with a significant family history of CAD, he has two risk factors for CHD. The therapeutic aim is reduction of LDL cholesterol (goal, ≤130 mg/dL) which should be attempted with the therapeutic lifestyle changes diet. If after 3 months of therapeutic lifestyle changes alone the LDL is less than 160 mg per dL, it should be continued. Drug therapy is not indicated because the patient is not at high short-term risk. Drug therapy should be initiated if the LDL is greater than or equal to 160 mg per dL.

31. A. Fenofibrate. Because the patient's TG is in the category of very high (greater than or equal to 500 mg/dL), the initial aim is to reduce the risk of pancreatitis by using a TG-lowering agent. Fibrates or nicotinic acid would be indicated due to their potential to reduce TGs 20% to 50%.

32. A. A > P > C > G. HMG-CoA reductase inhibitors decrease LDL by 18% to 55%. Atorvastatin is the most potent agent. Bile-acid sequestrants decreased LDL by 15% to 30%. Fibrates decrease LDL by 5% to 20%.

33. B. Forced diuresis with urine alkalinization and discontinuation of gemfibrozil and atorvastatin are indicated for this patient. Rhabdomyolysis secondary to the interaction of atorvastatin and gemfibrozil is responsible for this clinical picture. *Rhabdomyolysis* is defined as the disintegration of muscle, associated with the excretion of myoglobin in the urine. Clinical signs and symptoms include myalgias, elevated creatine kinase, elevated urine and serum myoglobin, and dark urine. Complications of rhabdomyolysis are numerous and may include renal failure, disseminated intravascular coagulation, metabolic acidosis, and cardiomyopathy. HMG-CoA reductase inhibitors (statins) can be considered direct myotoxins and may induce rhabdomyolysis when used alone. However, the risk of toxicity increases when statins are used in combination with fibric acid derivatives (gemfibrozil or fenofibrate), nicotinic acid, cyclosporin, itraconazole, or erythromycin, to name a few. Treatment of the underlying cause, in this case discontinuation of the offending agents, is necessary. In addition, renal failure due to products of tissue degradation must be combatted with urinary alkalinization and maintenance of a high urine volume.

34. D. ACE inhibitors have no effect on the lipid profile. Beta-blockers and thiazide diuretics typically have the most effect on raising TG levels. Beta-blockers may decrease HDL levels, whereas thiazide diuretics may increase LDL and total cholesterol. Protease inhibitors have the most effect on TGs and total cholesterol and cause adipose tissue redistribution.

35. C. Warfarin, with a target goal INR of 2.5. This patient is at high risk for a thromboembolic event. Recommendations for antithrombotic therapy include risk stratification. Risks are stratified into high, moderate, and low. High-risk patients include patients with prior stroke or TIA or systemic embolus, history of HTN, poor LV systolic function, age older than 75 years, rheumatic mitral valve disease, and a prosthetic heart valve. Moderate risk factors include age between 65 and 75 years, diabetes mellitus, and CAD with preserved LV systolic function. Low-risk patients are those younger than 65 years old with no clinical or TTE evidence of cardiovascular disease.

36. C. Warfarin with a target INR of 2.5 for 3 weeks before cardioversion and continued for 4 weeks after cardioversion. Recommendations from the Sixth ACCP Consensus Conference on Antithrombotic Therapy state that patients undergoing elective cardioversion for AFib should be initiated on PO anticoagulant therapy for 3 weeks before and at least 4 weeks after elective DC cardioversion. The grade of evidence is 1C+. Also, an alternative approach would to be initiate anticoagulation, have the patients undergo a TEE, and have the cardioversion performed if no thrombi are seen. Warfarin should be continued for at least 4 weeks, as long as the patient maintains NSR. This is a grade 1C recommendation.

37. C. Neutropenia. Ticlopidine causes neutropenia in 2.4% of patients who are initiated on therapy. Nearly 1% of patients develop severe neutropenia. Therefore, a complete blood count is required every 2 weeks during initiation of therapy for the first 3 months of therapy. Both agents can cause diarrhea and rash. Structurally, these two drugs are so similar that allergic cross-reactivity is expected. Thrombotic thrombocytopenic purpura has been reported with both agents. There have been more than 60 cases of thrombotic thrombocytopenic purpura with the use of ticlopidine and 11 cases reported with clopidogrel.

38. C. ADP inhibitor. ADP is released from red blood cells, activated platelets, and damaged endothelial cells, leading to platelet adhesion and aggregation. However, the precise mechanism of their action has not been identified. ADP blockade decreases the expression of the glycoprotein IIb/IIIa receptor. Platelet inhibition occurs at maximal effect within 3 to 5 days and produces approximately 40% to 50% platelet inhibition.

39. C. Tirofiban. Based on product information, tirofiban would be the best agent to use. The recommendation from the tirofiban product information states that when the creatinine clearance is less than 30 mL per minute, the dose should be reduced by one-half. Product information for eptifibatide states that it should not be given in patients with a serum creatinine greater than 4 mg per dL. Finally, results of the GUSTO-IV trial do not support the use of abciximab in patients presenting with acute coronary syndromes. The primary end point of death or MI at 30 days was not significantly different between the placebo, 24-hour infusion abciximab, and 48-hour abciximab groups.

40. A. Readministration of abciximab is not a contraindication. Concerns regarding the readministration of abciximab relate to the development of antibodies to abciximab. This may lead to increases in hypersensitivity reactions, decrease or loss of effectiveness, and the development of thrombocy-

topenia. Recently, published data from the ReoPro readministration registry show that the risk of thrombocytopenia is similar to that for abciximab-naïve patients. However, there was an increase in the number of patients who developed severe thrombocytopenia and also in cases of delayed-onset thrombocytopenia. There were no cases of hypersensitivity, and clinical outcomes were also unchanged.

41. B. Abciximab. All glycoprotein IIb/IIIa inhibitors may cause thrombocytopenia. However, abciximab has the highest rate of all, based on the clinical trials.

42. C. Abciximab. Abciximab has a serum half-life of 10 to 30 min; however, because of its high binding affinity to the glycoprotein IIb/IIIa receptor, it maintains its activity for many hours after discontinuation of therapy, and abciximab can be detected in the serum for longer than 2 weeks. The short-acting inhibitors have half-lives of approximately 2 hours, depending on renal function; however, because of their competitive inhibiting nature, once the infusion is discontinued, their effects wane relatively quickly.

43. A. Antithrombin. Heparin must first bind to antithrombin to exert is anticoagulant effect. This complex accelerates antithrombin effect. Heparin potentiates antithrombin's effect by binding to a glucosamine unit within a pentasaccharide sequence.

44. B. 50 mg. Every 1 mg of protamine will antagonize approximately 100 units of heparin. Because this patient just received the bolus, she would require 50 mg of protamine. If she had received the dose 30 to 60 min ago, then a dose of 0.50 to 0.75 mg of protamine per 100 units of heparin would be required. If she had been on a continuous infusion of heparin, then the dosing would be dependent on the time and dose of the last bolus of heparin and the rate of infusion. In this scenario, most patients require approximately 25 to 50 mg of protamine.

45. C. Use of regular insulin. Severe hypersensitivity reactions can occur with the administration of protamine. Patients at risk include those with fish allergies, who use NPH insulin, who have had prior protamine exposure (other than NPH insulin), and vasectomized men. Protamine is derived from fish. Originally, it was discovered in salmon testes. The commercially available product is still made from fish. Fifty percent of diabetic patients using NPH insulin may develop antibodies to protamine and are at risk of developing hypersensitivity reactions to protamine. Vasectomized males develop protamine antibodies approximately one-third of the time and are also at risk for developing a hypersensitivity reaction after the administration of protamine. Regular insulin does not contain protamine, and, therefore, diabetics just requiring regular insulin are not at risk.

46. C. Enoxaparin. Correlation of anti-Xa to anti-IIa for different LMWHs is a poor prediction of potency. However, for differentiation purposes, the ratio of anti-X to anti-IIa is commonly reported (Table 1). Danaparoid is not a LMWH and is a heparinoid. Danaparoid has a ratio greater than 20:1.

TABLE 1 *Anti-Xa:Anti-IIa Ratio for Low-Molecular-Weight Heparins*

Drug	Dalteparin	Enoxaparin	Tinzaparin
Anti-Xa:Anti-IIa	2.7	3.8	2.8

47. A. 90% to 100%. There have been several reports of patients who have heparin-induced thrombocytopenia being treated with LMWH. However, the cross reactivity *in vitro* approaches 100%. The use of LMWH should be considered a contraindication unless there is a documented negative test for antibodies against LMWH.

48. D. LMWHs are approximately one-third the size of unfractionated heparin. They have a consistent bioavailability in most patients and longer plasma half-life than unfractionated heparin. Because of their predictable ability to bind to factor Xa and consistent bioavailability, there is little need for laboratory monitoring for efficacy. However, there are limitations in pharmacokinetic data for administration of these agents in patients with renal dysfunction and in the very obese patient. Another limitation is the fact that the factor Xa activity is only partially neutralized by protamine.

49. C. Argatroban, 2 μg per kg per minute. Argatroban is hepatically cleared and, therefore, does not require dosing adjustment for patients with renal dysfunction and may be a safer alternative for anticoagulation. Lepirudin is reasonable as well; however, patients with significant renal dysfunction require appropriate dosing adjustments. Continuous infusion should not be used in patients with a creatinine clearance less than 15 mL per minute because of accumulation of drug. LMWHs have a high likelihood for *in vitro* and *in vivo* cross-reactivity of 80% to 100%, and there is a potential for an increase in thrombotic complications.

50. B. Lepirudin is not a reversible inhibitor of thrombin. Hirudin and recombinant derivatives bind to both the catalytic site and substrate-recognition site of thrombin irreversibly. Bivalirudin, a synthetic hirudin derivative, contains two covalently linked groups that bind to the catalytic site and the substrate site of thrombin. This bivalent binding is both reversible and transient. Argatroban and melagatran bind only to the catalytic site of thrombin. They bind by competitive inhibition and are reversible.

51. B. Cholestyramine is least likely to enhance the effects of warfarin. Amiodarone, metronidazole, and erythromycin all enhance warfarin's effects by decreasing the clearance of warfarin. Amiodarone may also alter protein binding of warfarin. Cholestyramine decreases the absorption and prevents the enterohepatic recycling of warfarin, thus decreasing the effectiveness of warfarin. It is recommended that the dose of warfarin be separated from the cholestyramine dose by at least 2 hours before or 2 hours after warfarin. In addition, more frequent monitoring should be done when initiating, discontinuing, or changing the dose of cholestyramine.

52. B. Mitral valve prolapse with documented unexplained TIAs does not require long-term systemic anticoagulation. The recommendations from the Sixth Consensus Conference on Antithrombotic Therapy from the ACCP state that patients with mitral valve prolapse and unexplained TIAs need only aspirin therapy. This is a grade 2C recommendation.

53. D. Diabetic retinopathy is not a contraindication to thrombolytic therapy. A review of large clinical trials did not show an increase in the rates of intraocular hemorrhage in patients with diabetic proliferative retinopathy. Other absolute contraindications include previous hemorrhagic stroke, other strokes or cerebrovascular events within 1 year, and active bleeding.

54. D. Time to presentation is not a risk factor for intracranial hemorrhage in patients receiving thrombolytic therapy. In clinical trials, the risks for intracranial hemorrhage included age older than 65 years, low body weight (less than 70 kg), HTN on hospital admission, and the use of alteplase. Also, the levels of concomitant anticoagulation can also increase the risk of intracranial hemorrhage.

55. C. 15-mg bolus; then 50 mg over 30 min; then 35 mg over 60 min. Based on the first GUSTO trial, the most effective dosing for acute ST segment–elevation MI is front-loaded t-PA. The maximum dose should be 100 mg and, therefore, answer B may increase the risk of major bleeding, specifically intracranial hemorrhage. Answer D is standard dosing of recombinant tissue-type plasminogen activator and was found inferior to front loading. Finally, answer A is the recommended dosing for acute ischemic stroke.

56. D. Furosemide. Loop diuretics can cause hypokalemic metabolic alkalosis with a coexisting chloride deficit. Loop diuretics enhance the renal secretion of K^+ and H^+, causing hypokalemic metabolic alkalosis. This is a function of the magnitude of the diuretic effect and can typically be reversed by K^+ replacement and correction of hypovolemia. Potassium chloride is the preferred potassium salt for replacement in this setting.

57. A. Ethacrynic acid is the only loop diuretic that is not a sulfonamide. It is used only in patients allergic to other either loop or thiazide diuretics. Disadvantages of ethacrynic acid include GI intolerance and a narrower dose response curve.

58. B. Hypocalcemia. Thiazide diuretics retain calcium by increasing reabsorption in the proximal tubule. Therefore, these agents need to be avoided in patients with hypercalcemia, in contrast to loop diuretics, which are used to treat hypercalcemia. Like loop diuretics, thiazide diuretics cause hypokalemia, hyperuricemia, and hypomagnesemia. Hyperuricemia is not typically problematic; however, it can produce gout attacks.

59. B. Amiodarone. Although amiodarone does not carry an FDA indication for the treatment of AFib, it can convert to and maintain NSR. The other agents listed are only used for rate control when used for AFib.

60. D. Flecainide is not an appropriate choice. In general, antiarrhythmic agents are proarrhythmic and possess myocardial-depressant effects. Flecainide, encainide, and moricizine were evaluated in the Cardiac Arrhythmia Suppression Trial I or II. These agents were evaluated in patients with multiple PVCs after MI. By suppressing ventricular ectopy, it was felt that there would be a decrease in mortality. However, there was an increase in mortality in all groups despite suppression of initial arrhythmia. At this time, class IC antiarrhythmics are indicated for life-threatening sustained VT and paroxysmal SVT, including Wolff-Parkinson-White syndrome and AFib or flutter in patients without structural heart disease.

61. B. Amiodarone. The most recent advanced cardiac life support guidelines recommend that amiodarone be the first-line agent in patients with pulseless VT/VF. This recommendation is based on the Amiodarone for Resuscitation After Out-of-Hospital Cardiac Arrest due to Ventricular Fibrillation (ARREST) trial, which showed that amiodarone increased the likelihood of admission to the hospital after an out-of-hospital arrest. This is further supported by the recently presented Amiodarone versus Lidocaine in Pre-Hospital Refractory Ventricular Fibrillation Evaluation (ALIVE) trial. Lidocaine is now considered Class Indeterminate based on the lack of controlled trials supporting its use in pulseless VT/VF. Procainamide administration is prolonged and not suitable for rapid administration. Bretylium is no longer available secondary to lack of raw materials.

62. A. Diltiazem is not contraindicated when coadministered with dofetilide. There are seven medications that are contraindicated to give with dofetilide; these include verapamil, trimethoprim, ketoconazole, itraconazole, cimetidine, hydrochorothiazine, and prochlorperazine. In general, medications that inhibit the cation transport system within the kidneys interfere with elimination of dofetilide. Dofetilide is primarily eliminated by the kidneys, and only 20% of elimination occurs via hepatic metabolism through the CYP3A4 enzyme system. Therefore, coadministration of contraindicated medications increases the risk of developing drug-induced arrhythmias, specifically torsades de pointes.

63. D. Diarrhea is not a side effect. Pulmonary toxicity in the form of pulmonary fibrosis and hypersensitivity pneumonitis occurs in approximately 3% to 17% of patients on amiodarone therapy. Pulmonary toxicity occurs primarily with doses greater than 400 mg q.d. and after several months to years. Pulmonary toxicity is very difficult to diagnose, because symptoms and signs are similar to HF and pneumonia. Patient self-reporting is the most effective way to identify pulmonary toxicity early. Thyroid dysfunction occurs in approximately 10% of patients on amiodarone. Patients can present with either hyper- or hypothyroidism and should be evaluated at baseline and every 6 months thereafter. Neuropathy and other neurologic side effects can occur in up to 20% of patients on chronic amiodarone therapy. Most frequently, amiodarone causes constipation in long-term administration.

64. A. Inhibition of the Na^+/K^+–adenosine triphosphatase. Digoxin inhibits the Na^+/K^+–adenosine triphosphatase pump on the myocardial cell surface. This inhibits the ability of the cell to exchange potassium for sodium and thus leads to an increase in intracellular sodium. This increase in intracellular sodium leads to exchange of sodium for calcium, increasing intracellular calcium concentrations. Increased intracellular calcium enhances contraction coupling.

65. B. Discontinue the digoxin and administer digoxin-specific antibodies. Digoxin-immune Fab is indicated for patients with life-threatening ventricular arrhythmias relating to digoxin toxicity. It is also indicated in patients with progressive bradyarrhythmias, such as severe sinus bradycardia or second- or third-degree heart block not responsive to atropine. It should not be used for milder forms of digoxin toxicity. Also, in the setting of hyperkalemia and digitalis intoxication, digoxin-immune Fab fragment is indicated. Digoxin-immune Fab fragment is ovine derived; there

is a potential for hypersensitivity reactions, and there are not data available in regards to readministration.

66. D. Milrinone. Milrinone is a phosphodiesterase inhibitor type III. It increases intracellular cAMP, leading to an increase in intracellular calcium by preventing the breakdown of cAMP. This would be the most reasonable inotropic agent because it does not rely on stimulation of the beta-receptors to improve cardiac index. There are limited data using phosphodiesterase inhibitors and beta-blockers; however, in patients with acute decompensation of HF and on beta-blockers, milrinone would bypass the beta-receptor.

67. C. The benefit of long-term IV inotropic therapy may outweigh the increased mortality risk in refractory patients unable to be weaned from IV inotropic support. Little evidence supports the practice of dosing digoxin according to serum levels. This is due to the lack of data exhibiting a relationship between digoxin serum concentrations and therapeutic effect. In addition, it is uncertain if higher doses of digoxin are more effective than lower doses when used in the treatment for HF.

In the RALES trial, spironolactone was shown to be associated with reduced mortality and morbidity. However, the patients who were included in this trial were patients with class IV HF. Therefore, it would only be prudent to consider spironolactone in patients with recent or current severe HF symptoms. Efficacy and safety of spironolactone's use in patients with mild to moderate HF is yet to be determined.

Because long-term IV positive inotropic therapy may cause an increased risk of death, such therapy is not regularly recommended. This risk, however, may be outweighed in patients who cannot be weaned from continuous support. Such patients with refractory HF may experience an improved quality of life due to the relative clinical stability afforded by the inotrope, therefore IV positive inotropic therapy may be considered as a palliative measure in end-stage HF.

The DIG (Digitalis Investigation Group) trial showed that digoxin's benefit in HF was the alleviation of symptoms and improvement in clinical status. These findings were associated with a decreased morbidity (fewer hospitalizations) but not mortality. Because digoxin has negligible effect on survival, it is recommended that digoxin be used in conjunction with diuretics, ACE inhibitors, and beta-blockers to decrease the clinical symptoms of HF.

68. C. Milrinone. Milrinone is a phosphodiesterase inhibitor classified as inodilator. Thus, milrinone produces positive inotropic effects and vasodilation. Milrinone inhibits the phosphodiesterase III enzyme, leading to an increase in intracellular cAMP, thus causing increased intracellular levels of calcium. In addition, milrinone will decrease pulmonary pressures and LV end-diastolic pressures more predictably than the other agents listed. These combined effects lead to minimal increases in myocardial O_2 consumption. Also, milrinone may be useful in this patient secondary to chronic metoprolol therapy.

69. E. No prophylaxis is recommended in this patient. This patient has only a negligible risk for endocarditis post–coronary artery bypass graft. In individuals with innocent heart murmurs or structurally normal hearts, prophylaxis is not required.

70. B. Ampicillin, 2 g IV every 4 hours for 4 to 6 weeks, plus gentamicin, 1 mg per kg IV every 8 hours for 4 to 6 weeks. Treatment of enterococcal endocarditis is complicated due to the high levels of resistance to penicillin, extended-spectrum penicillins, and vancomycin. However, penicillin, ampicillin, or vancomycin in combination with an aminoglycoside causes synergistic bactericidal effect on these organisms. Treatment with an aminoglycoside for the full 4 to 6 weeks at a synergistic dose (1 mg/kg IV every 8 hours) in addition to the penicillin agent or vancomycin is required.

SUGGESTED READING

Advisory Council to Improve Outcomes Nationwide in Heart Failure (ACTION HF). Consensus recommendations for the management of chronic heart failure. *Am J Cardiol* 1999;83(2A):1A–38A.

Albers GW, Dalen JE, Laupacis A, et al. Antithrombotic therapy in atrial fibrillation. *Chest* 2001;119:194S–206S.

Dajani AS, Taubert KA, Wilson W, et al. Prevention of bacterial endocarditis. *JAMA* 1997;277:1794–1801.

Expert Panel of Detection, Evaluation, and Treatment of High Blood Cholesterol in Adults. Executive summary of the third report of the National Cholesterol Education Program (NCEP) Expert Panel on Detection, Evaluation, and Treatment of High Blood Cholesterol in Adults (Adult Treatment Panel III). *JAMA* 2001;285:2486–2497.

Hansten PD, Horn JT. *Drug interactions analysis and management*. St. Louis: Facts and Comparison, 2000.

Johnson JA, Parker RB, Geraci SA, et al. *Pharmacotherapy: a pathophysiologic approach*, 4th ed. Stamford, Connecticut: Appleton & Lange, 1999:153–581.

McEvoy GK, ed. *AHFS drug information 2001*. Bethesda, MD: American Society of Health-System Pharmacists, 2001.

Ohman EM, Harrington RA, Cannon CP, et al. Intravenous thrombolysis in acute myocardial infarction. *Chest* 2001;119:252S–277S.

Reuning RH, Geraets DR, Rocci ML, et al. Digoxin. In: Evans WE, Schentag JJ, Jusko WJ, eds. *Applied pharmacokinetics: principles of therapeutic drug monitoring*. Vancouver, WA: Applied Therapeutics, 1992:20(1–48).

The Sixth Report of the National Committee on Detection, Evaluation, and Treatment of High Blood Pressure (JNC-VI). *Arch Intern Med* 1997;157:2413–2446.

CHAPTER 6

Aorta and Peripheral Vascular Disease

Craig R. Asher and Monica B. Khot

QUESTIONS

Case 1 (Questions 1–3)

A 72-year-old woman is referred to the cardiology clinic for further evaluation and management of aortic regurgitation. A review of systems is notable only for recent onset of headaches and myalgia. The patient has no cardiac risk factors, except mild hypertension (HTN), and has not previously undergone any cardiac testing.

Physical Examination

BP is 138/78 mm Hg in both arms.

Pulse is 62 bpm and regular.

The funduscopic examination reveals no changes consistent with hypertensive retinopathy.

The heart examination is notable for a normal S_1 and increased intensity S_2 (A_2). There was an S_4 gallop; a II/IV diastolic decrescendo murmur, heard best at the right sternal border; and a II/IV early-peaking systolic ejection murmur, heard at the left sternal border. There was no systolic ejection click.

The pulses were strong and equal in both the upper and lower extremities.

An ECG reveals sinus rhythm with nonspecific ST changes.

1. What is the most likely cause of the patient's heart murmur?

    A. a bicuspid aortic valve with aortic regurgitation
    B. degenerative severe aortic valve stenosis and regurgitation
    C. aortic dilation due to HTN
    D. aortic dilation due to an aortic aneurysm

Subsequently, a TTE is performed. It shows normal LV and RV size and function. The aortic valve anatomy could not be clearly determined. The aorta was dilated at the aortic sinuses to 4.0 cm, the sinotubular junction to 4.4 cm, and the ascending aorta to 4.5 cm. There was moderate effacement of the sinotubular junction. The peak and mean aortic gradients were 22/13 mm Hg, and there was grade 2+ aortic regurgitation. A small circumferential pericardial effusion was also detected. Laboratory tests revealed an erythrocyte sedimentation rate of 74.

2. What additional test would be most helpful in determining the etiology of the patient's aortic regurgitation?
   A. cardiac catheterization
   B. MRI of the aorta and magnetic resonance angiography (MRA) of the great vessels
   C. CT scan of the aorta
   D. CXR

MRI and MRA were performed. They showed enlargement of the aorta, as noted on the TTE, with uniform thickening of the aortic walls. There was sparing of the upper extremity branch vessels.

3. What is the most likely diagnosis for the patient's aortic regurgitation and aortic enlargement?
   A. Takayasu's arteritis
   B. annuloaortic ectasia
   C. hypertensive heart disease
   D. giant cell arteritis

Case 2 (Questions 4 and 5)

An 18-year-old woman presents for her annual physical examination. She had a brother with Marfan's syndrome who was 24 years old when he died suddenly. She also has a history of steroid-dependent asthma.

Physical Examination

The patient is 5' 7" and 150 lb.
Her span to height ratio is greater than 1.05.
The head and neck examination is notable for a high-arched palate, and a slit-lamp examination shows ectopia lentis.
The musculoskeletal examination is notable for a pectus carinatum and a positive wrist and thumb sign.
The cardiac examination is notable for a mitral valve click and a soft murmur of MR.

4. What additional testing is needed to determine whether this woman has Marfan's syndrome?
   A. a TTE
   B. an ECG
   C. a chest CT of the aorta
   D. no additional testing

A TTE is performed that shows mitral valve prolapse with 1+ MR. The aortic sinuses are dilated at 5.5 cm, with moderate effacement of the sinotubular junction. The ascending aorta is measured at 3.6 cm. There is no aortic regurgitation. See Figure 1 for the TEE from a patient with a similar finding.

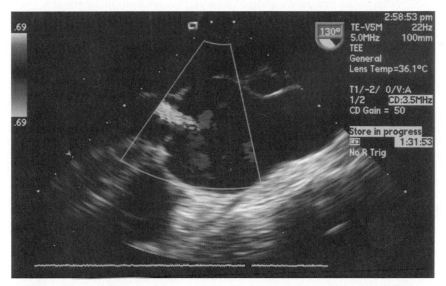

FIGURE 1 TEE. Long-axis view in a patient with Marfan's syndrome, showing dilation of the aortic sinuses, effacement of the sinotubular junction, and normal ascending aortic dimension. Mild aortic regurgitation is also seen due to annular dilation.

5. What is the most appropriate recommendation to be made to this patient after the TTE?

A. repeat the TTE in 6 months
B. initiate a beta-blocker
C. no treatment; avoid strenuous exertion or contact sports
D. elective aortic replacement surgery

Case 3 (Questions 6–8)

A 67-year-old man with long-standing HTN presents to the emergency room (ER) with sudden-onset chest pain, described as ripping in quality, which has subsided since its onset. He underwent a cardiac catheterization 1 year previously due to an abnormal treadmill ECG that showed only a 50% lesion in the mid–left anterior descending coronary artery. His medications include aspirin, gemfibrozil, and nifedipine. Other medical problems include O_2-dependent chronic obstructive pulmonary disease.

Physical Examination

He appears diaphoretic.
BP is 106/54 mm Hg in the right arm and 72/35 mm Hg in the left arm.
The jugular venous pressure is elevated.
The heart sounds are muffled, and there is no audible systolic or diastolic murmur.
The pulses are absent in the left arm.
The ECG on presentation shows ST elevation in the inferior leads and very low voltage.
The CXR shows cardiomegaly, with a globular-shaped heart and interstitial edema.

6. What is the first medication that should be given to this patient?

   A. thrombolytic therapy
   B. sodium nitroprusside
   C. IV ganglionic blocking agent
   D. none of the above

7. Which of the following is the first diagnostic test that should be performed?

   A. cardiac enzymes
   B. MRI of the aorta
   C. CT of the chest
   D. TTE or TEE
   E. cardiac catheterization

A TTE was performed, confirming a pericardial effusion and signs of cardiac tamponade.

8. What interventions should be performed next for the management of this patient?

   A. cardiac catheterization
   B. emergent aortic surgery
   C. Swan-Ganz catheterization
   D. pericardiocentesis

9. A 36-year-old man with a known bicuspid aortic valve develops sudden onset of headache, mental status changes, and unequal pupils. He is rushed to an ER, and a CT scan is done that shows an intracerebral bleed. Except for a known history of HTN, he has no known medical problems and no history of drug abuse. A visit to his physician's office 1 week before this event revealed a BP of 120/75 mm Hg on metoprolol and ramipril and a negative review of systems. What is the most likely reason for the patient's intracerebral bleed?

   A. hypertensive crisis
   B. aortic dissection
   C. cerebral aneurysm rupture
   D. mycotic aneurysm associated with endocarditis

Case 4 (Questions 10 and 11)

A 74-year-old man presents to the ER with lower back pain ongoing for 3 hours. The pain is described as sharp, occurring at rest. He has no associated symptoms of shortness of breath, chest pain, or presyncope. His past medical history is notable for a coronary artery bypass graft (CABG) 5 years ago, HTN, and continued tobacco use. At the time of his CABG, he was noted to have a 4.5-cm ascending aortic aneurysm. His medications include aspirin, an ACE inhibitor, and a beta-blocker.

Physical Examination

BP is 180/110 mm Hg.
Pulse rate is 90 bpm.
The lung and cardiac examinations are unremarkable, and no cardiac murmur is heard.
The abdomen is mildly tender.
No bruit is audible.
The pulses are equal but diminished in the lower extremities.

The ECG shows sinus rhythm with nonspecific ST changes and an old inferior MI.

A panel of laboratory tests, including liver function tests, amylase, and lipase, is normal.

10. What is the most appropriate diagnostic procedure to perform next?
    A. TTE
    B. TEE
    C. CT of the chest and abdomen
    D. aortography

The patient has presented to a community hospital that has access to a cardiac catheterization laboratory but not immediate access to a CT scan or TEE. Therefore, a cardiac catheterization and aortography are performed. The catheterization shows patent grafts and adequate filling of the distal native coronaries. Aortography demonstrates an ascending aortic aneurysm of 4.8 cm and a descending aortic aneurysm of 5.3 cm but no evidence of dissection. The patient continues to have ongoing pain despite high doses of beta-blockers and sodium nitroprusside as well as opioid analgesics.

11. What is most appropriate next decision for management?
    A. discharge, with no further interventions or testing required
    B. CT of the abdomen in the morning
    C. intensifying the medical regimen of beta-blockers and afterload reduction
    D. transfer the patient to a nearby facility for CT of the aorta, including the chest and abdomen

12. A 62-year-old man presents for a routine annual examination. He has a history of HTN that is managed with nifedipine. He is active and has no symptoms.

    BP is 162/88 mm Hg in both arms.
    Pulse rate is 70 bpm.
    The heart and lung examination is unremarkable.
    His abdominal examination reveals a pulsatile mass.
    An ECG shows sinus rhythm and a complete RBBB.
    An abdominal ultrasound finds an infrarenal abdominal aortic aneurysm of 3.9 cm.

    What is the most appropriate management step?
    A. initiate a beta-blocker and repeat ultrasound in 6 months
    B. refer for abdominal aortic aneurysm surgery
    C. refer for aortic stenting
    D. repeat ultrasound in 2 years

Case 5 (Questions 13–15)

A 76-year-old man presents to the ER with severe sharp chest pain that began 2 hours previously. He has a history of HTN; had CABG 2 years ago, after an MI; and continues to smoke. The CABG was performed off-pump due to severe atheroma of the ascending aorta seen by intraoperative TEE. The patient's pain has not subsided with the initiation of IV heparin, nitroglycerin, and beta-blockers. The pain is different in character from the pain before his MI.

Physical Examination

BP is 160/94 mm Hg.
Pulse is 76 bpm.
The lung and heart sounds are normal.
The pulses are diminished in the lower extremities.

The ECG shows a chronic left anterior hemiblock and RBBB.

The initial set of cardiac enzymes is negative.

13. What diagnostic test is *least* appropriate to perform next?
    A. cardiac catheterization
    B. aortogram
    C. TEE
    D. MRI

Despite the severe atheroma in the aorta, the physician taking care of the patient is not convinced that he does not have an acute coronary syndrome and so performs a cardiac catheterization. It shows that the grafts are patent, and there is no culprit lesion of the native vessels. He then decides to perform aortography, and a focal outpouching is seen in the aortic wall in the proximal ascending aorta at the site of a large atheroma (Fig. 2). Contrast dye collects slowly in this region. The patient's chest pain is intensifying.

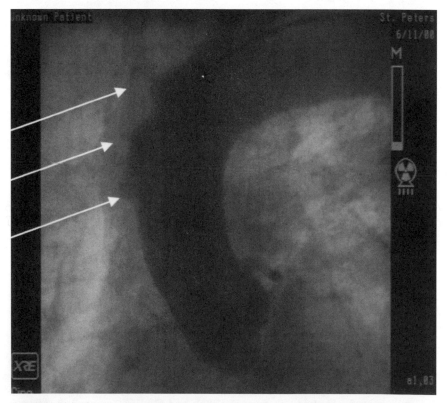

FIGURE 2 Aortogram in a patient with multiple penetrating aortic ulcers, seen as outpouching of the anterior surface of the ascending aortic wall. The arrows show three separate ulcers in the ascending aorta and in the aortic arch. (Image compliments of Dr. Wael Jaber, Cleveland Clinic Foundation.)

14. What is the most appropriate management step to take next?

   A. medical management with beta-blockers and afterload reduction only
   B. medical management and transfer to the operating room immediately; do intraoperative TEE
   C. medical management and obtain an MR or CT in the morning
   D. medical management and obtain a TEE in the morning

15. What is the most likely diagnosis?

   A. aortic dissection
   B. aortic aneurysm
   C. intramural hematoma
   D. penetrating aortic ulcer

Case 6 (Questions 16–18)

A 60-year-old European woman presents to her physician with new-onset claudication in her left leg, dizziness, headache, and a cold right hand. She has no chest pain or shortness of breath. There is no significant past medical history. She does not smoke and has no cardiac risk factors.

Physical Examination

BP is 170/82 mm Hg in the left arm and 140/68 mm Hg in the right arm.
Lung sounds are clear.
The cardiac examination is notable for a normal S_1 and S_2 and II/IV diastolic decrescendo murmur at the left sternal border. The right brachial pulse is diminished. A bruit is heard over the left carotid artery and right subclavian artery. The lower extremity pulses are diminished.

16. What is the best test for diagnosing the patient's condition?

   A. TEE
   B. carotid duplex ultrasound
   C. MRI of the head and carotid vessels
   D. angiography

Angiography is performed and shows a long segment of narrowing involving the right subclavian and left common carotid artery. There is also a segment of distal aorta and left iliac artery.

17. What medical therapy is *least* appropriate?

   A. warfarin
   B. methotrexate or cyclophosphamide
   C. corticosteroids
   D. antihypertensive agents

18. What is the most likely diagnosis?

   A. Behçet's disease
   B. relapsing polychondritis
   C. giant cell arteritis
   D. Takayasu's arteritis

Case 7 (Questions 19 and 20)

A 78-year-old man is seen by his primary care physician for a routine physical examination. He has a history of HTN and underwent CABG 7 years before. His cholesterol levels remain greater than 200, despite lipid-lowering agents. His medications include aspirin, gemfibrozil, atenolol, captopril, and hydralazine.

Physical Examination

BP is 188/94 mm Hg in the left arm.
The clinician performs a maneuver whereby the cuff is inflated to obliterate the brachial and radial pulse and palpates a rigid, noncompressible radial artery on the same side.

19. What is the most likely explanation for this finding?
    A. peripheral embolism
    B. noncompliant peripheral vessels
    C. brachial artery dissection with collateral circulation
    D. brachial artery occlusion with collateral circulation

20. What is the significance of this finding?
    A. overestimation of the intraarterial BP
    B. underestimation of the intraarterial BP
    C. no difference between the cuff and intraarterial BP

Case 8 (Questions 21 and 22)

A 45-year-old man is referred to a tertiary facility for elective mitral valve repair with severe MR. The referring TTE notes a possible cleft mitral valve. A repeat TTE is performed, and the cardiologist describes the anatomy as a congenitally corrected transposition of the great arteries.

21. Which of the following findings is *not* consistent with this anatomy?
    A. situs solitus
    B. AV discordance
    C. AV concordance
    D. ventriculoarterial discordance

22. What is the most likely explanation for the patient's MR?
    A. a cleft mitral valve
    B. Ebstein's anomaly of the tricuspid valve associated with the left-sided RV
    C. Ebstein's anomaly of the mitral valve associated with the left-sided RV
    D. mitral valve prolapse

Case 9 (Questions 23 and 24)

A 30-year-old man is referred to a cardiology clinic for evaluation of a heart murmur. He had an uneventful childhood, except that on two separate occasions he fractured his arm and leg. He has also developed hearing loss over the past year. He has no shortness of breath or chest pain.

Physical Examination

He is of normal stature.

The vital signs are normal.

The cardiac examination is notable for a decreased S_1 and normal S_2 with a III/IV diastolic decrescendo murmur. There are no gallops.

The pulses are normal, and the extremities are hypermobile.

There is no abnormality of the skin.

A TTE shows a dilated aortic root of 4.7 cm and severe aortic regurgitation with a dilated LV.

23. What other finding of the physical examination is most consistent with the patient's diagnosis?

    A. ectopia lentis
    B. blue sclerae
    C. high-arched palate
    D. thumb sign

24. What is the most likely diagnosis for this patient?

    A. Ehlers-Danlos syndrome
    B. Marfan's syndrome
    C. osteogenesis imperfecta
    D. homocystinuria

Case 10 (Questions 25–27)

A 65-year-old man presents to the ER with severe, tearing chest pain that started while he was shoveling snow. He has a history of HTN that is poorly regulated. He has a history of CAD, with a stent to the left anterior descending coronary artery 4 months ago.

Physical Examination

BP is 190/110 mm Hg.

Pulse is 90 bpm.

The cardiac examination is notable for a normal S_1 and S_2, with an S_4 gallop and II/IV systolic ejection murmur at the left sternal border.

An ECG shows sinus rhythm and no ST changes.

An initial set of cardiac enzymes is normal.

25. What is the most appropriate diagnostic test?

    A. cardiac catheterization
    B. TTE
    C. aortogram
    D. CT scan of the chest

A cardiologist in the ER seeing another patient offers to perform a TEE at the bedside. He sees an ascending aortic aneurysm measuring 6.2 cm, with a continuous crescentic area of wall thickening extending from the right coronary artery to the innominate artery. There are areas of echolucency within the walls. There is no intimal flap. There is intimal calcium that is displaced.

26. What is the most appropriate management?
    A. medical therapy with beta-blockers and nitroprusside
    B. urgent aortic replacement surgery
    C. medical therapy with beta-blockers and nitroprusside and repeat TEE or CT in 24 hours
    D. MRI to confirm findings and assess branch vessels

27. Which of the following is a *false* statement about the aortic disease of this patient?
    A. The prognosis is similar to an aortic dissection with an intimal tear.
    B. Controversy exists regarding the management of patients with this condition occurring after iatrogenic procedures.
    C. Surgery is only indicated when a concomitant intimal tear is seen.
    D. Aortography may miss the diagnosis.

Case 11 (Questions 28–30)

A 44-year-old man is admitted to the hospital due to a left hemisphere stroke with right arm and leg weakness. He has no known history of HTN or smoking, although his total cholesterol level is 314.

Physical Examination

The ECG shows sinus rhythm.
A carotid duplex ultrasound shows less than 20% obstruction bilaterally.
A head CT demonstrates an area of left cortical echogenicity consistent with an middle cerebral artery territory embolism.

28. Which test is most likely to elucidate the etiology of the patient's stroke?
    A. TTE with contrast injection
    B. telemetry monitoring
    C. MRI/MRA
    D. TEE

The patient is maintained on telemetry, and sinus rhythm without atrial arrhythmias is present. A TTE shows normal LV function and no valvular abnormalities. A contrast study is negative for right-to-left shunt. A TEE shows extensive aortic arch atheroma.

29. Which characteristic is *least* consistent with aortic atheroma resulting in the patient's stroke?
    A. size greater than or equal to 4 mm
    B. calcification of atheroma
    C. mobility of the atheroma
    D. absence of calcification of the atheroma

30. Which statement is *true* regarding performing CABG in a similar patient with aortic arch atheroma and focal areas of atheroma in the ascending aorta?
    A. Palpation of the aorta by the surgeon for calcified plaque correlates with findings of atheroma by TEE.
    B. Alternative sites of clamping or cannulation may reduce stroke risk.
    C. Aortic arch endarterectomy is recommended.
    D. Replacement of the ascending aorta is recommended due to increased likelihood of stroke.

Case 12 (Questions 31 and 32)

A 24-year-old Asian man presents to his primary care doctor with the report of claudication and shortness of breath. He was diagnosed with a patent ductus arteriosus as a child but has had infrequent follow-up visits, because he has felt well until the past year.

Physical Examination

He is normal in stature.
BP is 102/64 mm Hg in the right arm.
Pulse is 80 bpm.
There is no central cyanosis.
Lung sounds are clear.
The cardiac examination is notable for a normal S_1 and loud S_2 (P_2).
The feet bilaterally are cyanotic.

31. Which additional physical examination finding is *not* consistent with the patient's abnormality?

    A. pink hands
    B. decreased BP in the lower extremities
    C. a continuous heart murmur
    D. an RV heave

32. Which diagnosis best describes the patient's condition?

    A. Eisenmenger's physiology
    B. coarctation of the aorta
    C. patent ductus arteriosus without Eisenmenger's physiology
    D. Takayasu's arteritis

Case 13 (Questions 33 and 34)

A 28-year-old man is referred to a cardiologist for exertional dyspnea and a cardiac murmur. As a child, he was evaluated by a pediatrician for congenital heart disease due to mild mental retardation. No specific diagnosis was made.

Physical Examination

His vital signs are normal.
The cardiac examination is notable for a III/IV systolic ejection murmur radiating to the neck. The left brachial pulse is diminished relative to the right brachial pulse.

33. What diagnosis best explains the patient's disorder?

    A. patent ductus arteriosus
    B. coarctation of the aorta
    C. supravalvular pulmonary stenosis
    D. Williams syndrome

34. What additional finding on physical examination is *not* consistent with the patient's diagnosis?

    A. decreased BP in the left arm relative to the right arm
    B. decreased (A_2) component of S_2
    C. small chin and wide-spaced eyes

35. What abnormal protein is produced due to the genetic defect associated with Marfan's syndrome?

    A. procollagen
    B. elastin
    C. fibrillin

36. Which are the most common arteries affected by peripheral vascular disease (PVD) in patients younger than 40 years?

    A. aorta, popliteal
    B. iliac, femoral
    C. femoral, aorta
    D. aorta, iliac

37. A 65-year-old man (twin 1) reports pain in his calves while walking that is relieved with rest. His identical twin brother (twin 2) reports pain in his buttocks and hips while walking that is relieved with rest. Which of the two brothers is most likely to have PVD based on the history?

    A. twin 1
    B. twin 2
    C. both twins
    D. neither twin

38. Which of the following statements regarding claudication is *true*?

    A. Claudication is a progressive cramping or aching sensation that begins when one is standing.
    B. Claudication always affects both lower extremities.
    C. Pseudoclaudication is claudication that affects the arms and not the legs.
    D. Claudication is a cramping sensation that affects a muscle group that is distal to an obstruction in an artery and that is relieved with rest.

39. Which of the following statements about the ankle-brachial index (ABI) is *true*?

    A. The ABI gives only an indication whether PVD is present or absent.
    B. Patients with high ABI values (greater than 1.3) have no concern for PVD.
    C. A patient with an ABI of 0.9 has more severe PVD than a patient with an ABI of 0.3.
    D. There is a higher associated mortality in patients with severe PVD as assessed by ABI than in patients with mild PVD.

Case 14 (Questions 40–42)

A 72-year-old man with a history of HTN for 5 years and current smoking is seen in a cardiology clinic. He reports that after walking 0.5 mile, he develops shortness of breath and pain in his right lower thigh and calf. If he stops walking, both the pain and shortness of breath subside. He denies any chest pain.

Physical Examination

The BP in his left arm is 200/100 mm Hg and in his right arm is 180/92 mm Hg. His BP in his right ankle is 180/80 mm Hg, and the BP in his left ankle is 200/90 mm Hg.

40. What is the ABI of his right leg?

    A. 0.9
    B. 1.0
    C. 0.95
    D. 0.1

41. What recommendation should be made regarding management of this patient?

    A. referral to a vascular surgeon for consideration of revascularization
    B. referral for a peripheral angiogram and recommendation to stop walking
    C. referral to a smoking cessation clinic, advice to continue walking, and initiation of antihypertensive therapy
    D. prescription for antiinflammatory medications

42. Laboratory tests on the same patient reveal a HgbA$_1$C of 4.5, an LDL of 125 mg per dL, and an HDL of 45 mg per dL. Which of the following should you add to your recommendations?

    A. nothing, because the laboratory tests are all normal
    B. prescribe a statin
    C. order a pharmacologic stress test due to exertional dyspnea
    D. prescribe an aspirin
    E. B, C, and D

43. Which of the following is a *true* statement regarding PVD?

    A. Patients with PVD who are asymptomatic are similar to patients without PVD with regard to their lifespan.
    B. There is a high risk of limb amputation in patients with PVD.
    C. Symptomatic PVD carries only a 5% increased risk of death within 5 years.
    D. Most patients with PVD need surgery or angioplasty.
    E. None of the above is true.

44. In which of the following patients should revascularization be considered?

    A. a 55-year-old man who develops leg pain after walking 5 miles
    B. a 45-year-old diabetic woman with intermittent claudication and an ulcer in her left third toe
    C. a 90-year-old man with a history of HTN and hypercholesterolemia who develops calf pain after climbing two flights of stairs
    D. a 65-year-old woman who develops pain in both of her legs when standing or walking

45. A 65-year-old postmenopausal woman with a strong family history of CAD is referred to you for BP management. On review of systems, she states that she develops severe lower-thigh and calf pain (worse in her right leg) after walking one block, but this is relieved with rest.

    BP is 160/100 mm Hg in the right arm, 160/90 mm Hg in the left arm, 120/80 mm Hg in her right ankle, and 140/80 mm Hg in her left ankle.
    She is on no medications.

    Which medication should you consider starting?

    A. ACE inhibitor
    B. calcium channel blocker
    C. alpha$_1$-blocker
    D. alpha$_2$-blocker

46. A 40-year-old man presents to his physician with a report of severe inter-mittent claudication with limited exertion. An angiogram reveals a focal lesion in his right iliac artery that is 3 cm long with a 90% stenosis. What management should you recommend?

    A. pentoxifylline (Trental)
    B. percutaneous angioplasty and stenting
    C. peripheral bypass surgery
    D. none of the above

47. A 65-year-old woman with diabetes and a long history of PVD is referred for evaluation. Five years ago, she underwent percutaneous angioplasty for a lesion in her right superficial femoral artery. She had relief for 2 years, after which she underwent stenting of the area. Again, she was pain free until 6 months ago. A repeat angiogram revealed a long, 12-cm narrowing in the proximal portion of her right superficial femoral artery, involving the stented region. Which of the following statements is *not* true?

    A. Stenting has failed, so bypass surgery should be recommended.
    B. Bypass surgery is the best option, because there is a long segment of severe atherosclerosis.
    C. Medical therapy should be recommended, because angioplasty and stenting have failed, and she is at high risk for surgery.

48. A 67-year-old man with CAD is seen emergently in your office because of sudden, severe pain and numbness in his right leg that started 1 hour before. On physical examination, his right dorsalis pedis pulse could not be pal-pated. Which of the following should *not* be done?

    A. start IV heparin with partial thromboplastin time goals of 60 to 80
    B. start IV thrombolytics
    C. perform an angiogram of his right leg
    D. perform intraarterial thrombolysis using a catheter to deliver the lytic agent to the thrombus

49. Which of the following is *not* a predictor for a good result from percutane-ous peripheral vessel angioplasty?

    A. The stenosis is in a large artery.
    B. The stenosis is 13 cm long.
    C. There is good proximal and distal circulation (run-off).
    D. There is no history of diabetes.

50. The ABI may *not* be reliable in which of the following scenarios?

    A. severe PVD affecting both upper and lower extremities
    B. patients with noncompressible ankle arteries (ankle systolic BP greater than 300 mm Hg)
    C. a diabetic patient with a foot ulcer with an ABI of 1.4
    D. all of the above

51. In the scenario in which an ABI is not decreased but PVD is highly suspected, which of the following tests should *not* be used to assess for PVD?

    A. duplex ultrasonography
    B. pulse volume recording (PVR)
    C. MRA
    D. exercise testing
    E. CT scan

52. A 72-year-old woman is seen for evaluation in a cardiology clinic. She has a history of HTN, hypercholesterolemia, and current smoking. For the past 6 months, she has noticed that she gets left arm pain when brushing her hair with her left arm but has no pain using her right arm. What test should you most likely recommend first?

    A. duplex ultrasonography
    B. ABI
    C. MRA
    D. dipyridamole (Persantine) stress test

53. For infrapopliteal arterial disease, under what circumstances should revascularization be attempted?

    A. if the patient is a diabetic
    B. if the patient has poor distal run-off on angiogram
    C. if the lesion is long
    D. if there is rest pain or an ischemic limb

54. Which of the following statements is *true* regarding the various techniques to diagnose renal artery stenosis?

    A. Renal artery duplex ultrasonography is an excellent screening test for renal artery stenosis, with both a high sensitivity and specificity.
    B. A renal angiogram is the gold standard and should be done on all patients initially.
    C. An MRA is the gold standard but has a high false-negative rate.
    D. Captopril renal scintigraphy is most useful when there is significant renal dysfunction.

55. Which of the following statements regarding percutaneous transluminal renal angioplasty (PTRA) is *true*?

    A. When PTRA is performed on nonostial renal artery stenosis, which is caused by fibromuscular dysplasia, good results are obtained.
    B. PTRA of atherosclerotic ostial renal artery stenosis has excellent results.
    C. In patients with Takayasu's arteritis, lesions are usually very amenable to PTRA.
    D. The use of stents has not changed the rate of restenosis in patients with atherosclerotic renal artery stenosis.

56. What is the approximate risk of stroke and death associated with carotid endarterectomy (CEA)?

    A. less than 1%
    B. 6%
    C. 20%
    D. 50%

57. A 60-year-old man is referred for evaluation of a 70% stenosis of his right internal carotid artery. He has had no strokes, TIAs, or other neurologic symptoms. What should you recommend?

A. medical management
B. a CEA in a hospital with significant experience
C. angioplasty of his right internal CEA

58. Which of the following drugs has been shown to be most effective for treating claudication?

A. papaverine
B. pentoxifylline
C. cilostazol
D. all of the above

59. An 82-year-old woman with diabetes and a gangrenous left first toe is seen in consultation for PVD. Which of the following test results is consistent with her presentation?

A. ABI = 1.0, normal PVR
B. ABI = 1.5, normal PVR
C. ABI = 1.4, significantly decreased amplitude on PVR
D. ABI = 0.7, significantly high amplitude on PVR

60. In the general population, which of the following is the most prevalent cause of renal artery stenosis?

A. fibromuscular dysplasia
B. atherosclerosis
C. neither
D. both have similar prevalence

61. A 70-year-old man with three-vessel CAD has planned to undergo CABG surgery. You do a physical examination, and his neck examination reveals no carotid bruits. What percentage of patients with significant internal carotid artery stenosis has an audible bruit?

A. 0%
B. 10%
C. 40%
D. 100%

62. Which of the following is *not* a symptom or sign of PVD?

A. disuse atrophy of the lower extremity
B. pain at rest
C. nonhealing ulcers
D. dry gangrene after minor trauma
E. none of the above may be symptoms or signs of PVD

Case 15 (Questions 63–65)

A 38-year-old man is seen by his primary care physician for an ulcer on his left toe. He has been generally healthy and takes no medications. He drinks alcohol and has smoked for 15 years. For the past 4 months, he has had pain in his left calf with ambulation, which for the past week now occurs at rest.

Physical Examination

His vital signs are normal.
The cardiac and lung examinations are normal.
The pulse examination is notable for a positive Allen-test and reduced left dorsalis pedis, posterior tibial, and radial pulse.

63. Which of the following test results would be *inconsistent* with the likely diagnosis?

   A. a normal sedimentation rate and C-reactive protein
   B. a normal cryoglobulin, antiphospholipid antibody, and complement level
   C. a HgbA$_1$C of 11.2
   D. a normal TTE

64. Which of the following tests would *not* be important to confirm the diagnosis?

   A. TEE
   B. arteriography of the involved limbs
   C. biopsy of the involved limb vessel

65. Which of the following treatment options is most likely to benefit this patient?

   A. infusion of prostaglandins
   B. use of calcium channel blockers
   C. discontinuation of smoking
   D. intraarterial thrombolytic therapy
   E. surgical revascularization

66. A 62-year-old woman presents for evaluation of Raynaud phenomenon. Over the past year, she has noticed triphasic discoloration of her right hand that is precipitated by exposure to cold weather. She has also noticed difficulty swallowing. Her examination is unremarkable except for edematous fingertips. Which of the following features is *not* consistent with secondary Raynaud phenomenon?

   A. systemic manifestations
   B. asymmetric involvement
   C. ischemic changes
   D. pulse deficits
   E. all are consistent

67. What treatment recommendation is *least* appropriate for this patient?

   A. ergotamine, as needed, for episodes of discoloration
   B. trial of prazosin
   C. trial of a calcium channel blocker
   D. trial of reserpine
   E. avoidance of cold weather, stress, and tobacco

Case 16 (Questions 68 and 69)

A 78-year-old man is referred to a cardiology clinic for evaluation of edema. He has a history of HTN but no other medical or surgical history. His only medication is amlodipine.

Physical Examination

He has no symptoms.

His vital signs are normal.

His cardiac examination is notable for normal heart sounds and normal jugular venous pressure. His right lower extremity is edematous from the thigh down to the toe.

68. What additional findings on physical examination would *not* be consistent with the type of edema detected in this patient?

   A. edema involving the toes
   B. superficial varicose veins
   C. nonpitting character

69. Which of the following tests is of *least* use in determining the cause of this patient's edema?

   A. abdominal CT scan
   B. prostate-specific antigen and prostate examination
   C. lymphoscintigraphy
   D. venogram

70. A patient is rushed to the ER after a motor vehicle accident between two cars. The CXR shows widening of the mediastinum. What cardiac or aortic structure is *least* likely to be injured?

   A. aortic isthmus
   B. aortic cusp tear with aortic regurgitation
   C. right atrial rupture
   D. LV rupture

ANSWERS

1. D. Aortic dilation due to aortic aneurysm. The clinical history, examination, and ECG do not suggest long-standing HTN as a contributing factor to valvular heart disease. There is no systolic ejection click to suggest a bicuspid valve, and the patient is older than most patients who present with aortic stenosis due to a bicuspid valve. The murmur is not consistent with severe aortic stenosis because it is early peaking and S_2 (A_2) is audible. Therefore, the most likely etiology of the heart murmur is aortic dilation with associated aortic regurgitation. This type of murmur associated with an abnormality of the aorta is often heard along the right sternal border.

2. B. MRI of the aorta and MRA of the great vessels. The presence of aortic dilation, sinotubular effacement, a pericardial effusion, and an elevated erythrocyte sedimentation rate suggests an inflammatory etiology for aortic dilation. Aortic aneurysms can be classified as due to (a) arteriosclerosis, (b) connective tissue disorders, (c) trauma, (d) infectious diseases, (e) inflammatory diseases or "aortitis," and (f) annuloaortic ectasia. Inflammatory aortitis includes numerous systemic diseases that may involve the aorta, including systemic lupus erythematosus, rheumatoid and psoriatic arthritis, systemic sclerosis, relapsing polychondritis, the rheumatoid factor–negative spondyloarthropathies, and other primarily vascular disorders, such as

Takayasu's and giant cell arteritis. MR of the aorta may distinguish characteristic thickening and tissue characteristics that are consistent with inflammatory aortitis.

3. D. Giant cell arteritis. The presence of systemic symptoms, such as headaches and myalgia, as well as pericardial effusion and an elevated sedimentation rate, is consistent with giant cell arteritis as the cause of the aortic aneurysm and secondary aortic regurgitation. Headaches suggest the associated problem of temporal arteritis. The disease affects women twice as often as it does men and is most commonly seen after age 55 years.

   The MRI showed sparing of the branch vessels and uniform thickening of the walls that is consistent with giant cell arteritis and not Takayasu's arteritis. Takayasu's arteritis generally involves younger patients with pulse differences and signs of arterial insufficiency. The MRI typically shows stenosis of branch vessels of the upper or lower extremity. Annuloaortic ectasia is a primary disease of the aorta that morphologically looks similar to Marfan's syndrome and pathologically involves cystic medial necrosis, as in Marfan's syndrome. However, there are no other noncardiovascular systems involved with annuloaortic ectasia.

4. D. No additional testing. The current diagnostic criteria revised by Gent require major criteria in one organ system and minor criteria in a different organ system for diagnosis of Marfan's syndrome when a family history of the disease is present. If no family history is present, two major criteria are required in separate organ systems and one minor criterion in a third organ system. Organ involvement affects the skeletal, ocular, cardiovascular, pulmonary, neurologic, and dermatologic systems. The patient had a major criterion of ectopia lentis and multiple musculoskeletal criteria, including pectus carinatum, a span to height ratio of greater than 1.05, wrist and thumb sign, and high-arched palate. She also has mitral valve prolapse, which is a minor criterion.

5. D. Elective aortic replacement surgery. The most widely cited study of beta-blockade and Marfan's syndrome was performed by Shores and colleagues. This study was an open-label study of adult patients with mild or moderate aortic dilatation and Marfan's syndrome who were randomized to propanolol or no treatment. Patients with asthma were excluded. The follow-up was near 10 years. Patients randomized to propanolol had less aortic dilatation and aortic complications, although the numbers were small for the latter end point.

   The timing of surgery for patients with aortic dilatation due to Marfan's syndrome remains controversial. Surgical morbidity and mortality for elective surgery has decreased over the years, and, therefore, there has been an impetus toward earlier surgery. In addition, the potential for valve-sparing surgery has favored an earlier time of intervention. Current criteria consider the rate of change of aortic size, the presence of aortic regurgitation, the family history of dissection or sudden cardiac death, and the extent of aortic involvement. Most centers consider 5.5 cm an absolute criterion for surgery for aortic root involvement. In general, surgery would be considered for any patient with an aortic size larger than 5 cm and in high-risk patients (e.g., anticipated pregnancy, family history of dissection or sudden death) as early as 4 cm or more. Importantly, aortic size should be adjusted for body size, and some centers use a ratio of greater than 10:1 for the cross-sectional area of the aorta to height ratio for timing surgery.

6. D. None of the above. The clinical history and examination suggest an acute proximal aortic dissection with involvement of the right coronary artery and left subclavian artery. According to the examination, ECG, and CXR, there are signs of CHF that suggest a pericardial effusion and cardiac tamponade. In this setting, thrombolytic therapy would be contraindicated because it is likely that the patient's inferior ECG injury pattern is due to dissection involving the right coronary artery and not coronary thrombosis. Sodium nitroprusside should not be used due to hypotension and the possibility of cardiac tamponade. Furthermore, it should not be used as a sole agent before the use of medications that will decrease dP/dt, such as beta-blockade or nondihydropyridine calcium channel blockers. Sodium nitroprusside results in reflex tachycardia that results in increased force of LV contraction. Ganglionic blocking agents (e.g., trimethaphan) are an option for patients who have contraindications to beta-blockers, such as severe chronic obstructive pulmonary disorder. These medications are not commonly used currently due to the availability of medications with fewer side effects and greater ease of use. In addition, this agent causes hypotension and should not be used in this patient. Therefore, none of these medications should be used in this patient.

7. D. TTE or TEE. A diagnostic test should be performed immediately in this patient. Cardiac enzymes may determine the presence of myocardial injury but not reveal the cause. The advantages, disadvantages, and pitfalls of CT, MRI, and TEE have been reviewed extensively. Each of these tests has high diagnostic accuracy, but their use must be determined based on the relative expertise of each institution, the rapid availability of the test, and the specific individual circumstances of a patient. Given the likelihood of a proximal aortic dissection and the possibility of cardiac tamponade, a TTE or a TEE is best suited for this patient. In institutions that have cardiac surgery, the patient could be taken immediately to the operating room, and a TEE could be performed as the patient is prepared for possible surgery. Otherwise, a limited TTE could assess whether a pericardial effusion and cardiac tamponade are present. Figure 3 shows a TEE in a patient with a dissection but without a pericardial effusion. An example of a cardiac MRI in a patient with an aortic dissection is seen in Figure 4.

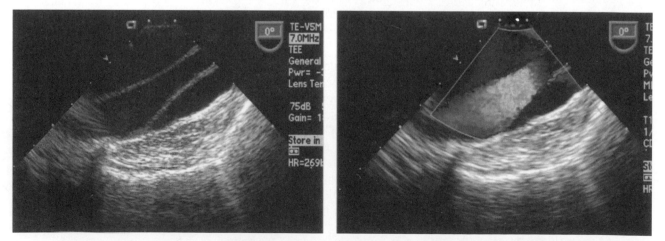

FIGURE 3 TEE (long-axis view) with and without color Doppler, showing the presence of both a true and false lumen in a patient with an aortic dissection.

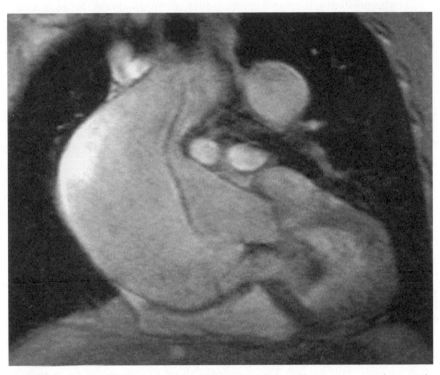

FIGURE 4 Cardiac MRI in a patient with an ascending aortic aneurysm and an aortic dissection.

8. B. Emergent aortic surgery. A proximal aortic dissection with hypotension or cardiac tamponade should be treated by emergent aortic surgery. As noted above, a rapid confirmatory test can be performed on the way to or awaiting the preparation of the operating room. Small retrospective reviews have raised some concerns regarding pericardiocentesis in patients with cardiac tamponade and aortic dissection. Rapid decompensation and death can occur in some patients. Most important, the presence of cardiac tamponade with aortic dissection should mandate immediate surgery. Pericardiocentesis can be performed if the patient is deteriorating rapidly and surgical assistance is not readily available.

Controversy also exists regarding cardiac catheterization for patients with proximal aortic dissection. Proponents of cardiac catheterization argue that patients with severe obstructive CAD require grafting at the time of surgery and that failure to do so will increase the risk for perioperative and postoperative cardiac events. Those who favor not performing cardiac catheterization argue that any delay may increase the risk of death and that an invasive procedure will add further risk of dissection, tamponade, or rupture. Therefore, most centers carefully select those patients who undergo coronary angiography, including those with known CAD, recent unstable coronary symptoms, and new regional wall-motion abnormalities. One study comparing outcomes of patients undergoing surgery for aortic dissection found that those not undergoing cardiac catheterization had similar mortality to those undergoing this procedure.

9. C. Cerebral aneurysm rupture. The history of HTN requiring therapy in a young man with a bicuspid valve suggests the possibility of an aortic coarctation. Given his recent well being and well-controlled BP, aortic dissection,

hypertensive crisis, and endocarditis are unlikely. A known association between aortic coarctation and cerebral aneurysms has been described. Screening for this abnormality with MRI or MRA is often performed for patients when any neurologic symptoms are present or before major surgery, such as cardiac surgery.

10. C. CT of the chest and abdomen. The patient's history is most suggestive of a distal aortic dissection. He has a known thoracic aortic aneurysm, atherosclerosis, and presents hypertensive, with back pain and diminished pulses. Although TEE may be accurate for diagnosis of aortic dissection above the diaphragm, CT scanning may extend imaging to the entire aorta, including the abdominal aorta, and provide information regarding the involvement of branch vessels. Therefore, if both tests were available with equal rapidity and expertise for interpretation, CT would be preferable. Aortography is invasive and could cause further injury to the aorta, although it could provide useful information along with angiography regarding the patency of the patient's bypass grafts and native circulation.

11. D. Transfer the patient to a nearby facility for CT of the aorta, including the chest and abdomen. The patient is experiencing ongoing pain, and the clinical history is still suggestive of an aortic dissection. Although aortography is accurate for diagnosis of an intimal flap with communication with the false lumen, it may not be accurate in detection of an intramural hematoma, because it provides information only about flow within the lumen. CT scanning may reveal a descending thoracic aortic intramural hematoma, and although management is generally medical therapy for distal involvement, the presence of ongoing pain requires diagnosis and could be a reason for surgical consideration. Therefore, immediate transfer and CT imaging should be undertaken.

12. A. Initiate a beta-blocker and repeat ultrasound in 6 months. A noninflammatory abdominal aortic aneurysm of less than 4 cm has a 0% to 2% risk of rupture over 2 years. Therefore, surgery or stenting is usually performed when the size is larger than 5 cm, although consideration is given to early elective surgery for aneurysms in the range of 4.5 to 5.0 cm. To determine the stability of an aortic aneurysm once it is detected, a follow-up ultrasound is usually performed in 6 months. The rate of change is also considered as a strong indicator of the risk of rupture. Beta-blockers have been shown to delay the rate of aneurysm enlargement and would be indicated for this patient with HTN.

13. A. Cardiac catheterization is the least appropriate. The character of the pain that is different from a prior MI, the lack of relief with antianginal therapy, and the absence of ECG changes or positive enzymes suggest that an acute coronary syndrome is not the cause of the patient's discomfort. Other considerations include an aortic dissection. Less invasive imaging modalities are preferred to make this diagnosis. At most institutions, a TEE can be done with less time delay with an equal accuracy to an MRI.

14. B. Medical management and transfer to the operating room immediately; do intraoperative TEE. The finding on the aortogram is highly suggestive of a pseudoaneurysm of the aortic wall due to inward rupture of atheroma into the aortic wall. This finding is an indication for immediate surgical correc-

tion because of the potential for aortic rupture. Further confirmation of the diagnosis is not required. Two views of the TEE in this patient are shown in Figure 5.

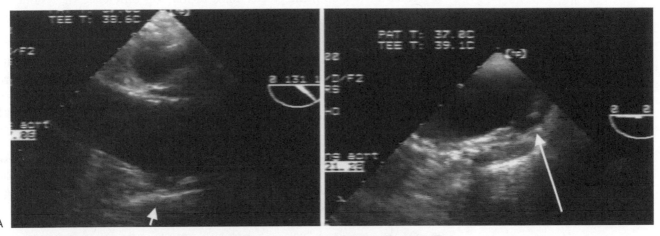

FIGURE 5 TEE (two views at different levels) in the same patient as in Figure 2. The images show extensive calcific aortic atheroma and two penetrating aortic ulcers. **A:** The arrow points to an ulcer in the ascending aorta. **B:** The arrow points to a second ulcer in the aortic arch. (Images compliments of Dr. Wael Jaber, Cleveland Clinic Foundation.)

15. D. Penetrating aortic ulcer. Aortic dissections can be broadly categorized into typical and variant forms. Svennson proposed a classification description as follows: (a) classic dissection or dual lumens, (b) intramural hematoma, (c) limited dissection, (d) penetrating aortic ulcer, and (e) iatrogenic or traumatic dissection. A penetrating aortic ulcer occurs when aortic atheroma ruptures into the aortic media through the internal elastic lamina. Subsequently, an aneurysm, pseudoaneurysm, localized dissection, hematoma, or aortic rupture may develop.

Penetrating ulcers can be diagnosed by aortography, CT, MRI, or TEE. Typical findings include a focal outpouching and ulcer crater in the region of severe, calcified atheroma. A limited or a dissection flap may also be present. Localized flow can be seen by contrast opacification or color or pulsed Doppler. The presence of ongoing pain and the possibility of a pseudoaneurysm would be a definite indication for surgery in this patient.

16. D. Angiography. The patient presents with pulse deficits, bruits, or arterial insufficiency in multiple distributions, including the upper and lower extremity, suggesting a systemic disease. Angiography or aortography would most directly define the site and extent of arterial disease. The appearance of the lesions may also help with determining the etiology of the vascular disease (i.e., atherosclerotic vs. vasculitic).

17. A. Warfarin is least appropriate. The findings are suggestive of a vasculitis and not arteriosclerosis. Therefore, antiinflammatory and immunosuppressive therapy is indicated. Antihypertensive therapy may also be considered. There is no definite role for anticoagulation.

18. D. Takayasu's arteritis. This is an inflammatory disease of large and medium-sized arteries that generally occurs in middle-aged patients. Although most commonly described in Japanese patients, it has been described in many

continents. A diagnostic classification proposed by the American College of Rheumatology includes the necessity for three of six criteria: (a) age older than 40 years, (b) claudication on an extremity, (c) decreased brachial artery pulse, (d) greater than 10-mm Hg difference in systolic BP between arms, (e) bruit over the subclavian arteries or the aorta, or (f) angiographic narrowing or occlusion of the aorta or branches.

19. B. Noncompliant peripheral vessels. This is Osler's maneuver. The radial artery remains rigid and noncompressible, despite obliteration of the brachial and radial pulses. The explanation for this is a stiff and noncompliant arterial system due to atherosclerosis. This is considered a positive Osler's sign.

20. A. Overestimation of the intraarterial BP. A positive Osler's sign suggests that the cuff pressures by sphygmomanometer may overestimate the intraarterial BP due to the increased pressure required to compress the stiff vessels. The patient is considered to have pseudohypertension.

21. C. AV concordance is not consistent with this anatomy. Congenitally corrected transposition of the great arteries is an uncommon form of congenital heart disease in the adult. The basic anatomy includes (a) situs solitus (normal viscera location, systemic veins to the right-sided right atrium, and pulmonary veins to the left-sided left atrium), (b) AV discordance (right atrium to right-sided LV, left atrium to left-sided RV), and (c) ventriculoarterial discordance (LV to posterior rightward PA, RV to anterior leftward aorta).

22. B. Ebstein's anomaly of the tricuspid valve associated with the left-sided RV. The AV valve follows the ventricle so that the tricuspid valve is the left-sided valve associated with the left-sided RV. A cleft mitral valve is trileaflet and was confused with the tricuspid valve because it was not initially recognized that the patient had congenitally corrected transposition of the great arteries. Ebstein's anomaly of the tricuspid valve occurs frequently in these patients. Therefore, the patient's MR is actually tricuspid regurgitation due to an abnormal tricuspid valve with Ebstein's malformation.

23. B. Blue sclerae. The patient has a connective tissue disorder affecting the aortic root and resulting in aortic regurgitation. Marfan's syndrome is the most common connective tissue disorder affecting the aorta and is associated with ocular and skeletal abnormalities, including ectopia lentis and a high-arched palate. It is not associated with hearing loss, recurrent fractures, or blue sclerae.

24. C. Osteogenesis imperfecta. Osteogenesis imperfecta is a heritable disease of the connective tissue with mutations in procollagen that is associated with bone fragility, ocular changes (most notably blue sclerae), abnormal dentition, and hearing loss. Some patients have cardiovascular manifestations similar to Marfan's syndrome, with aortic root dilatation, aortic regurgitation, and mitral valve prolapse.

25. D. CT scan of the chest. The presence of tearing chest pain and HTN suggests an aortic dissection. Recent revascularization on the left anterior descending coronary artery, without ECG changes or cardiac enzyme elevation, makes an acute coronary syndrome less likely. CT of the chest to determine whether an aortic dissection is present is noninvasive and can be

performed rapidly, without the risks of further disruption of the aorta if a dissection is present.

26. B. Urgent aortic replacement surgery. The TEE description is consistent with an intramural hematoma. There is a continuous crescentic mural thickening without the presence of an intimal flap and dual lumens. The intimal calcium is displaced, differentiating an intramural hematoma from aortic atheroma. There are echolucent regions, with flow consistent with intramural blood vessels, likely due to ruptured vessels within the vasa vasorum. An example of this is seen in Figure 6.

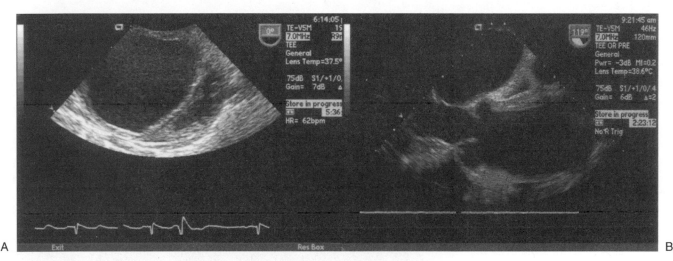

FIGURE 6 TEE (**A:** short-axis view; **B:** long-axis view) in a patient with an intramural hematoma of the ascending aorta. Typical features include (a) continuous crescentic mural thickening without the presence of either an intimal flap or dual lumens, (b) displacement of intimal calcium, and (c) echolucent regions.

There is controversy regarding whether this variant form of aortic dissection is as fatal as the classic form with an intimal flap. Most natural history studies of unoperated patients have shown an equally poor prognosis. In this patient, the hematoma is extensive and associated with a large ascending aortic aneurysm. Generally, surgery is considered in atherosclerotic ascending aortic aneurysms in the range of 5.5 to 6.0 cm in size.

27. C. As noted in the explanation of question 26, intramural hematomas involving the ascending aorta are generally managed similarly to aortic dissections with intimal tears because the natural history is similar. An exception may be those due to iatrogenic procedures, such as a percutaneous coronary intervention or cardiac catheterization. Often, these may be limited, retrograde dissections, and many believe that conservative management can be undertaken in select patients. Those with intimal flaps may thrombose spontaneously. A pitfall of aortography is that it visualizes only the lumen and may miss the presence of an intramural hematoma.

28. D. TEE. With the absence of significant carotid artery disease and the location of the stroke in the middle cerebral artery territory, an embolic source is likely. Therefore, a TEE would be the more likely technique to reveal the etiology of the patient's event. It is possible that the patient has small-vessel intracranial disease that could be demonstrated by MRA, although, given

his age and the absence of significant carotid artery disease, a cardioembolic source seems more likely.

29. **B.** Calcification of atheroma is least consistent with aortic atheroma resulting in the patient's stroke. Factors that are most highly associated with embolic risk include mobility, size greater than or equal to 4 mm, and the absence of calcification. It is speculated that those plaques without calcification are more likely vulnerable plaques that may have superimposed thrombus. Some studies have also shown that ulcerated plaques are more often associated with embolic events.

30. **B.** Alternative sites of cross clamping and cannulation, such as femoral or axillary arteries, may reduce the risk of stroke. Aortic arch endarterectomy has been found to increase the risk of perioperative stroke and is seldom recommended. Replacement of the ascending aorta in this patient would be unlikely to reduce the risk of stroke due to the presence of severe atheroma in the ascending aorta. Palpation of the aorta by the surgeon is usually not accurate in finding noncalcified atheroma that may be detected by TEE. Figure 7 shows aortic atheroma as seen by the TEE.

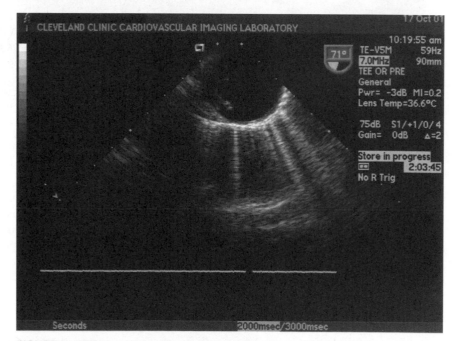

FIGURE 7 TEE of a patient with severe protruding atheroma in the aorta.

31. **B.** Decreased BP in the lower extremities is not consistent with the patient's abnormality. The presence of cyanotic feet in a patient with a patent ductus arteriosus and pink upper extremities suggests the onset of pulmonary HTN and right-to-left shunting. Concomitant findings would include a loud P_2 and an RV heave. The classic machinery murmur of a patent ductus arteriosus may not be heard; technically, if it extends through S_2 uninterrupted, it is still considered a continuous murmur. The blood flow to the lower extremities will be deoxygenated blood, although the BP in the lower extremities would not necessarily be reduced.

32. A. Eisenmenger's physiology. The scenario described is most consistent with Eisenmenger's physiology with right-to-left shunting through a patent ductus arteriosus. The patient has severe pulmonary HTN, with pulmonary pressures greater than systemic pressures.

33. D. Williams syndrome. The patient has a clinical examination consistent with supravalvular aortic stenosis, with a systolic ejection murmur and associated decreased left brachial pulse. Patent ductus arteriosus and severe coarctation of the aorta more typically have continuous murmurs and would not have the pulse differences. Supravalvular pulmonary stenosis would also not have a pulse difference. The association of supravalvular aortic stenosis and mental retardation is found with Williams syndrome.

34. B. Decreased (A_2) component of S_2 is not consistent with the patient's diagnosis. Because the aortic stenosis is supravalvular, S_2 (A_2) is preserved and would not be diminished. Other findings consistent with Williams syndrome include a reduced BP or pulse in the left upper extremity due to preferential deflection of flow to the right side of the body, a small chin and wide-spaced eyes, and hypercalcemia.

35. C. Fibrillin. A mutation in the fibrillin-1 protein is the defect associated with the autosomal-dominant inheritance of Marfan's syndrome. Defects in procollagen are associated with osteogenesis imperfecta and Ehlers-Danlos syndrome.

36. D. Aorta, iliac. Patients who are older than 40 years most commonly have the femoral and popliteal arteries affected (65%), whereas younger patients most commonly have the aorta and iliac arteries affected.

37. C. Both twins. Suspected patients should be asked about claudication of all muscle groups in both upper and lower extremities. Claudication in the calves is the most common site of symptoms due to occlusion or atherosclerosis of the superficial femoral artery. The thighs, hips, and buttocks can be affected if the disease is in the aortoiliac segment or the internal iliac artery. If only the feet are affected, then small vessel occlusive disease should be suspected.

38. D. Claudication is a cramping sensation that affects a muscle group that is distal to an obstruction in an artery and that is relieved with rest. Claudication and pseudoclaudication are often confused. Claudication is caused by vascular disease, whereas pseudoclaudication is caused by neurologic compromise, such as with lumbar spinal canal stenosis. Claudication is usually a cramping or aching sensation that begins with exertion (usually walking) and that is relieved with rest and even standing. Pseudoclaudication is usually of a sharp, paresthetic nature and occurs while standing or walking and is relieved with sitting or leaning forward. Claudication may or may not affect extremities of both sides, depending on whether there is bilateral vascular disease; in contrast, pseudoclaudication usually affects the extremities bilaterally.

39. D. There is a higher associated mortality in patients with severe PVD as assessed by ABI than in patients with mild PVD. When the severity of PVD is assessed by the ABI or by symptoms of PVD, patients with more severe symptoms or lower ABIs have a higher mortality rate. In general, patients with a lower ABI have more severe PVD, and values greater than 0.9 are

considered normal. However, ABI values greater than 1.3 are also abnormal and suggest medial wall calcification and noncompressible vessels, which may reflect severe PVD.

40. A. 0.9. The ABI is determined by dividing the systolic pressure in the ankle by the higher of the two systolic pressures in the arms. Therefore, in this patient, the ABI = 180/200 = 0.9.

41. C. Referral to a smoking cessation clinic, advice to continue walking, and initiation of antihypertensive therapy. By ABI, this patient has mild PVD at rest. Most patients can be managed medically, with emphasis on modifying risk factors, especially smoking cessation. In addition, patients should have a walking regimen, stopping when they get severe pain and then restarting after the pain subsides. Most (65% to 70%) patients will improve with time as collateral vessels develop.

42. E. B, C, and D. The patient has multiple cardiovascular risk factors, including his gender, age, HTN, and smoking, and also has exertional symptoms. Patients with PVD are more likely to have CAD, and those with CAD have higher mortality rates (4 to 6 times higher), primarily from cardiovascular causes, compared to people without PVD. Because the increased mortality and morbidity in patients with PVD is due primarily to cardiovascular disease or events, a functional stress test should be performed. Furthermore, all risk factors should be modified. An LDL of less than 100 mg per dL should be the goal, and, thus, a statin should be started. All patients with PVD should be on an aspirin if there is no contraindication.

43. E. None of the above is true. PVD patients without symptoms have a two- to fivefold higher risk of cardiovascular events compared to patients without PVD, and the average lifespan is shortened by 10 years. The mortality risk for symptomatic patients with PVD is approximately 30% within 5 years and almost 50% within 10 years, primarily due to MI (60%) or stroke (12%). There is a low risk of limb-threatening ischemia, requiring amputation, involving only 1.4% of patients per year; however, both diabetics and smokers have an increased risk. Less than 25% of patients with PVD require surgery or angioplasty.

44. B. A 45-year-old diabetic woman with intermittent claudication and an ulcer in her left third toe. Revascularization is indicated for claudication that affects quality of life in nondiabetics and for diabetics, owing to the potential for limb loss in the latter group. Other indications are rest pain, ulcers, or gangrene. Medical treatment should be attempted in all the other patient scenarios. Patient D likely has pseudoclaudication (lumbar spinal canal stenosis).

45. A. ACE inhibitor. The ABI in her right ankle is 0.75, consistent with moderate PVD. The Heart Outcomes Prevention Evaluation (HOPE) trial studied patients who were at high risk for cardiovascular events (patients with a history of CAD, cerebrovascular accident, PVD, or diabetes with one other cardiovascular risk factor) and determined that ramipril reduced the incidence of death, MI, and stroke compared to placebo (14.0% vs. 17.8%). Based on this data, an ACE-inhibitor should decrease her risk of cardiovascular events. In addition, an aspirin should be started.

46. B. Percutaneous angioplasty and stenting. Patients with severe intermittent claudication should be considered for revascularization. Patients with aortic or iliac disease have the highest success rate for percutaneous interventions, with a procedural success rate of 90% and angiographic patency rates of greater than 70% at 2-year follow-up. Short lesions of less than 5 cm in the iliac artery are most amenable to percutaneous interventions such as angioplasty and stenting. The mechanism of action of pentoxifylline is not well understood but is known to have several actions. It inhibits cyclic adenosine monophosphate phosphodiesterase, thus relaxing smooth muscle and having a vasodilatory effect. It also stimulates the formation of prostacyclin, which can decrease platelet aggregation. Further, it increases the deformability of both red and white blood cells, thus decreasing the viscosity of the blood. Despite these actions, pentoxifylline provides symptomatic benefit in only 20% patients with PVD, which is only slightly better than placebo.

47. C. Diabetics with severe PVD have a high risk of limb loss. Revascularization is thus indicated. Surgery is indicated because angioplasty was not successful, and she has restenosis of the stent. A preoperative cardiac stress test should be performed before vascular surgery, and the patient should be treated with perioperative beta-blockers if there are no contraindications.

48. B. In 1998, a consensus report was published with recommendations for treating patients with acute arterial occlusions. This report stated that IV thrombolytics should no longer be used because they were not effective. More localized delivery (i.e., intrathrombus lysis via a catheter delivery system) should be attempted. In addition, IV heparin at full dose should be given and imaging, either via angiography or via duplex ultrasound, should be done.

49. B. In general, the shorter the lesion, the better the result from percutaneous angioplasty. For aortic or iliac disease, angioplasty is the preferred treatment of choice over surgery if the lesion is smaller than 5 cm. Smaller than 2 cm is the ideal length of the focal stenosis for percutaneous intervention to the tibial artery. For the superficial femoral artery, if the lesion is smaller than 10 cm, angioplasty and stenting are preferred once medical therapy has failed. However, percutaneous intervention of the femoropopliteal arteries has been plagued with high restenosis rates, and so, currently, stenting should only be performed if there is a flow-compromising dissection or if angioplasty does not give an optimal result for a focal lesion.

50. D. All of the above. Patients with PVD of all four extremities may erroneously have a normal ABI secondary to decreased BP in both the arms and legs. Patients with noncompressible ankle arteries usually have significant medial wall calcification and usually have significant PVD, but the ABI is indeterminable. Similarly, for diabetic patients with a foot ulcer, severe PVD is usually present. An ABI greater than 1.3 suggests medial calcification.

51. E. CT scan should not be used to assess for PVD. Duplex ultrasonography can identify the narrowed segment of the artery and then can measure the velocity of the blood flow at various points to estimate the severity of the lesion. PVRs are especially useful when the ABI is falsely elevated secondary to medial wall calcification. Exercise testing is used to determine if the

ankle systolic BP drops with walking certain distances. MRA provides a noninvasive assessment of the arteries but can overestimate the severity of the lesion. CT has no role in assessing the severity of PVD.

52. A. Duplex ultrasonography. The patient likely has left subclavian stenosis, and a duplex ultrasound is the first step to assess flow. MRA can also be done but is more expensive and should not be done as the initial test. The ABI is not indicated because it is used to assess PVD in the lower extremities. A dipyridamole (Persantine) stress test does not need to be done if she is asymptomatic and is not to undergo any major surgery.

53. D. If there is rest pain or an ischemic limb. Long-term medical therapy is appropriate for infrapopliteal arterial disease because only one patent infrapopliteal artery is sufficient to prevent limb ischemia, despite severe disease in multiple other infrapopliteal arteries. Percutaneous angioplasty is associated with a high restenosis rate, as high as 40% to 60%, primarily due to the diffuse disease, calcification, and the small caliber of vessels. Bypass surgery has a moderate (10%) risk for subacute occlusion and has a higher risk of amputation compared to surgery for other arterial segments. Only *in situ* grafting or saphenous vein grafts are now used due to the high early occlusion rates associated with synthetic grafts. Because of these limitations, revascularization should only be done when there is rest pain or an ischemic limb.

54. A. Renal artery duplex ultrasonography is an excellent screening test for renal artery stenosis, with both a high sensitivity and specificity. Renal angiograms are the gold standard but carry a significant risk of increased renal failure in patients with diabetes and severe renal insufficiency. Thus, in these patients, screening should be done first with a duplex ultrasound. MRA is not the gold standard, because older studies have shown an overestimation of lesion severity. In addition, it is less reliable for examining the distal segments. It is also not as useful as invasive angiography in diagnosing fibromuscular dysplasia. Captopril renal scintigraphy is difficult to interpret when there is renal insufficiency.

55. A. When PTRA is performed on nonostial renal artery stenosis, which is caused by fibromuscular dysplasia, good results are obtained. The results of PTRA are more favorable in medial fibromuscular dysplasia than in the intimal or adventitial forms of dysplasia. The rates of long-term patency are approximately 80% to 90%. Most patients with fibromuscular dysplasia are young and healthy, and so PTRA complications in these patients are low. Most patients with atherosclerotic renal artery stenosis are older, with more comorbidities, and so the risk for PTRA is greater, and 20% to 40% of these patients do not respond favorably to PTRA. Ostial lesions have worse results than nonostial lesions. Stent placement has improved results. In patients with Takayasu's arteritis, the renal artery stenotic lesions are generally fibrotic and long, and favorable results may not be obtained.

56. B. 6%. The combined risk of stroke and death is between 5% and 8% but can be as high as 18% in patients with CAD. In the Asymptomatic Carotid Atherosclerosis Study (ACAS), the risk of ipsilateral stroke or any perioperative stroke or death was 5% in the surgically treated patients. In the North American Symptomatic Carotid Endarterectomy Trial (NASCET), there was a 9% risk for ipsilateral stroke in patients surgically treated during the

2-year follow-up, compared to 26% of those medically treated. However, current event rates are declining, and current recommendations suggest CEA may be considered earlier in centers with event rates less than 3%.

57. B. A CEA in a hospital with significant experience. Based on ACAS, the largest randomized trial to date to assess CEA in asymptomatic patients, which included patients who were younger than 80 years old and who had carotid stenoses greater than or equal to 60% (as diagnosed by Doppler), the recommendation is to surgically manage asymptomatic patients if the medical center is experienced and has a low surgical morbidity rate (less than 3%). However, most community centers do not carry this low risk for carotid endarterectomies. In this study, CEA reduced the risk for stroke or death by 53% compared to medical therapy in asymptomatic patients with a carotid stenosis of greater than 60%. In the multicenter North American Cerebral Percutaneous Transluminal Registry, symptomatic patients with a greater than 70% stenosis who were refractory to medical treatment and deemed poor surgical candidates but qualified for angioplasty were followed. Angioplasty reduced the stenosis significantly and had a combined rate of stroke and death of 9%, similar to CEA results. Carotid stenting is now being performed in patients ineligible for CEA, with similar procedure-related stroke and death rates as with CEA.

58. C. Cilostazol. Cilostazol, a phosphodiesterase type 3 inhibitor, inhibits platelet aggregation, the formation of arterial thrombi, and vascular smooth-muscle proliferation. Its exact mechanism for improving claudication is unknown. In placebo-controlled trials, cilostazol improved claudication and walking distance. It is contraindicated in patients with a decreased ejection fraction. There is no evidence of efficacy for papaverine or other vasodilatory drugs. Pentoxifylline was found to have only a small, if any, benefit compared to placebo.

59. C. ABI = 1.4, significantly decreased amplitude on PVR. The history suggests severe vascular insufficiency. An ABI greater than 1.3 is not normal and implies medial wall calcification. A PVR with a decreased amplitude is consistent with severe PVD.

60. B. Atherosclerosis. Although fibromuscular dysplasia is the most common cause of renal artery stenosis in young patients, atherosclerosis is more common in the general population. Fibromuscular dysplasia typically occurs in young or middle-aged women who present with secondary HTN. The pathologic process involves the distal two-thirds of the renal artery and branches compared to atherosclerosis, which more commonly involves the ostium.

61. C. 40%. Because only 40% of patients with significant carotid artery disease have a bruit, patients with significant CAD or with a history of claudication should also have duplex ultrasonography performed on their carotids preoperatively.

62. E. None of the above. Answers A through D are all potential symptoms or consequences of PVD. Once PVD worsens to a critical level of leg ischemia, the typical symptom of intermittent claudication progresses to rest pain, which usually occurs at night when the patient is supine or when the patient raises his legs. As the disease progresses, ulcers can occur, and

dry gangrene can present. In addition, once patients have severe PVD and are unable to walk, they may lose significant muscle mass of the lower extremity.

63. C. A HgbA$_1$C of 11.2 is inconsistent with the likely diagnosis. The presence of claudication, a leg ulcer, and positive Allen test in a male smoker younger than age 40 to 45 years is highly suggestive of thromboangiitis obliterans (Buerger's disease). Several diagnostic criteria have been proposed to make this diagnosis. The criteria of Olin includes the presence of distal-extremity ischemia (claudication, rest pain, gangrene, or ulcers) confirmed by vascular testing in a smoker younger than 45 years of age with the exclusion of sources of emboli, diabetes mellitus, and hypercoagulable or autoimmune diseases.

64. C. Biopsy of the involved limb vessel is not important to confirm the diagnosis. Both a TEE and arteriography are important to exclude a source of peripheral emboli. Although arteriography in general may not show specific findings of Buerger's disease, the classic angiographic demonstration is that of multiple occlusions with "corkscrew collaterals." A biopsy is usually not required and not part of the diagnostic criteria.

65. C. Discontinuation of smoking. Many treatment strategies have been attempted for management of Buerger's disease, including prostaglandins and intraarterial thrombolytic therapy, but the data are inconclusive. Iloprost (a prostaglandin analogue) has shown promising results in relieving pain and healing ulcers. The data regarding thrombolytic therapy are very limited. Calcium channel blockers are not used for treatment of Buerger's disease. Surgical revascularization is of limited benefit due to the diffuse nature of the disease and the involvement of small and distal vessels. Therefore, only smoking discontinuation has been shown to be of definite benefit.

66. E. All are consistent. The patient has secondary Raynaud phenomenon due to systemic sclerosis and probable CREST (calcinosis, Raynaud phenomenon, esophageal involvement, sclerodactyly, telangiectasia) syndrome. Secondary Raynaud phenomenon generally involves men older than 40 years of age with other systemic manifestations and evidence of arterial insufficiency. They may not have the bilateral and symmetric involvement that is generally seen with the more benign primary disease of younger females.

67. A. Ergotamine, as needed, for episodes of discoloration is least appropriate. Patients with Raynaud phenomenon should avoid cold weather, stress, and tobacco because these factors will promote vasoconstriction. In addition, medications such as ergotamine, beta-blockers, and some chemotherapeutic agents may promote Raynaud phenomenon. Alleviating agents include alpha-adrenergic blocking drugs, such as prazosin and reserpine, as well as calcium channel blockers.

68. B. Superficial varicose veins would not be consistent. The patient likely has lymphedema, because he is elderly, without jugular venous distention, and has unilateral edema. Features consistent with lymphedema in contrast to venous insufficiency include asymmetric involvement, absence of superficial venous changes, nonpitting character, and involvement of the toes.

69. D. Venogram is of least use. Lymphedema can be primary or secondary. Primary lymphedema generally occurs in pregnant women. Secondary lymphedema can be obstructive or inflammatory in nature. The finding of lymphedema in an elderly man suggests neoplasm until proven otherwise, with prostate cancer being most likely. The appropriate testing should assess lymphatic drainage and potential causes of malignancy.

70. D. LV rupture is least likely to occur. Common sites of injury of the heart and great vessels involve anterior structures, thin-walled structures, and those with some degree of tethering. The aortic isthmus is a common site of rupture, as are the innominate artery and subclavian artery. Cardiac structures most often injured include the right atrium and RV and, less commonly, the left-sided chambers.

SUGGESTED READING

Bajwa TK, Shalev YA, Gupta A, et al. Peripheral vascular disease, part 1. *Curr Probl Cardiol* 1998;23(5):245–304.

Bajwa TK, Shalev YA, Gupta A, et al. Peripheral vascular disease, part 2. *Curr Probl Cardiol* 1998;23(6):305–352.

Case 38-1991. Case records of the Massachusetts General Hospital. *N Engl J Med* 1991;325:874–882.

Celermajer DS, Cullen S, Deanfield JE, et al. Congenitally corrected transposition and Ebstein's anomaly of the systemic atrioventricular valve: association with aortic arch obstruction. *J Am Coll Cardiol* 1991;18:1056–1058.

Coady MA, Rizzo JA, Hammond GL, et al. What is the appropriate size criterion for resection of thoracic aortic aneurysms? *J Thorac Cardiovasc Surg* 1997;113:476–491.

DePaepe A, Devereux RB, Dietz HC, et al. Revised diagnostic criteria for Marfan syndrome. *Am J Med Genet* 1996;62:417–426.

Garasic JM, Creager MA. Percutaneous interventions for lower-extremity peripheral atherosclerotic disease. *Rev Cardiovasc Med* 2001;2(3):120–125.

Hansen KJ, Tribble RW, Reavis SW, et al. Renal duplex sonography: evaluation of clinical utility. *J Vasc Surg* 1990;12:227–236.

Hiatt WR. Medical treatment of peripheral arterial disease and claudication. *N Engl J Med* 2001;344:1608–1621.

Isselbacher EM, Cigarroa JE, Eagle KA. Cardiac tamponade complicating proximal aortic dissection: is pericardiocentesis harmful? *Circulation* 1994;90:2375–2378.

Maraj R, Rerkpattanapipat P, Jacobs LE, et al. Meta-analysis of 143 reported cases of aortic intramural hematomas. *Am J Cardiol* 2000;86:664–668.

McCready RA, Vincent AE, Schwartz RW, et al. Atherosclerosis in the young: a virulent disease. *Surgery* 1984;96:863–869.

McDaniel MD, Cronenwett JL. Basic data related to the natural history of intermittent claudication. *Ann Vasc Surg* 1989;3:273–277.

Mukherjee D, Yadav JS. Update on peripheral vascular diseases: from smoking cessation to stenting. *Cleve Clin J Med* 2001;68(8):723–733.

Nienaber CA, Von Kodolitsch Y, Nicolas V, et al. The diagnosis of thoracic aortic dissection by noninvasive imaging procedures. *N Engl J Med* 1993;328:1–9.

Olin JW. Thromboangiitis obliterans (Buerger's disease). *N Engl J Med* 2000;343:864–869.

Penn MS, Smedira N, Lytle B, et al. Does coronary angiography before emergency aortic surgery affect in-hospital mortality? *J Am Coll Cardiol* 2000;35:889–894.

Pretre R, Chilcott M. Blunt trauma to the heart and great vessels. *N Engl J Med* 1997;336:626–632.

Sacco RL. Extracranial carotid stenosis. *N Engl J Med* 2001;345(15):1113–1118.

Safian RD, Textor SC. Renal-artery stenosis. *N Engl J Med* 2001;344(6):431–442.

NOTES

Sharma BK, Jain S, Suri S, et al. Diagnostic criteria for Takayasu's arteritis. *Int J Med* 1996;54(suppl):S141–S147.

Shores J, Berger KR, Murphy EA, et al. Progression of aortic dilatation and the benefit of long-term beta-adrenergic blockage in Marfan's syndrome. *N Engl J Med* 1994;330:1335–1341.

Song JK, Kim HS, Kang DH, et al. Different clinical features of aortic intramural hematoma versus dissection involving the ascending aorta. *J Am Coll Cardiol* 2001;37:1604–1610.

Svennson LG, Labib SB, Eisenhauer AC, et al. Intimal tear without hematoma: an important variant of aortic dissection that can elude current imaging techniques. *Circulation* 1999;99:1331–1336.

Tierney S, Fennessy F, Hayes DB. ABC of arterial and vascular disease. Secondary prevention of peripheral vascular disease. *BMJ* 2000;320:1262–1265.

Tunick PA, Kronzon I. Atheromas of the thoracic aorta: clinical and therapeutic update. *J Am Coll Cardiol* 2000;35:545–554.

Vilacosta I, San Roman JA, Aragoncillo P, et al. Penetrating atherosclerotic aortic ulcer: documentation by transesophageal echocardiography. *J Am Coll Cardiol* 1998;32:82–89.

Winslow CM, Solomon DH, Chassin MR, et al. The appropriateness of carotid endarterectomy. *N Engl J Med* 1988;318:721–727.

Working Party on Thrombolysis in the Management of Limb Ischemia. Thrombolysis in the management of lower limb peripheral arterial occlusion—a consensus document. *Am J Cardiol* 1998;81:207–218.

Yusuf S, Sleight P, Pogue J, et al. Effects of an ACE inhibitor, ramipril, on cardiovascular events in high-risk patients. The Heart Outcomes Prevention Evaluation Study Investigators. *N Engl J Med* 2000;342:145–153.

CHAPTER 7

Congestive Heart Failure

Gary S. Francis and Leslie Cho

QUESTIONS

1. Which of the following characterizes heart failure?

   A. downregulation of β_1- and β_2-receptors
   B. downregulation primarily of β_1-receptors with little change in β_2-receptors
   C. downregulation of G proteins and β_1- and β_2-receptors
   D. increase in myocardial norepinephrine stores
   E. intact baroreceptor function

2. Which of the following treatments most consistently improves EF in patients who have systolic heart failure?

   A. diuretics
   B. beta-blockers
   C. ACE inhibitors
   D. vasodilators
   E. all of the above

3. When used chronically, all of the following drugs increase mortality *except*

   A. milrinone
   B. dobutamine
   C. vesnarinone
   D. xamoterol
   E. amlodipine

4. In the Veterans Administration Heart Failure Trial II (V-HeFT II), which combination of medications improved LV function and exercise tolerance?

   A. ACE inhibitors
   B. hydralazine plus nitrates
   C. ACE inhibitor plus hydralazine plus nitrates
   D. ACE inhibitor plus nitrates

5. A 56-year-old man presents to your clinic for follow-up after being discharged from the hospital 6 weeks ago. He underwent a successful primary angioplasty for acute anterior MI; however, his EF is now 40%. He is currently taking simvastatin (Zocor), acetylsalicylic aspirin, clopidogrel bisulfate (Plavix), metoprolol tartrate (Lopressor), and losartan (Cozaar). He states that he cannot afford all of these medications. He would like to know which medications are essential for a longer life. Which medications should you tell him are essential?

A. all of them
B. all of them except clopidogrel bisulfate
C. all of them except losartan
D. all except clopidogrel bisulfate and losartan

6. A 23-year-old woman presents to your clinic 8 weeks after delivery for a second opinion. She was diagnosed with peripartum cardiomyopathy, and her EF is 25%. She has been doing well and wants to know her prognosis. She is currently on an ACE inhibitor and a beta-blocker. She is not breastfeeding. What advice should you give her?

A. Her EF will be 25%. She will need life-long ACE inhibitors and beta-blockers.
B. She is likely to make a full recovery and will not need any intervention.
C. She has a 50% chance of recovery. If a TTE in 8 weeks shows abnormal EF, then she most likely will not recover.
D. None of the above is your advice.

7. A 78-year-old woman with CHF (EF, 25%), chronic AFib, gastroesophageal reflux disease, hypertension (HTN), hyperlipidemia, diabetes, and osteoporosis takes 12 different pills. At the recent senior citizen day at the local church, a nurse told her that she does not need to take digoxin because she is on amiodarone. She wants to eliminate digoxin from her medication regimen, and she wants to know why you put her on it in the first place. What is your answer?

A. Digoxin improves survival.
B. Digoxin reduces hospitalization.
C. Digoxin improves contractility.
D. Digoxin decreases the volume of distribution of amiodarone.
E. Digoxin reduces sympathetic nervous system activity.

8. Recently, a 43-year-old lawyer received heart transplantation. His hospital course was unremarkable, and he was discharged. He found out from the heart failure nurses that allograft vasculopathy is the leading cause of long-term morbidity and mortality in transplant patients. He wants to know what proven treatments prevent allograft vasculopathy. Which of the following treatments should you recommend?

A. annual cardiac catheterization, intravascular ultrasound, and percutaneous coronary intervention (PCI), as needed
B. annual stress test
C. biannual stress test
D. statins
E. no known treatment

9. The following neurohormones are associated with vasoconstriction, cell growth, hypertrophy, and sodium retention *except*

A. angiotensin II
B. norepinephrine
C. brain natriuretic peptide (BNP)
D. endothelin
E. arginine vasopressin

10. BNP has which of the following properties?

A. Urine volume increases.
B. Sodium excretion is enhanced.
C. More BNP is secreted.
D. A decrease in plasma aldosterone concentration occurs.
E. All of the above occur.
F. None of the above occurs.

11. A 34-year-old woman with dilated cardiomyopathy is admitted to the coronary care unit (CCU) for heart failure exacerbation. On examination, her respiratory rate is 25 with distended neck vein and prominent S_3. In addition to aggressive diuresis, a decision was made to start nesiritide (Natrecor). After the infusion, you notice hemodynamic changes. Which of the following changes is not related to the effects of nesiritide?

A. decrease in heart rate (HR)
B. decrease in BP
C. reduction in pulmonary capillary wedge pressure (PCWP)
D. no change in stroke volume index
E. all of the above
F. none of the above

12. A 72-year-old woman is transferred from another hospital. She was initially admitted with palpitation, diagnosed with AFib, and treated with amiodarone. A TTE showed an EF of 10% with a regional wall motion abnormality. She underwent cardiac catheterization and was found to have a heavily calcified 80% lesion in the mid–left anterior descending artery (LAD), a 40% lesion in a nondominant circumflex, and an 80% lesion in the posterior descending artery. Her children want to know what you plan to do for her. What should you recommend?

A. She has terrible EF and should be on medication only because coronary artery bypass graft (CABG) would be too high risk.
B. She should undergo PCI because she is too high risk for CABG.
C. She should undergo CABG because this is the definitive treatment.
D. She should have a positron emission tomography (PET) scan to assess the area of viability before proceeding with CABG or PCI.

13. A 53-year-old woman with a history of CHF presents to the emergency room (ER). She is cool and clammy. She reports being short of breath. Her BP is 71/40 mm Hg, her HR is 110 bpm, and her respiratory rate is 30. She has elevated neck veins and a prominent S_3. Her ECG shows sinus tachycardia. She is admitted to the CCU with heart failure. A PA catheterization is performed, and her hemodynamics are as follows: right atrial pressure, 12 mm Hg; PA pressure, 62/30 mm Hg; cardiac output, 1.9 L per minute per m^2; PCWP, 36 mm Hg; and systemic vascular resistance (SVR), 2,000 dyne per second per cm^5. Which of the following is your next step?

A. Start furosemide (Lasix).
B. Start dopamine.
C. Insert IABP.
D. Begin dobutamine.
E. Start nesiritide.

14. This patient continues to deteriorate after your initial treatment. Her BP is 64/32 mm Hg, and her HR is 132 bpm. She is now intubated on maximal pressor support and has an IABP in place. Which of the following should be your next therapeutic option?

    A. There is no option. She is on maximal therapy.
    B. Consider emergent cardiac transplant.
    C. Consider LV assist device.
    D. Consider cardiopulmonary bypass.

15. A 35-year-old man with a history of HTN presents to the ER in respiratory distress. He is intubated in the ER for respiratory distress. His BP is 73/48 mm Hg, his HR is 130 bpm, and his respiratory rate is 20. He is taken to the medical ICU, and a PA catheterization is performed. His hemodynamics are as follows: RA pressure, 22 mm Hg; PA pressure, 20/10 mm Hg; cardiac output, 3.5 L per minute per m^2; PCWP, 12 mm Hg; and SVR, 1,690 dyne per second per cm^5. What is your diagnosis?

    A. pulmonary embolism
    B. cardiogenic shock
    C. acute RV failure
    D. decompensated heart failure
    E. hypovolemic shock

16. You receive a call from a cardiologist in a small community hospital regarding a patient in heart failure. She states that the patient was admitted last night with heart failure and was started on IV nitroglycerin; IV furosemide infusion; captopril, 12.5 mg t.i.d.; and digoxin. There has been no improvement; therefore, the cardiologist placed a Swan-Ganz catheter this morning. The patient's hemodynamics are as follows: BP, 120/89 mm Hg; HR, 89 bpm; cardiac output, 2.0 L per minute per m^2; PCWP, 29 mm Hg; and SVR, 1,766 dyne per second per cm^5. The cardiologist also added dobutamine. Which of the following additional therapies should you recommend to the cardiologist for this patient?

    A. Begin patient transfer arrangement.
    B. Suggest nitroprusside.
    C. Suggest nesiritide.
    D. Suggest dopamine.
    E. Suggest IABP.

17. A 57-year-old woman, who experienced inferior wall MI in 1992, has an EF of 30% and was diagnosed with nonsustained VT (4 beats of VT) at another hospital on a routine ECG that she needed before cataract surgery. She has been in excellent health and has never been hospitalized for CHF. She has never had palpitation or syncopal episodes. Her doctors advised her that she would need an implantable defibrillator. She does not agree and wants a second opinion. She wants to know if there is any evidence to support the implantable defibrillators. What is your advice?

A. Place an implantable defibrillator.

B. Do not place an implantable defibrillator: A single episode is probably insignificant.

C. Perform an EP study.

D. Begin beta-blockers with amiodarone.

18. A 49-year-old man is admitted with new-onset heart failure. He is diagnosed with dilated cardiomyopathy with an EF of 20%. On hospital day 1, he is diuresed and started on a regimen of furosemide, digoxin, acetylsalicylic aspirin, captopril, and simvastatin. A medical student wants to know why you did not start him on a beta-blocker. What is your explanation?

A. Beta-blockers have not been shown to decrease mortality in dilated cardiomyopathy patients. Only ischemic cardiomyopathy patients have derived benefit.

B. There have been several conflicting results from randomized trials; therefore, beta-blockers are not recommended as the first line of therapy.

C. Beta-blockers have been shown to improve survival but should only be used in patients with an EF greater than 25%.

D. Beta-blockers should be started in stable CHF patients.

19. The same medical student wants to know whether the patient should also be started on calcium channel blockers. What is your answer?

A. There has never been a study to demonstrate the benefit of calcium channel blockers.

B. Diltiazem has proved to be of small but significant benefit in nonischemic cardiomyopathy patients and should be started.

C. Calcium channel blockers should be started after discharge once the patient has stabilized.

D. Felodipine has proved to be of small benefit only in ischemic cardiomyopathy patients. This patient does not fit this criterion.

E. Amlodipine proved to be of small benefit in a New York Heart Association (NYHA) class III or IV patient with an EF less than 30%. This benefit was seen more in dilated cardiomyopathy patients.

20. A 24-year-old female medical student presents to urgent care with 5 days of fever and shortness of breath. She is diagnosed with a viral infection and sent home. Five months later during her physical examination class, she is found to have an S_3 by her fellow students. She presents to your office for a second opinion. On examination, she appears healthy and in no distress. Her BP is 96/50 mm Hg, with an HR of 71 bpm and a respiratory rate of 12. Her neck veins are not distended, and her examination is unremarkable except for an enlarged heart. You do not appreciate an S_3. You order a TTE, which shows an EF of 20% with a dilated heart. There is no valvular abnormality. Which of the following is your recommendation?

A. Begin ACE inhibitor, beta-blockers, and steroid.

B. Begin ACE inhibitor and beta-blockers.

C. Begin ACE inhibitor, beta-blockers, diuretics, and digoxin.

D. Begin ACE inhibitor, beta-blockers, diuretics, and spironolactone.

E. She is well compensated; nothing needs to be done.

21. A 79-year-old man with diabetes, HTN, chronic renal insufficiency, and ischemic cardiomyopathy was recently admitted with CHF exacerbation. At home, he takes captopril, 75 mg t.i.d.; digoxin, 0.125 mg per day; furo-

semide, 60 mg b.i.d.; aspirin; and atorvastatin calcium (Lipitor). When admitted, he was in heart failure with elevated neck veins and S_3. During his admission, he was diuresed with IV furosemide and metolazone. His baseline creatinine was 1.7 and now is 2.5, with a BUN of 100. What is your next step?

A. Stop captopril.
B. Stop diuretics.
C. Rule out renal artery stenosis.
D. Stop aspirin and ACE.

22. The severity of symptomatic exercise limitation in heart failure
    A. is due to elevated PCWP
    B. is due to reduced blood flow to skeletal muscles
    C. bears little relation to the severity of LV dysfunction
    D. can be reversed by inotropic therapy
    E. is related to markers of central hemodynamic disturbance

23. A 59-year-old woman with CHF and an EF of 30% comes to your office for follow-up. She is on carvedilol (Coreg), enalapril, aspirin, atorvastatin calcium, digoxin, and furosemide. She has been doing well without any rehospitalization. However, she wants to improve her exercise tolerance. What should you recommend?
    A. cardiac transplantation
    B. IV dobutamine
    C. higher doses of ACE inhibitor
    D. adding spironolactone
    E. enrolling her in an exercise training program

24. Prognosis in heart failure correlates best with which of the following?
    A. peak $\dot{V}O_2$ during exercise
    B. $\dot{V}E/\dot{V}O_2$ slope during exercise
    C. EF at rest
    D. blood gases during exercise
    E. myocardial contractility measurements

25. An 86-year-old woman is transferred from a nursing home in respiratory distress. She was found to be short of breath. On examination, she has labored breathing, and her BP is 62/34 mm Hg with an HR of 60 bpm. She is intubated in the ER and admitted to the CCU. She is started on norepinephrine and dopamine at high doses without significant effect. Her ECG shows sinus bradycardia but is otherwise unremarkable. Her CXR shows pulmonary edema. The nursing home calls and says that she has mistakenly received 100 mg IV metoprolol tartrate. Which of the following should be your next step?
    A. glucagon and milrinone
    B. glucagon and dobutamine
    C. IABP
    D. fluid resuscitation
    E. transvenous pacemaker

26. A 62-year-old man with an EF of 20% and chronic renal insufficiency presents to your office for follow-up. He has non–insulin-dependent diabetes mellitus and has developed worsening renal failure due to diabetes. His medi-

cation regimen includes a beta-blocker that is significantly affected by reduced renal function. Which of the following beta-blockers is he taking?

A. propanolol
B. atenolol
C. carvedilol
D. metoprolol
E. sotalol

27. A 38-year-old patient with CHF is transferred from another hospital. You are doing rounds in the CCU while the clinicians are performing a TTE. They ask you to assess his LV function. You notice the E:A wave ratio is greater than 1.5, with an E-wave deceleration time of 120 msec. Which of the following do you guess is his PCWP?

A. PCWP is 12 mm Hg.
B. PCWP is 18 mm Hg.
C. PCWP is 26 mm Hg.
D. You cannot tell from the E:A wave ratio and deceleration time.

28. For the patient in the previous question, the E:A wave ratio and the E-wave deceleration time indicate which of the following?

A. low filling pressure and reduced LV compliance
B. high filling pressure and increased LV compliance
C. low filling pressure and increased LV compliance
D. high filling pressure and reduced LV compliance

29. A 67-year-old patient with HTN, hyperlipidemia, and an EF of 45% comes to your office for a second opinion. He had an exercise test and was told that his HR recovery was abnormal. His physician told him not to worry *unless* his heart function deteriorates. He is not convinced and wants your opinion and treatment. What should you recommend?

A. Abnormal HR recovery does not predict mortality in patients with an EF greater than 35%; therefore, no treatment is needed.
B. Abnormal HR recovery predicts mortality only in patients after MI; therefore, no treatment is needed.
C. Abnormal HR recovery predicts mortality in all patients; however, there is no treatment.
D. Abnormal HR recovery predicts mortality in all patients, and exercise training is the treatment of choice.

30. All of the following are indications for heart transplantation *except*

A. dilated cardiomyopathy
B. diabetes
C. hypertrophic cardiomyopathy
D. age
E. amyloid heart disease

31. A 41-year-old man presents to the CCU with CHF symptoms. On examination, he has elevated neck veins, severe peripheral edema, and S_3 gallop. He is started on medication and has improvement in all of his symptoms. He has a PET scan, which shows a large area of hibernating myocardium. His cardiac catheterization reveals mild disease in the right coronary artery, a focal 80% lesion in the circumflex, and a focal 70% lesion in the LAD. All of his lesions

are type A American College of Cardiologists/American Heart Association score. His EF is 15%. According to randomized clinical trials, which of the following is the best treatment for this patient?

A. percutaneous transluminal coronary angioplasty (PTCA)/stent with abciximab and clopidogrel bisulfate
B. PTCA/stent with cardiothoracic surgery backup
C. CABG
D. PTCA/stent with abciximab and IABP

32. A 28-year-old woman comes to your office for a second opinion. She had peripartum cardiomyopathy and wants to get pregnant again. You obtain a TTE, which shows a normal LV. What should you recommend?

A. She should not have another pregnancy because she is likely to have recurrent cardiomyopathy.
B. She may conceive again because her LV is normal. Her chance of having recurrent cardiomyopathy is less than 5%.
C. She may conceive again because her LV is normal. However, her chance of having recurrent cardiomyopathy is 30% to 50%.
D. She should undergo exercise testing for better assessment.

33. Primary causes of diastolic heart failure include all of the following *except*

A. hypertrophic cardiomyopathy
B. dilated cardiomyopathy
C. HTN
D. MI
E. infiltrative cardiomyopathy

34. A 78-year-old retired federal judge comes to your office for follow-up. He has long-standing HTN and has undergone PTCA/stent for a mid-LAD lesion. He has normal LV function and is active and healthy. Currently, he is on ramipril (Altace), atorvastatin, and aspirin. He heard on television that the combination of aspirin and ramipril increases mortality. He wants your opinion. What is your answer?

A. These are only observational studies, and they have not been proven. Continue the current regimen.
B. There are randomized studies to support this; however, the sample size was too small to make any conclusive recommendations. Continue the current regimen.
C. This has been shown in large trials; we should change aspirin to clopidogrel bisulfate or ramipril to metoprolol tartrate.
D. Although this has been seen in retrospective trials, it has not been validated in a randomized trial; therefore, continue the current regimen.

35. A 56-year-old man with dilated cardiomyopathy with an EF of 15% comes to your office for an opinion regarding medication. He is in NYHA class II and wants to know about biventricular pacing. He heard on television news that this may save lives. His ECG shows a sinus rate of 71, a PR interval of 210 msec, a QRS duration of 188 msec, and a QT/QT$_C$ of 364:427 msec. What should you recommend?

A. Refer the patient for biventricular pacing based on PR interval.
B. Refer the patient for biventricular pacing based on QRS duration.
C. Refer the patient for biventricular pacing based on QT/QT$_C$ interval.
D. Refer the patient for exercise test to further assess.

36. A 31-year-old woman with hypertrophic cardiomyopathy presents to your office for follow-up. She has been doing well. She denies any palpitation or syncope. She has researched her disease on the Web and found out that most people die of arrhythmia. She would like to have an EP study. Which of the following is the predictive value of the EP study for ventricular arrhythmia?

    A. 20%
    B. 40%
    C. 50%
    D. 80%
    E. 100%

37. A 61-year-old woman with an EF of 50% is admitted with an AFib with rapid ventricular response. She is started on metoprolol tartrate with excellent rate control and heparin. Her daughter, who is a nurse, wants to know why you did not start her on dofetilide because this is the best new drug. What is your response?

    A. Dofetilide showed increased mortality when compared to amiodarone and would be a bad choice for her mother.
    B. Dofetilide had safety and efficacy comparable to those of beta-blockers.
    C. Dofetilide was used in patients with an EF less than 35%.
    D. Dofetilide has safety and efficacy comparable those of to calcium channel blockers.
    E. Dofetilide is reserved for patients with chronic renal insufficiency.

38. A 79-year-old woman with HTN and non–insulin-dependent diabetes mellitus comes to your office for a second opinion. She is doing well and is currently on enalapril, aspirin, simvastatin, glipizide, and metformin. She read in her monthly American Association of Retired Persons newsletter that losartan is better than enalapril. She wants you to change her prescription. Based on trial data, which of the following is your recommendation?

    A. Losartan did not show mortality benefit but did show reduced hospitalization; because she has no history of CHF, there is no reason to change her medication.
    B. Losartan showed neither mortality benefit nor reduced hospitalization.
    C. Losartan did not show mortality benefit but decreased the risk of MI; therefore, she should have her prescription changed.
    D. Losartan did show mortality benefit—but only in patients younger than 60 years.

39. A 77-year-old man presents to the ER with shortness of breath. He is found to have an HR of 90 with a respiratory rate of 26. His BP is 110/63 mm Hg. His examination is remarkable for distended neck vein, S_3 gallop, edema, and ascites. His CXR shows pulmonary congestion. His ECG shows sinus rhythm and an old anterior MI. He is diuresed; on hospital day 4, he has a TTE. His TTE shows abnormal LV and RV diastolic function. Also, there is thickened myocardium, which appears to sparkle. He is diagnosed with amyloidosis. Which of the following is the treatment of choice for this patient?

    A. melphalan, prednisone, and colchicine
    B. cardiac transplantation
    C. pacer
    D. calcium channel blockers
    E. no known treatment available

In Table 1 (questions 40–42), interpret the echocardiographic diastolic filling pattern:

TABLE 1 *Echocardiographic Diastolic Filling Patterns*

Question	40	41	42
E:A wave ratio	1.3	2.7	1.7
Mitral deceleration time (msec)	200	110	167
Systolic:diastolic ratio	1.6	0.5	0.9
Isovolemic relaxation time (msec)	80	40	82

A. pseudonormal filling pattern
B. restrictive filling pattern
C. normal filling pattern

43. A 61-year-old woman with CHF and an EF of 25% is admitted with CHF exacerbation to your partner's service. On the day of discharge, your partner is sick, and you must explain her discharge medications. You explain to her the benefits of lisinopril, simvastatin, aspirin, digoxin, and furosemide. Finally, you want to explain the benefit of spironolactone (Aldactone) to her. What is your explanation?

A. Spironolactone in addition to standard therapy (ACE inhibitor, diuretic) does not decrease mortality or morbidity.
B. Spironolactone in addition to standard therapy only decreases rehospitalization—it does not improve NYHA functional class.
C. Spironolactone in addition to standard therapy decreases mortality and rehospitalization.
D. Spironolactone only benefits those not on standard therapy.

44. A 63-year-old man with non–insulin-dependent diabetes mellitus, HTN, hyperlipidemia, and chronic renal insufficiency is admitted with acute anterior wall MI 10 hours after symptom onset. He is taken emergently to the cardiac cathctcrization laboratory. He is noted to have proximal LAD occlusion, and he undergoes a successful PTCA/stent to the LAD with abciximab and heparin. His EF is noted to be 30% on a TTE performed 3 days later. On hospital day 4, he reports chest pain and is found to be in AFib with an HR of 121. His BP is 90/44 mm Hg, and he is short of breath and anxious. Which of the following should you administer next?

A. procainamide
B. lidocaine
C. amiodarone
D. metoprolol tartrate
E. cardioversion

45. Common precipitating causes of acute decompensated heart failure include all of the following *except*

    A. exercise
    B. nonsteroidal antiinflammatory drug use
    C. noncompliance with diet and medication
    D. infection
    E. trastuzumab (Herceptin)

46. An LV pressure volume loop is shown in Figure 1. Label A, B, C, and D.

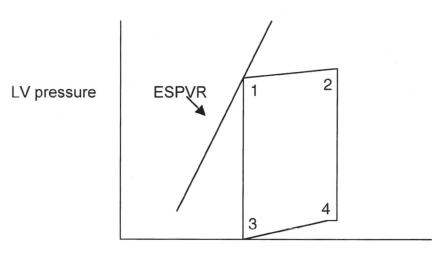

LV volume

FIGURE 1 ESPVR, end-systolic pressure-volume relation. (From Little WC, Braunwald E. Assessment of cardiac function. In: Braunwald E, ed. *Heart disease: a textbook of cardiovascular medicine*, 5th ed. Philadelphia: WB Saunders, 1997, with permission.)

    A. mitral valve opening
    B. end-diastole
    C. aortic valve opening
    D. end-systole

47. A 57-year-old man with a history of CHF presents with acute pulmonary edema. His BP is 110/60 mm Hg with an HR of 92 bpm. His examination is consistent with heart failure. His hemodynamics are as follows: PA pressure, 62/27 mm Hg; PCWP, 12 mm Hg; cardiac output, 1.8 L per minute per m^2; and SVR, 1,968 dyne per second per cm^5. Which way should the LV pressure volume loop be shifted?

    A. to the right
    B. to the left
    C. up
    D. down

48–52. In Figure 2, identify which drugs would have this effect on the same patient during hospitalization:

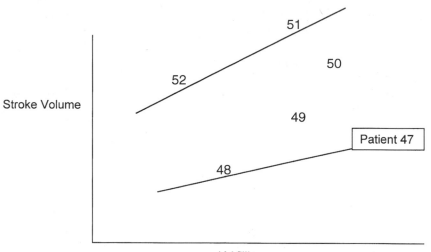

FIGURE 2 (From Smith TW, Kelly RA, Stevenson LW, et al. Management of heart failure. In: Braunwald E, ed. *Heart disease: a textbook of cardiovascular medicine*, 5th ed. Philadelphia: WB Saunders, 1997, with permission.)

A. diuretic only
B. vasodilator only
C. inotropic agent only
D. inotropic agent with vasodilator
E. inotropic agent, vasodilator, and diuretic

Figures 3 to 7 are schematic illustrations of the carotid pulse. Match the diagnosis with the pulse.
A. normal
B. aortic stenosis
C. aortic regurgitation
D. hypertrophic cardiomyopathy
E. severe CHF decompensation

53.

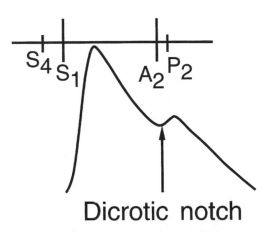

FIGURE 3 (From Chatterjee K. Physical examination. In: Topol EJ, ed. *Textbook of cardiovascular medicine*, 2nd ed. Philadelphia: Lippincott Williams & Wilkins, 2002: Fig. 15.2, with permission.)

54.

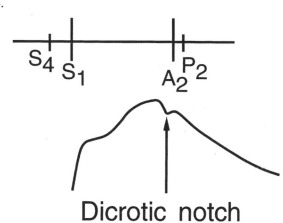

Dicrotic notch

FIGURE 4 (From Chatterjee K. Physical examination. In: Topol EJ, ed. *Textbook of cardiovascular medicine*, 2nd ed. Philadelphia: Lippincott Williams & Wilkins, 2002: Fig. 15.2, with permission.)

55.

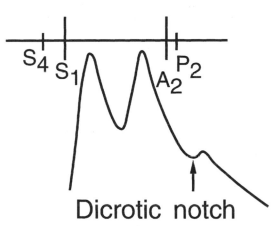

Dicrotic notch

FIGURE 5 (From Chatterjee K. Physical examination. In: Topol EJ, ed. *Textbook of cardiovascular medicine*, 2nd ed. Philadelphia: Lippincott Williams & Wilkins, 2002: Fig. 15.2, with permission.)

56.

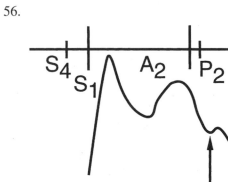

Dicrotic notch

FIGURE 6 (From Chatterjee K. Physical examination. In: Topol EJ, ed. *Textbook of cardiovascular medicine*, 2nd ed. Philadelphia: Lippincott Williams & Wilkins, 2002: Fig. 15.2, with permission.)

57.

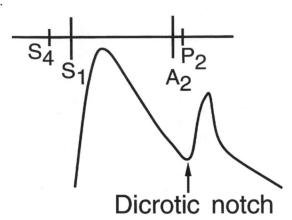

Dicrotic notch

FIGURE 7 (From Chatterjee K. Physical examination. In: Topol EJ, ed. *Textbook of cardiovascular medicine*, 2nd ed. Philadelphia: Lippincott Williams & Wilkins, 2002: Fig. 15.2, with permission.)

58. During physical examination, you notice an elevated systemic *venous* pressure with sharp *y* descent Kussmaul's sign and quiet pericardium. What might the patient have?

   A. constrictive pericarditis
   B. restrictive myocardial disorder
   C. tricuspid regurgitation
   D. pulmonary HTN
   E. tamponade

59. During another physical examination, you notice a prominent *v* wave with a sharp *y* descent. What condition does the patient have?

   A. constrictive cardiomyopathy
   B. restrictive cardiomyopathy
   C. tricuspid regurgitation
   D. pulmonary HTN
   E. tamponade

60. Again you notice an elevated systemic *venous* pressure without obvious *x* or *y* descent and quiet precordium and pulsus paradoxus. What does the patient have?

   A. constrictive cardiomyopathy
   B. restrictive cardiomyopathy
   C. tricuspid regurgitation
   D. pulmonary HTN
   E. tamponade

ANSWERS

1. B. Downregulation primarily of β_1-receptors with little change in β_2-receptors.

2. B. Beta-blockers. Although ACE inhibitors have been shown to improve survival, they have not consistently been shown to improve EF in patients with systolic heart failure. Vasodilators and diuretics have not been shown to improve EF.

3. E. Amlodipine. Vasopressors have been found to increase mortality when taken chronically. Amlodipine did not increase mortality in the Prospective Randomized Amlodipine Survival Evaluation trial.

4. B. Hydralazine plus nitrates. In the V-HeFT II, although ACE inhibitors improved survival, it was hydralazine in combination with nitrates that had greater improvement in LV function and exercise tolerance.

5. C. All of them except losartan. There is no trial evidence that angiotensin II-receptor blocker improved mortality in post-MI patients. The Studies of Left Ventricular Dysfunction (SOLVD) prevention used ACE inhibitors in patients with an EF less than 35%.

6. D. None of the above is your advice. Approximately 50% of patients spontaneously recover in 6 months. Improvement after that time is unlikely. While the patient is waiting, she should be placed on the usual CHF medications, including ACE inhibitors and beta-blockers, and discouraged from breast-feeding.

7. B. Digoxin reduces hospitalization. In the large Digitalis Investigation Group study, digitalis only improved hospitalization. It had no effect on survival.

8. E. No known treatment. Allograft vasculopathy is the leading cause of long-term morbidity and mortality for cardiac transplant patients. Routine cardiac catheterization has been advocated for these patients but has not shown survival benefit with revascularization. Statin therapy appears to improve long-term survival in these patients and should be used for all heart transplant patients. However, its effect on allograft vasculopathy is unknown.

9. C. BNP. The release of BNP is due to increased myocardial stretch in the ventricle. Plasma levels of BNP mainly reflect the degree of LV overload. Like atrial natriuretic factor, both C-type natriuretic peptide and BNP can elicit vasorelaxant activity.

10. E. All of the above occur. BNP has all of the above characteristics in addition to being a vasorelaxant.

11. A. Decrease in HR. BNP increases HR. All of the others are effects of BNP on hemodynamic parameters.

12. D. She should have a PET scan to assess the area of viability before proceeding with CABG or PCI. This patient is at high risk for any type of intervention due to her low EF. However, if there are areas of viability on the PET scan, her EF might improve with complete revascularization. Studies have consistently shown that patients with low EF do better with CABG than with PCI.

13. B. Start dopamine. This patient is in cardiogenic shock. She needs BP support before all else. In these patients, dopamine is the first line of choice, followed by norepinephrine. If there is no change with dopamine and norepinephrine, then dobutamine may be added while the patient is being prepared for IABP placement.

14. C. Consider LV assist device. This is a relatively young patient with no contraindication to cardiac transplant. However, in the current state, she is not eligible for transplantation. LV assist device as a bridge to transplant has been performed with success.

15. C. Acute RV failure. His hemodynamic pressures are characteristic of acute RV failure. He needs aggressive fluid resuscitation.

16. B. Suggest nitroprusside. This patient is in heart failure and needs to have her BP and SVR lowered. BP is adequate and does not need vasopressor or IABP support. Although nesiritide has been approved for use in acute heart failure, it only mildly lowers the BP.

17. A. Place an implantable defibrillator. She fits the criteria of the initial Multicenter Automatic Defibrillator Trial (MADIT). Therefore, based on randomized clinical trial data, she would benefit from an implantable defibrillator. Also, secondary prevention trials such as the Antiarrhythmics Versus Implantable Defibrillators Trial, the Canadian Implantable Defibrillator Study, and the Cardiac Arrest Study Hamburg trial also support an implantable defibrillator in this patient.

18. D. Beta-blockers should be started in stable CHF patients. They should not be started when the patient is congested. Although nonselective agents with vasodilating effects may be preferred, this is not clear at this time.

19. E. In the Prospective Randomized Amlodipine Survival Evaluation Trial, in which NYHA class III or IV patients with an EF less than 30% were enrolled, there was a statistically insignificant reduction in the combined mortality and morbidity in the amlodipine group. However, the benefit appeared to be greater in patients with nonischemic cardiomyopathy.

20. B. Begin ACE inhibitor and beta-blockers. She has well-compensated cardiomyopathy. Only medication that prolongs her life needs to be started. She does not need medication for symptom relief; therefore, ACE inhibitor and beta-blockers should be started.

21. B. Stop diuretics. This patient has prerenal azotemia due to aggressive diuresis. His renal function should recover.

22. C. Bears little relation to the severity of LV dysfunction. Short-term administration of positive inotropic agents and vasodilators does not improve maximal exercise capacity in patients with CHF; moreover, ACE inhibitors have failed to show consistent improvement in exercise tolerance. Numerous studies have not shown a correlation between LV function and exercise tolerance.

23. E. Enrolling her in an exercise training program. As stated, there is no medication that has consistently shown improvement in exercise tolerance; exercise training is the only method that has shown consistent improvement in these patients.

24. B. $\dot{V}E/\dot{V}O_2$ slope during exercise. This is the best correlate of prognosis. There is a higher ventilation for any given CO_2 production ($\dot{V}E/\dot{V}O_2$ slope), which reflects the severity of heart failure and prognosis.

25. A. Glucagon and milrinone. Milrinone is a second-generation phosphodiesterase inhibitor. It has no beta effect; therefore, it is an ideal vasopressor in the setting of beta-blocker overdose. Although a pacer is a good idea and should be placed, giving medication is faster and should be instituted first.

26. B. Atenolol. Atenolol is most affected by reduced renal function. Depending on how severe his creatinine clearance is, he should have his medication dose or frequency adjusted.

27. C. PCWP is 26 mm Hg. Restrictive mitral inflow pattern in the presence of a short E-wave deceleration time has been shown to correlate with high pulmonary capillary pressure, impaired functional class, and bad prognosis in postinfarction patients.

28. D. High filling pressure and reduced LV compliance. These conditions are indicated by a restrictive mitral inflow pattern with short E-wave deceleration time.

29. C. Abnormal HR recovery predicts mortality in all patients; however, there is no treatment. A delayed decrease in HR after exercise or an abnormal HR recovery predicts all-cause mortality in healthy adults and in patients referred for exercise testing—independent of ischemia. However, at this time, there is no treatment to improve abnormal HR recovery.

30. E. Amyloid heart disease. Although severe diabetes and age older than 70 years are exclusion criteria for transplantation, diabetes without end-organ damage and age from 60 to 70 years are not.

31. C. CABG. This patient has left main trunk equivalent with low EF. He is a candidate for CABG with left internal mammary artery to the LAD. CABG will prolong his long-term survival compared to PTCA/stent.

32. D. She should undergo exercise testing for better assessment. Recurrent peripartum cardiomyopathy occurs in 20% of patients with normal resting LV function but abnormal stress ventricular response. Recurrent peripartum cardiomyopathy with decompensation occurred in 41% of patients with abnormal resting LV function.

33. B. Dilated cardiomyopathy. All of the others may cause diastolic heart failure, whereas dilated cardiomyopathy causes systolic heart failure.

34. D. Although this has been seen in retrospective trials, it has not been validated in a randomized trial; therefore, continue the current regimen. In a substudy done by the Gruppo Italiano per lo Studio della Sopravvivenza nell'Infarto Miocardico, aspirin did not decrease the mortality benefit of lisinopril after MI or increase the risk of adverse clinical events. There have been some retrospective studies to assess this question that have had conflicting results; therefore, it is best to stay with the current regimen.

35. B. Refer the patient for biventricular pacing based on QRS duration. Patients with QRS duration greater than 150 to 160 msec derived the greatest benefit from biventricular pacing.

36. A. 20%. There is no role for routine EP study in the asymptomatic hypertrophic cardiomyopathy patient.

37. C. Dofetilide was used in patients with an EF less than 35%. The study compared dofetilide to amiodarone. Dofetilide did not increase mortality. It has not been studied against beta-blockers or calcium channel blockers in patients with normal EF.

38. B. In the large Evaluation of Losartan in the Elderly II study, losartan did not show mortality benefit or reduced hospitalization. Losartan was better tolerated than captopril. Because the patient has no side effects with enalapril, her prescription should not be changed.

39. E. No known treatment available. There have been two randomized trials of chemotherapy showing benefit in amyloid patients with melphalan, prednisone, and colchicine when the major features were not cardiac or renal. For patients with cardiac manifestation, no treatment has shown clear benefit.

40. C. Normal filling pattern.

41. B. Restrictive filling pattern.

42. A. Pseudonormal filling pattern.

43. C. Spironolactone in addition to standard therapy decreases mortality and rehospitalization. In the Randomized Aldactone Evaluation Study, patients with NYHA class III or IV with an EF less than 35% had improvement in mortality, reduction in hospitalization, and improvement in functional class when spironolactone was taken in addition to standard therapy (ACE inhibitor and diuretic).

44. E. Cardioversion. This patient has post-MI AFib. He has LV dysfunction and renal insufficiency. Procainamide should be used in patients with normal LV and renal clearance. Amiodarone would take too long to work, and he is already in distress. Lidocaine is not used in AFib. Metoprolol tartrate would exacerbate his heart failure; therefore, cardioversion is the only choice.

45. A. Exercise. Exercise is recommended in patients with stable heart failure. Nonsteroidal antiinflammatory drugs, trastuzumab (Herceptin), infection, and noncompliance are well-known causes of acute decompensated heart failure.

46. An LV pressure volume loop.
    A. = 1. mitral valve opening
    B. = 2. end-diastole
    C. = 3. aortic valve opening
    D. = 4. end-systole

47. C. Up. The response of the LV to increased afterload is to shift the loop up. Increased preload would shift the loop to the right.

48. A. Diuretic only. This loop represents a Frank-Starling ventricular function curve in a heart failure patient due to systolic dysfunction.

49. B. Vasodilator only.

50. C. Inotropic agent only.

51. D. Inotropic agent with vasodilator.

52. E. Inotropic agent, vasodilator, and diuretic.

53. A. Normal.

54. B. Aortic stenosis.

55. C. Aortic regurgitation.

56. D. Hypertrophic cardiomyopathy.

57. E. Severe CHF decompensation.

58. A. Constrictive pericarditis.

59. C. Tricuspid regurgitation.

60. E. Tamponade.

SUGGESTED READING

Braunwald E, Coluccci WS, Grossman W. Clinical aspects of heart failure: high output heart failure: pulmonary edema. In: Braunwald E, ed. *Heart disease: a textbook of cardiovascular medicine*, 5th ed. Philadelphia: WB Saunders, 1997.

Chatterjee K. Physical examination. In: Topol EJ, ed. *Textbook of cardiovascular medicine*, 2nd ed. Philadelphia: Lippincott Williams & Wilkins, 2002.

Francis G. Pathophysiology of the heart failure clinical syndrome. In: Topol EJ, ed. *Textbook of cardiovascular medicine*, 2nd ed. Philadelphia: Lippincott Williams & Wilkins, 2002.

Haas GJ, Young JB. Acute heart failure management. In: Topol EJ, ed. *Textbook of cardiovascular medicine*, 2nd ed. Philadelphia: Lippincott Williams & Wilkins, 2002.

Smith TW, Kelly RA, Stevenson LW, et al. Management of heart failure. In: Braunwald E, ed. *Heart disease: a textbook of cardiovascular medicine*, 5th ed. Philadelphia: WB Saunders, 1997.

Young JB. Chronic heart failure management. In: Topol EJ, ed. *Textbook of cardiovascular medicine*, 2nd ed. Philadelphia: Lippincott Williams & Wilkins, 2002.

CHAPTER 8

Adult Congenital Heart Disease

Sasan Ghaffari and Raymond Q. Migrino

QUESTIONS

1. What is the most common coexisting congenital anomaly in patients with coarctation of the aorta?

    A. cleft mitral valve
    B. bicuspid aortic valve
    C. Ebstein's anomaly
    D. VSD
    E. patent ductus arteriosus (PDA)

2. All of the following are characteristic findings of ostium primum atrial septal defect (ASD) *except*

    A. precordial heave
    B. fixed split S_2
    C. right-axis deviation
    D. systolic ejection murmur
    E. prominent pulmonary vascular markings on CXR

3. All of the following are complications of unrecognized coarctation of the aorta *except*

    A. aortic dissection
    B. cerebrovascular aneurysms
    C. CHF
    D. LV hypertrophy
    E. SVT

4. All of the following statements are true regarding bicuspid aortic valve *except*

   A. In approximately 20% of cases, there are associated congenital conditions, such as coarctation of the aorta.
   B. A coexisting abnormality in the medial layer of the aorta causes dilatation of the aortic root.
   C. It is associated with diminished life expectancy.
   D. It is more common in males than females.
   E. With aortic valve stenosis, percutaneous balloon valvotomy has good short-term results in children but not in adults.

5. All of the following statements regarding pulmonary stenosis are true *except*

   A. Balloon valvuloplasty is the procedure of choice and has good long-term results.
   B. The majority of cases are subvalvular or supravalvular in location.
   C. Valve replacement is usually reserved for dysplastic and calcified leaflets or for cases with significant regurgitation.
   D. Among patients with valvular stenosis, only approximately 10% to 15% of cases have dysplastic leaflets.
   E. Adults are usually asymptomatic when first diagnosed.

6. A 19-year-old man seeks your advice regarding profound dyspnea on exertion. He was born cyanotic, and he has not had regular follow-up. On examination, there is significant clubbing and cyanosis of all digits. There is RV lift, with a loud systolic ejection murmur in the left upper sternal border with a thrill. P_2 is absent. CXR demonstrates RV enlargement and pulmonary oligemia. His ECG reveals sinus rhythm with RV hypertrophy. Which of the following two-dimensional TTE findings will *not* be seen in this condition?

   A. pulmonary stenosis
   B. apical displacement of tricuspid leaflets
   C. RV hypertrophy
   D. overriding aorta
   E. VSD

7. The above patient undergoes surgical repair. Which of the following statements regarding long-term post-repair follow-up is *false*?

   A. The survival rate is 86% 32 years after surgery.
   B. Ventricular arrhythmias and sudden death pose long-term health hazards.
   C. On 12-lead ECG, a QRS duration of longer than 180 msec is associated with VT.
   D. A palliative shunt is the preferred surgical strategy.
   E. He is at increased risk of infective endocarditis.

8. All of the following statements regarding PDA are true *except*

   A. The majority of cases close spontaneously after infancy.
   B. There is a higher incidence in mothers who acquired rubella during pregnancy.
   C. A decrease in the duration and intensity of the murmur has a poor prognostic implication.
   D. LV hypertrophy precedes RV hypertrophy.
   E. If it is uncorrected, approximately one-third of patients die by the age of 40 years.

9. All of the following are found in cor triatriatum *except*

   A. pulmonary hypertension
   B. increased mitral orifice inflow velocity by pulsed-wave Doppler
   C. a double-chamber left atrium
   D. diastolic fluttering of the mitral leaflet
   E. a fibromuscular diaphragm inferior to the left atrial appendage

10. A 20-year-old asymptomatic man is referred for further evaluation of uncontrolled hypertension. He has a strong family history of premature hypertension. His vital signs reveal a left upper extremity BP of 150/100 mm Hg and a right lower extremity BP of 130/94 mm Hg. Heart rate is 88 bpm. His cardiac examination is remarkable for a 2/6 systolic ejection murmur in the right upper sternal border and an S_4 gallop. There is brachial-femoral pulse delay. The rest of the physical and neurologic examinations are within normal limits. A TTE confirmed a diagnosis of coarctation of the aorta, with a maximum gradient of 26 mm Hg. He has a bicuspid aortic valve with peak/mean gradients of 12/6 mm Hg and trivial aortic insufficiency. Cardiac catheterization reaffirms the transcoarctation gradient and demonstrates a narrowed segment in the descending aorta distal to origin of the subclavian artery. What is the most appropriate management strategy?

    A. surgical repair with end-to-end anastomosis
    B. percutaneous balloon angioplasty
    C. BP control that includes a beta-blocker agent
    D. EP testing for risk stratification
    E. repeat cardiac catheterization in 6 months

11. Congenital MR is commonly encountered in all of the following conditions *except*

    A. cor triatriatum
    B. ostium primum ASD
    C. coarctation of the aorta
    D. congenitally corrected transposition of the great arteries
    E. subaortic stenosis

12. Which of the following is the most common coronary artery anomaly?

    A. Bland-Garland-White syndrome (left main coronary artery arising from the PA)
    B. coronary arteriovenous fistula
    C. left circumflex artery arising from the right coronary artery
    D. left coronary artery arising from the right sinus of Valsalva
    E. coronary cameral fistula

13. Which of the following differentiates valvular aortic stenosis from subvalvular aortic stenosis?

    A. male preponderance
    B. surgical risk of repair
    C. dilatation of the ascending aorta
    D. aortic regurgitation
    E. valvular calcification

14. Besides pulmonary valve stenosis, which of the following is the most common associated cardiac defect present in patients with PA stenosis?

    A. VSD
    B. ASD
    C. coarctation of the aorta
    D. PDA
    E. bicuspid aortic valve

15. The following cardiovascular malformations are all associated with congenital rubella *except*

    A. PDA
    B. PA stenosis
    C. Ebstein's anomaly
    D. tetralogy of Fallot
    E. coarctation of the aorta

16. Which of the following statements about coronary arteriovenous fistula is *true*?

    A. The left coronary artery is most commonly involved.
    B. The fistula most commonly empties into the LV.
    C. Despite the success of surgical closure, the prognosis is still poor.
    D. Spontaneous closure rarely occurs.
    E. A large right-to-left shunt may cause CHF.

17. A 20-year-old asymptomatic man was diagnosed to have a subaortic membrane. The peak gradient across the membrane is 20 mm Hg. The aortic valve remains mobile, but there is associated moderate aortic valve insufficiency. What should you advise this patient?

    A. Elective surgical resection should be considered.
    B. TTE should be performed twice per year, and surgical correction is performed when the peak gradient across the membrane becomes greater than 40 mm Hg.
    C. Transluminal balloon dilatation should be performed, because the long-term results are superior to surgical treatment.
    D. Endocarditis prophylaxis is not necessary.
    E. Surgical resection is rarely curative.

18. Which of the following syndromes is associated with pulmonary arteriovenous fistula?

    A. Williams syndrome
    B. Weber-Osler-Rendu syndrome
    C. Bland-Garland-White syndrome
    D. Kartagener's syndrome
    E. Crouzon's syndrome

19. In which of the following cases is surgical correction recommended?

    A. asymptomatic small VSD to decrease risk of endocarditis
    B. PDA with severe pulmonary hypertension
    C. asymptomatic subaortic stenosis with severe aortic valve insufficiency
    D. coarctation of the aorta with a transcoarctation gradient of 20 mm Hg
    E. small ASD to prevent paradoxical embolization

20. All of the following statements regarding anomalous pulmonary venous drainage are true *except*

    A. It is frequently associated with the secundum-type ASD.
    B. The degree of pulmonary hypertension depends on the number of anomalous veins involved.
    C. Oximetry is of limited value if the pulmonary vein drains into the inferior vena cava.
    D. It may be associated with VSD.
    E. TTE frequently misses this finding.

21. Which of the following is an indication for aortic surgical repair in patients with coarctation of the aorta?

    A. 50-mm Hg transcoarctation pressure gradient
    B. headaches
    C. chest pain
    D. presyncope
    E. right upper extremity claudication

22. All of the following statements regarding Ebstein's anomaly are true *except*

    A. The majority of patients have interatrial communication with potential for right-to-left shunting.
    B. There may be widely split S_1 and S_2 with triple or quadruple rhythm and a holosystolic murmur at the left lower sternal border.
    C. Approximately 20% of patients have ventricular preexcitation or other forms of tachyarrhythmias.
    D. There is displacement of mitral leaflets into the LV.
    E. With valve replacement, bioprosthetic durability compares favorably with other cardiac valve positions.

23. A patient with congenitally corrected transposition may present with all of the following clinical features *except*

    A. CHB
    B. platypnea-orthodeoxia
    C. heart failure
    D. AV valve regurgitation
    E. supraventricular arrhythmias

24. Patients with Eisenmenger's syndrome should avoid all of the following *except*

    A. dehydration
    B. high altitude
    C. heavy exertion
    D. vasodilators
    E. phlebotomy

25. With which of the following adult congenital heart conditions can the following ECG tracing be seen (Fig. 1)?

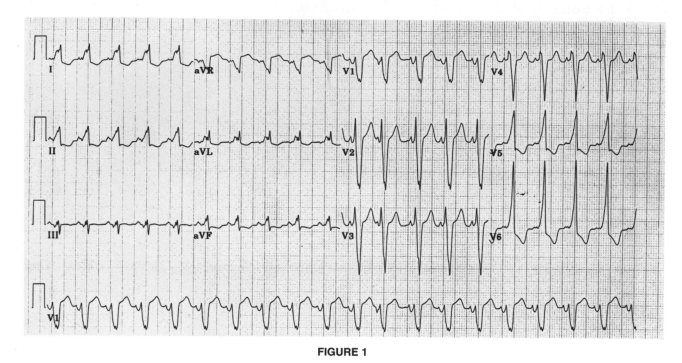

FIGURE 1

A. primum ASD
B. congenitally corrected transposition
C. Ebstein's anomaly
D. VSD
E. coarctation of the aorta

26. A 25-year-old man is referred to you for an abnormal heart sound. The patient is asymptomatic and very active. He has a continuous murmur at the left upper sternal border. A TTE reveals a small PDA with normal LV and RV and normal pulmonary pressures. How would the patient be best managed?

A. ligation or closure of the PDA
B. repeat TTE in 1 year
C. stress TTE to determine LV enlargement or dysfunction postexercise
D. endocarditis prophylaxis
E. TEE

27. All of the following statements are consistent with the natural history of ASD *except*

A. In the sixth decade, the mortality rate can approach 10%.
B. Most patients are minimally symptomatic in the first three decades.
C. LV dysfunction is unusual (less than 5%) in patients older than 50 years.
D. The majority of patients are symptomatic by the fifth decade.
E. Approximately one-half of patients older than 40 years develop pulmonary hypertension.

28. A 30-year-old man with Eisenmenger's syndrome and irreversible pulmonary hypertension due to untreated VSD is at risk for developing symptoms and signs of hyperviscosity. All of the following are associated with hyperviscosity syndrome *except*

    A. coronary artery ectasia
    B. erythrocytosis
    C. visual disturbances
    D. paresthesias
    E. iron-deficiency anemia

29. Bacterial endocarditis prophylaxis is indicated in all adults who have the following congenital heart diseases *except*

    A. VSD
    B. coarctation of the aorta
    C. secundum ASD
    D. hypertrophic obstructive cardiomyopathy
    E. PDA

30. Pregnancy should be avoided in which of the following adult congenital heart diseases?

    A. Eisenmenger's syndrome
    B. Marfan's syndrome with an enlarged aortic root
    C. severe pulmonary hypertension
    D. congenital aortic stenosis with New York Heart Association class III heart failure
    E. all of the above

31. All of the following are indications for surgical closure of an ASD *except*

    A. significant symptoms in a 65 year old
    B. RV dysfunction
    C. pulmonary vascular resistance greater than 15 Wood units that does not diminish with vasodilators
    D. an asymptomatic 20 year old with a Qp/Qs of 1.7 with no pulmonary hypertension
    E. RV enlargement

32. All of the following statements regarding PDA are true *except*

    A. The pulmonic bed is usually dilated.
    B. The most common location is distal to the left subclavian artery.
    C. Infectious endocarditis frequently occurs at the pulmonary end.
    D. The risk of endocarditis is less in patients with inaudible PDA.
    E. Transcatheter-device closure or coil occlusion is the procedure of choice for closure in adults.

33. All of the following physical examination findings are usually associated with ostium secundum ASD *except*

    A. precordial heave
    B. fixed split S_2
    C. lateral and inferior displacement of the apex beat
    D. soft systolic ejection murmur in the second left intercostal space
    E. normal S_1

34. Which of the following is an absolute contraindication to pregnancy?
    A. surgically corrected transposition of great arteries
    B. congenitally corrected transposition of great arteries
    C. Ebstein's anomaly
    D. Eisenmenger's syndrome
    E. status post Fontan operation

35. A 45-year-old man with known Ebstein's anomaly seeks your advice with regard to optimal management. He is asymptomatic and has an active lifestyle without any limitations. His physical examination is remarkable for the absence of cyanosis. He has a loud holosystolic murmur at the left lower sternal border that is accentuated with respiration. He has no organomegaly or peripheral edema. His TTE reveals moderately severe 3+ tricuspid regurgitation with an RV systolic pressure of 46 mm Hg and normal LV and RV systolic functions. There is no evidence of interatrial communication. Which of the following should you recommend?
    A. furosemide and digoxin
    B. tricuspid valve repair
    C. tricuspid valve replacement
    D. dual-chamber pacemaker
    E. regular follow-up with repeat TTE in 6 months

Match the following conditions with their corresponding surgical procedures. There may be more than one answer for each question.
    A. Ross
    B. Blalock-Taussig
    C. Senning or Mustard
    D. arterial switch
    E. Fontan
    F. Rashkind
    G. none of the above

36. Pulmonary atresia

37. Transposition of great vessels

38. Tricuspid atresia

39. Congenitally corrected transposition

40. Aortic stenosis

Match the following disease conditions with their gender preponderance.

    A. predominantly male
    B. predominantly female
    C. equal preponderance

41. VSD

42. ASD

43. Bicuspid aortic valve

44. Coarctation of the aorta

45. Pulmonary atresia with an intact ventricular septum

Match the following cardiac catheterization still-frame slides (Figs. 2 through 6) to their respective diagnoses.

    A. coarctation of the aorta
    B. PDA
    C. hypertrophic cardiomyopathy
    D. pulmonic stenosis
    E. VSD

46.

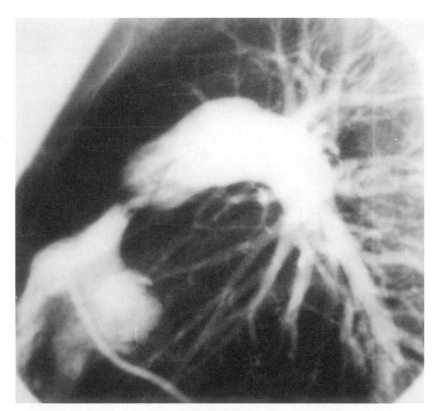

FIGURE 2

NOTES

47.

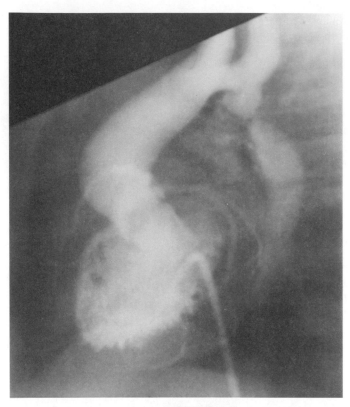

FIGURE 3

48.

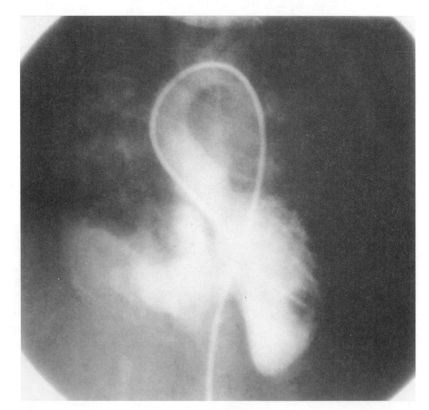

FIGURE 4

49.

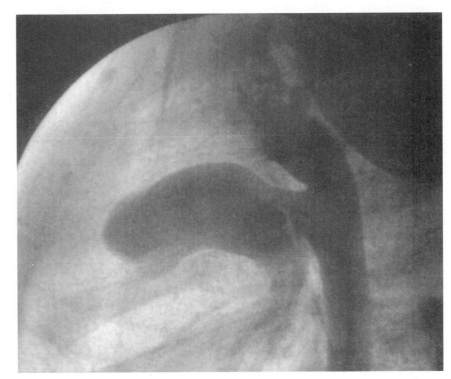

FIGURE 5

50.

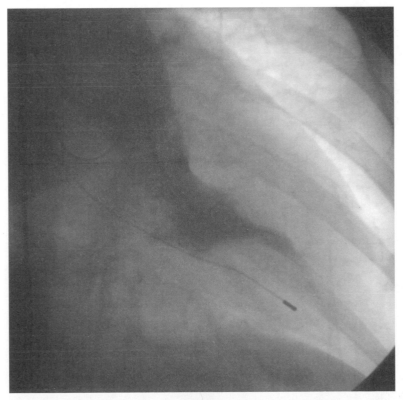

FIGURE 6

Match the adult congenital heart disorder with the corresponding physical examination findings.

    A. Eisenmenger's syndrome
    B. coarctation of the aorta
    C. PDA
    D. Ebstein's anomaly
    E. tetralogy of Fallot

51. RV lift with a loud systolic ejection murmur along the left sternal border, with a single S_2

52. Loud S_1, holosystolic murmur in left lower sternal border, systolic ejection click, and hepatomegaly

53. Weak or delayed femoral arterial pulses, harsh systolic ejection murmur in the back, and a systolic ejection click in the aortic area

54. Cyanosis, digital clubbing, loud P_2, and a variable Graham-Steell murmur

55. Wide pulse pressure, prominent LV impulse, and a continuous machinery murmur enveloping S_2

Match the following congenital defects with their associated disease conditions.

    A. supravalvular aortic stenosis
    B. supravalvular pulmonic stenosis
    C. cleft mitral valve
    D. anomalous pulmonary venous drainage
    E. persistent left superior vena cava

56. Ostium primum ASD

57. Noonan's syndrome

58. Coronary sinus ASD

59. Williams syndrome

60. Sinus venosus ASD

Match the characteristic chest radiography findings with the corresponding congenital disorder.

    A. Eisenmenger's syndrome
    B. coarctation of the aorta
    C. PDA
    D. Ebstein's anomaly
    E. tetralogy of Fallot

61. Prominent central PAs (possible calcifications) and peripheral PA pruning

62. Right aortic arch, RV enlargement, and a "boot-shaped" heart

63. Marked cardiomegaly, severe right atrial enlargement, and normal lung fields

64. Posterior rib notching and a "reverse E" or "3" sign

65. Pulmonary plethora, prominent ascending aorta, proximal PA dilatation, and opacity at the confluence of the aortic knob and descending aorta

Match the following congenital cardiac disorder with the characteristic TTE finding (Figs. 7 through 11).

A.

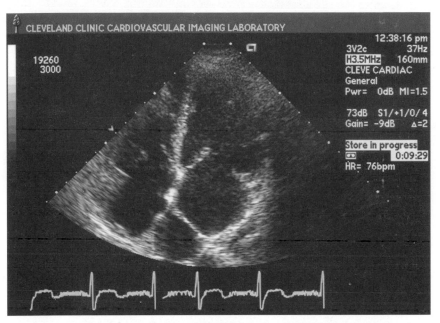

FIGURE 7

B.

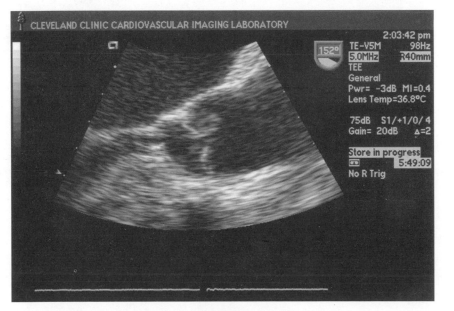

FIGURE 8

C.

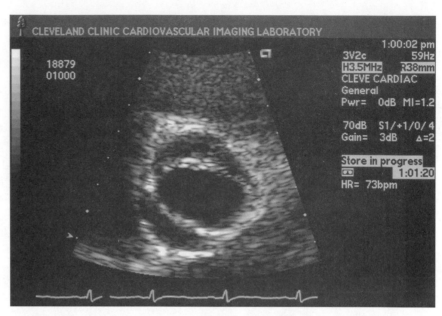

FIGURE 9

D.

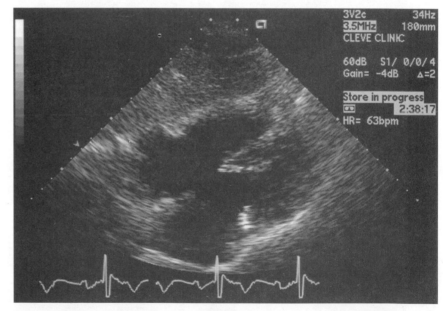

FIGURE 10

E.

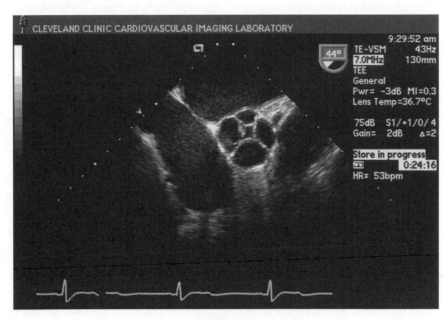

FIGURE 11

66. Bicuspid aortic valve

67. Cor triatriatum

68. Ostium primum ASD

69. Quadricuspid aortic valve

70. Subaortic valve stenosis

ANSWERS

1. B. Bicuspid aortic valve. Aortic coarctation is a common congenital defect that consists of a constriction just distal to the left subclavian artery at the site of residual ligamentum arteriosus. Bicuspid aortic valve is the most common coexisting anomaly. However, the presence of VSD, PDA, and malformations of the mitral valve apparatus is well documented. There is no association between aortic coarctation and Ebstein's anomaly.

2. C. Right-axis deviation is not a characteristic finding. Ostium primum ASD is usually associated with left-axis deviation. The other findings are characteristic physical and radiologic findings of ASD.

3. E. Unrecognized and untreated aortic coarctation causes premature death, with mean survival of 35 years and 75% mortality by age 50. Ninety percent of patients with this condition die before they reach the age of 60 years. Complications of aortic coarctation include systemic hypertension with LV hypertrophy, aortic dissection, premature CAD with MI, cerebral vascular

complications, infective endocarditis, and CHF. SVT is most commonly associated with other congenital diseases, such as Ebstein's anomaly, ASD, or tetralogy of Fallot.

4. C. Asymptomatic adult patients have normal life expectancy. Bicuspid aortic valve has a male preponderance. In approximately 20% of cases, this condition is associated with congenital conditions, such as coarctation of the aorta and PDA. It is frequently associated with dilatation of the aortic root because of a congenital abnormality in the medial layer of the aorta. Percutaneous balloon valvotomy for congenital aortic stenosis has demonstrated good short-term results in children but not in adults.

5. B. Approximately 90% of cases are valvular in nature. Balloon valvuloplasty is the procedure of choice and has excellent long-term results. In approximately 10% to 15% of cases, the valve leaflets are dysplastic and may be thickened, immobile, or myxomatous. Valve replacement is reserved for dysplastic leaflets or if significant regurgitation is present. Adults are usually asymptomatic, and the condition is discovered through routine auscultation.

6. B. Apical displacement of tricuspid leaflets will not be seen in this condition. The most common cyanotic congenital heart defect is tetralogy of Fallot. The characteristic signs that are confirmed by two-dimensional TTE are obstruction of RV outflow tract (pulmonary stenosis), RV hypertrophy, an aorta that overrides the LV and RV, and a large VSD. Apical displacement of tricuspid leaflets is the hallmark of Ebstein's anomaly.

7. D. Surgical repair is recommended to patients with tetralogy of Fallot to relieve symptoms and improve survival. In one series, performed by Murphy et al., the rate of survival 32 years after surgery was 86% among patients with repaired tetralogy and 96% in an age-matched control population. Both supraventricular and ventricular arrhythmias are commonly seen in patients post-repair and are a significant cause of morbidity and mortality. Complete surgical correction with closure of VSD and relief of RV outflow obstruction is the preferred surgical strategy in the appropriate setting. Palliative shunting is performed in severely ill infants or in those patients who have underdeveloped PAs. Palliative surgery does not correct the underlying anatomic defects and is associated with long-term risk.

8. A. A PDA, unlike VSD, rarely closes spontaneously after infancy. It is associated with maternal rubella, perinatal hypoxemia, premature births, or births at high altitude. It causes left atrial and LV hypertrophy. With development of pulmonary hypertension, RV hypertrophy may develop, and the duration and intensity of the machinery murmur may diminish. Uncorrected, one-third of patients die of heart failure, pulmonary hypertension, or endocarditis by the age of 40 years, and two-thirds die by the age of 60 years.

9. E. Fibromuscular diaphragm inferior to the left atrial appendage is not found in cor triatriatum. Cor triatriatum is a congenital disease that is characterized by the presence of a fibromuscular diaphragm in the left atrium that divides the left atrium into two chambers. It arises from the failure of resorption of the common pulmonary vein. There may be significant obstruction between the posterosuperior chamber that receives the pulmo-

nary veins and the anteroinferior chamber that encompasses the left atrial appendage and the mitral valve. Pulmonary hypertension may result. The increased velocity across the diaphragm may cause diastolic fluttering of the mitral valve and increased flow through the distal atrial chamber and at the mitral orifice. The diaphragm arises superior to the left atrial appendage, unlike the supravalvular mitral ring.

10. C. BP control that includes a beta-blocker agent. This young man's aortic coarctation is mild to moderate and does not warrant surgical repair at this time. Surgical repair is indicated when the transcoarctation pressure gradient exceeds 30 mm Hg. Percutaneous balloon angioplasty is associated with a higher rate of recurrent coarctation and increased risk of subsequent aortic aneurysm and, therefore, is not the first therapeutic choice. Because this patient has hypertension and is at risk for aortic dissection, tight BP control with beta-blockers is advised. There is no role for EP study, and repeat cardiac catheterization is not indicated due to its invasive nature. A follow-up TTE every 6 months is recommended.

11. A. Congenital MR is associated with multiple congenital heart diseases, including ostium primum septal defect, coarctation of the aorta, congenitally corrected transposition of the great arteries, subaortic stenosis, hypertrophic obstructive cardiomyopathy, endocardial fibroelastosis, and anomalous pulmonary origin of the coronary artery. Cor triatriatum produces symptoms and findings similar to mitral stenosis but is not associated with congenital MR.

12. C. Left circumflex artery arising from the right coronary artery.

13. E. Valvular calcification. Both valvular and subvalvular aortic stenosis have male preponderance and may be associated with dilatation of the ascending aorta. The indications and risk of operation are similar. Although aortic regurgitation is more common in subvalvular aortic stenosis, it may also occur in valvular aortic stenosis. Valvular calcification is usually not observed in subvalvular aortic valve stenosis.

14. A. VSD. Two-thirds of patients with PA stenosis, also known as *supravalvar pulmonic stenosis*, have associated cardiac anomalies. The most common are valvular pulmonic stenosis and VSD. PDA and ASD are common, especially in mothers with rubella. Tetralogy of Fallot is also seen.

15. C. Ebstein's anomaly is not associated with congenital rubella. The most common malformations associated with congenital rubella are PA stenosis and PDA. Other malformations include pulmonary valve stenosis, systemic arterial stenosis, hypoplasia of the abdominal aorta, VSD, ASD, tetralogy of Fallot, coarctation of the aorta, aortic valvular or supravalvar stenosis, transposition of the great arteries, tricuspid atresia, and multiple valvular sclerosis.

16. D. Spontaneous closure rarely occurs. The most common origin of coronary arteriovenous fistula is the right coronary artery, with a fistulous communication into the RV, right atrium, or coronary sinus. Less commonly, it empties into the LV, left atrium, or PA. Complications may include CHF from left-to-right shunt, bacterial endocarditis, coronary ischemia, and rupture or thrombosis of the fistula. Surgical closure is associated with a good outcome. A fistula rarely closes spontaneously.

17. A. Elective surgical resection should be considered. Subaortic valve stenosis involves the presence of a membranous diaphragm in the LVOT that creates a turbulent flow across the LVOT. This frequently causes damage to the aortic valve and may cause aortic valve insufficiency, aside from creating LVOT obstruction. Because of the potential damage to the aortic valve, elective surgical resection is advised even with mild stenosis, especially if damage to the aortic valve is already established. Although recurrences occur, surgical resection is frequently curative. Transluminal balloon dilatation may be appropriate in carefully selected patients, but the relief of obstruction is frequently not as durable or complete as surgical resection. Trauma to the aortic valve predisposes to bacterial endocarditis, and endocarditis prophylaxis should be advised.

18. B. Weber-Osler-Rendu syndrome. Pulmonary arteriovenous fistula involves direct communication between PAs and veins. Most patients have associated Weber-Osler-Rendu syndrome, a condition associated with the presence of multiple telangiectasias. Williams syndrome is associated with mental retardation, elfin facies, and supravalvular aortic and pulmonic stenosis. Bland-Garland-White syndrome involves the anomalous origin of the left coronary artery from the PA. Kartagener's syndrome is associated with situs inversus, sinusitis, and bronchiectasis. Crouzon's syndrome is associated with PDA and aortic coarctation.

19. C. Asymptomatic subaortic stenosis with severe aortic valve insufficiency. In subaortic stenosis, a high-velocity jet damages the aortic valve. Thus, even in the absence of symptoms, surgery is recommended because of progressive valve destruction. In VSD, surgical correction does not entirely eliminate the risk of endocarditis. In ASD, closure is not recommended solely for the purpose of preventing paradoxical embolization. In PDA, high pulmonary vascular resistance connotes poor survival, and surgical correction is not recommended. In coarctation of the aorta with a small transcoarctation gradient of 20 mm Hg or less, surgical treatment has not been proven to be superior to medical treatment.

20. A. It is not frequently associated with secundum-type ASD. Anomalous pulmonary venous drainage is frequently associated with sinus venosus–type ASD. In addition, in approximately 20% of cases, there is an associated cardiac anomaly, such as VSD or tetralogy of Fallot. The physiologic consequence increases with the number of pulmonary veins involved. TTE may miss this finding, and TEE may be needed for identification of the defect. Because of the contribution of oxygenated blood from the renal arteries, oximetry may be limited if the pulmonary vein drains into the inferior vena cava.

21. A. 50-mm Hg transcoarctation pressure gradient. A greater than 30-mm Hg transcoarctation gradient is a definite indication for surgical repair. Symptoms such as headaches, chest pain, and presyncope are nonspecific and by themselves do not warrant surgical repair. The site of discrete narrowing is commonly distal to the left subclavian artery; it should not cause right upper extremity claudication.

22. D. Ebstein's anomaly involves the tricuspid valve, with displacement of tricuspid leaflets (mainly posterior) into the RV, resulting in an "atrialized" small RV. Approximately 80% of patients with this form of congenital anomaly have an interatrial communication, with potential for right-to-left

shunting of blood. On physical examination, there are widely split S_1 and S_2. S_3 and S_4 gallop sounds are often heard. Because of the incompetency of the tricuspid leaflets (deformed and abnormal attachments), a loud tricuspid regurgitation murmur can be heard, a holosystolic murmur at the left lower sternal border that accentuates in intensity with respirations. Approximately 20% of patients with Ebstein's anomaly develop Wolff-Parkinson-White syndrome with preexcitation and supraventricular tachyarrhythmias. When surgical repair is indicated, replacement of the deformed tricuspid leaflets with a bioprosthetic valve has been shown to compare favorably with bioprosthesis durability in other cardiac valve positions.

23. B. Platypnea-orthodeoxia. In congenitally corrected transposition, there is AV discordance as well as ventriculoarterial discordance. Systemic and pulmonary circulations are in series, just like normal cardiopulmonary circulation, and in the absence of a shunt, the patient is acyanotic. Morphologic RV and tricuspid valves are aligned with the aorta and perform life-long systemic work. Other accompanying defects include perimembranous VSD, pulmonary stenosis, and Ebstein's anomaly. Clinical features that manifest themselves in adulthood include CHB, significant AV valve regurgitation with heart failure, and supraventricular arrhythmias. Platypnea (dyspnea induced by assumption of the upright position and relieved by assumption of a recumbent position) and orthodeoxia (O_2 desaturation and hypoxemia in the upright position) can be seen with aortic elongation and patent foramen ovale and is not a common presentation of congenitally corrected transposition.

24. E. Patients with Eisenmenger's syndrome develop irreversible pulmonary vascular disease, pulmonary hypertension, and right-to-left shunting with cyanosis. Erythrocytosis and hyperviscosity syndrome is a significant source of morbidity and increases risk of mortality. Dehydration, high altitude with lower partial O_2 pressure, heavy exertion, and vasodilators tend to worsen this condition and result in greater right-to-left shunting and hypoxemia. On the contrary, phlebotomy is therapeutic when patients present with hematocrit greater than 60 and symptoms of hyperviscosity.

25. C. Ebstein's anomaly. The ECG demonstrates a short PR interval, presence of delta waves, and wide QRS interval that are all consistent with preexcitation and Wolff-Parkinson-White syndrome. Wolff-Parkinson-White syndrome is most commonly associated with Ebstein's anomaly.

26. A. Ligation or closure of the PDA. There is no evidence by clinical or TTE examination of elevated pulmonary vascular resistance. The mortality rate for ligation and division of the PDA is exceedingly low, but the risk of endarteritis with unrepaired ductus is significant enough (0.45%/year after the second decade of life) that authorities recommend closure or ligation even with small PDA. Endocarditis prophylaxis is recommended but does not definitely address the problem. Direct visualization with TTE may be difficult, but if good visualization is achieved, a TEE is rarely needed.

27. C. LV dysfunction is unusual in the young, but the incidence is as high as 15% in patients older than age 50. The annual mortality rate increases to 10% in the sixth decade. Most patients are minimally symptomatic in the first three decades of life, but by the fifth decade, more than 70% are symptomatic. Pulmonary hypertension is unusual in patients younger than 20

years, but approximately 50% of patients older than 40 years of age develop it.

28. A. Coronary artery ectasia is not associated with hyperviscosity syndrome. Chronic hypoxemia and cyanosis lead to compensatory erythrocytosis and significant rise in hematocrit. Symptoms and signs of hyperviscosity syndrome include visual disturbances, headache, dizziness, fatigue, hemoptysis, thrombosis and bleeding, and paresthesias. Cerebral catastrophes may occur as a result of venous thrombosis of cerebral vessels, intracranial hemorrhage, or paradoxical embolization.

29. C. Secundum ASD is a very low-risk lesion and, therefore, does not require endocarditis prophylaxis. Current guidelines for prevention of bacterial endocarditis apply to most congenital heart lesions, with the exception of isolated secundum ASD and surgically repaired atrial and ventricular or ductal shunt without residual shunt beyond 6 months after repair.

30. E. All of the above. The conditions that result in greatest risk to the mother or the fetus, or both, include Eisenmenger's syndrome, severe pulmonary hypertension, severe LV outflow obstruction, Marfan's syndrome with an enlarged aortic root, and New York Heart Association class III or IV heart failure.

31. C. Pulmonary vascular resistance greater than 15 Wood units that does not diminish with vasodilators is not an indication for surgical closure. Surgery is not recommended in patients with ASD with elevated pulmonary vascular resistance, which is irreversible.

32. A. Dilatation at the aortic end is found in 65% of patients. Constriction of the PDA starts at the pulmonary end, where endocarditis frequently originates. Patients with clinically silent PDA detected by TTE do not appear to be at risk for endocarditis. PDA is most commonly located distal to the origin of the left subclavian artery. The fetal ductus is derived from the sixth aortic arch, the same origin as that of the left and right PAs.

33. C. Lateral and inferior displacement of the apex beat are not associated with ostium secundum ASD. Lateral and inferior displacement of the apex beat occur with LV enlargement. In secundum ASD, the major hemodynamic consequences occur to the RV and not to the LV. An RV impulse or precordial heave as well as pulmonary arterial impulse may be palpable. There is fixed splitting of the S_2 because the phasic changes in the systemic venous return that occurs with respiration and that is responsible for physiologic splitting are minimized by the accompanying reciprocal changes in shunted blood from the left atrium to the right atrium.

34. D. Eisenmenger's syndrome. Eisenmenger's syndrome is one of few conditions that pose an absolute contraindication to pregnancy. Pregnancy in patients with Eisenmenger's syndrome is associated with mortality rates of up to 50%.

35. E. Regular follow-up with repeat TTE in 6 months. The patient has moderately severe tricuspid regurgitation and mild pulmonary hypertension, with preserved RV systolic function. He has no symptoms and no evidence of CHF. There is no need to intervene at this time, and regular follow-up with TTE should suffice.

36. B,E. Blalock-Taussig and Fontan.

37. C,D,F. Senning or Mustard, arterial switch, and Rashkind.

38. E,F. Fontan and Rashkind.

39. G. None of the above.

40. A. Ross. Please refer to Table 1, which provides a complete overview of common surgical procedures for congenital heart disease.

TABLE 1 *Common Surgical Procedures for Congenital Heart Disease*

Procedure	Description	Intent	Result
Blalock-Taussig	Subclavian artery to PA anastomosis	PAL	Increases pulmonary blood flow
Central shunt	Conduit or anastomosis between aorta and PA	PAL	Increases pulmonary blood flow
Damus-Kaye-Stansel	PA end-to-side anastomosis to aorta, valved conduit between RV and main PA	COR	Increases blood flow to aorta and PA when there is aortic stenosis and two ventricles; reestablishes RV to PA continuity
Fontan	Anastomosis or conduit between right atrium and PA	PAL	Increases pulmonary blood flow in cases of univentricular heart or tricuspid atresia
Glenn (bidirectional Glenn)	SVC to PA anastomosis	PAL	Increases pulmonary blood flow
Arterial switch or Jatene	Transection of aorta and PA with reimplantation onto the proper ventricles, coronary arteries reimplanted	COR	Creates normal relationship between the ventricles and great arteries in transposition
Hemi-Fontan	SVC to PA anastomosis with baffle placed in right atrium so that inferior vena cava blood flow goes across ASD to left heart	PAL	Increases pulmonary blood flow and sets the stage for eventual complete Fontan
Konno	Replacement of aortic valve with aortic valve annular enlargement	COR	Alleviates subaortic obstruction and replaces abnormal aortic valve
Mustard	Atrial switch with intraatrial baffle made of pericardium	COR	Reestablishes proper flow sequence to PA and aorta in D-transposition of the great arteries
Norwood (first stage)	PA anastomosis to aorta, conduit from aorta to main PA	PAL	Increases flow to aorta for subaortic obstruction with single ventricle
Potts	Descending aorta-to-PA shunt	PAL	Increases pulmonary flow (rarely done anymore)
PA band	Constrictive band around main PA	PAL	Decreases pulmonary flow
Rashkind	Atrial septostomy with catheter balloon	PAL	Increases mixing of blood for transposition of the great arteries or tricuspid atresia
Rastelli	Valved conduit from RV to PA, closure of VSD	COR	Increases pulmonary flow, may reestablish proper sequence of flow to aorta and PA
Ross	Pulmonary autograft to aorta, pulmonary homograft	COR	Correction for aortic stenosis; avoids mechanical and bioprosthetic valve
Senning	Atrial switch with intraatrial baffle made of atrial wall flaps	COR	Reestablishes proper flow sequence to PA and aorta in transposition of the great arteries
Waterston	Ascending aorta to right pulmonary anastomosis	PAL	Increases pulmonary blood flow (rarely done anymore)

ASD, atrial septal defect; COR, total correction; PAL, palliation; SVC, superior vena cava.
From *ACC Current Journal Review* March/April 1996:46, with permission.

41. C. Equal preponderance.

42. B. Predominantly female.

43. A. Predominantly male.

44. A. Predominantly male.

45. C. Equal preponderance.

46. D. Pulmonic stenosis. A left lateral right ventriculogram demonstrates pulmonic stenosis with dilatation of the proximal main PA.

47. A. Coarctation of the aorta. Left lateral view of the LV and aorta. The catheter was advanced from the femoral vein and crossed a large patent foramen ovale to reach the left side of the heart. A discrete area of narrowing (coarctation) is seen in the upper descending aorta.

48. E. VSD. A left ventriculogram obtained in the left anterior oblique view allows optimal visualization of the interventricular septum and demonstrates a large VSD and a large left-to-right shunt.

49. B. PDA. An aortogram in straight lateral view. There is a large abnormal communication between the upper descending aorta and the main PA, confirming the diagnosis of PDA.

50. C. Hypertrophic cardiomyopathy. A left ventriculogram in right anterior oblique projection demonstrates a small ventricle with marked ventricular hypertrophy and narrow LVOT.

51. E. Tetralogy of Fallot. On cardiac palpation and auscultation, patients with tetralogy of Fallot demonstrate RV lift (RV hypertrophy) and a systolic ejection murmur over the pulmonic region due to RV outflow tract obstruction. A soft, short systolic ejection murmur suggests severe obstruction. The intensity and severity of the ejection murmur are inversely related to the severity of RV obstruction. P_2 is absent, and only the aortic component of S_2 is audible.

52. D. Ebstein's anomaly. Patients with Ebstein's anomaly have widely split S_1 and S_2, with loud T_1 and extra heart sounds and ejection clicks. A tricuspid regurgitation murmur is usually present. Hepatomegaly due to passive congestion and elevation right atrial pressure may be present.

53. B. Coarctation of the aorta. Patients with coarctation of the aorta have systolic hypertension and higher BP in their arms than in their legs, resulting in delayed femoral arterial pulses. Because many patients also have bicuspid aortic valve, a systolic ejection click is frequently present, and the aortic component of S_2 is accentuated. A harsh systolic ejection murmur is audible along the left sternal border and radiates to the back, especially over the point of discrete coarctation.

54. A. Eisenmenger's syndrome. Patients with Eisenmenger's syndrome demonstrate cyanosis and digital clubbing, the severity of which depends on the magnitude of right-to-left shunting. An RV lift and loud P_2 due to pulmonary hypertension are usually present. The murmur caused by ASD, VSD, or PDA is no longer present when Eisenmenger's syndrome develops. Many patients can have a tricuspid or pulmonary regurgitation murmur, or both.

55. C. PDA. Patients with PDA exhibit hyperdynamic LV impulse with wide pulse pressure. A continuous machinery murmur, heard best in the pulmonic region, is a characteristic finding.

56. C. Cleft mitral valve.

57. B. Supravalvular pulmonic stenosis.

58. E. Persistent left superior vena cava.

59. A. Supravalvular aortic stenosis.

60. D. Anomalous pulmonary venous drainage.

61. A. Eisenmenger's syndrome.

62. E. Tetralogy of Fallot.

63. D. Ebstein's anomaly.

64. B. Coarctation of the aorta.

65. C. PDA.

66. C. Figure 9. This is a parasternal short-axis view at the aortic valve level using TTE. Two leaflets showing a "fish-mouth" opening during systole are seen instead of three leaflets.

67. A. Figure 7. This is an apical four-chamber view using TTE. There is a membrane separating the left atrium into a posterior chamber, usually where the pulmonary veins empty, and an anterior chamber that contains the mitral valve.

68. D. Figure 10. Subcostal TTE view showing the ASD in the lower atrial septum, with downward displacement of the AV valve.

69. E. Figure 11. This is a parasternal short-axis view at the aortic valve level, using TTE. There are four visible leaflets.

70. B. Figure 8. A magnified TEE long-axis view of the LVOT, aortic valve, and ascending aorta. There is a membrane visible in the LVOT, consistent with a subaortic membrane.

SUGGESTED READING

Brickner ME, Hillis LD, Lange RA. Congenital heart disease in adults. *N Engl J Med* 2000;342:256–263, 334–342.

Gregoratos G, ed. *Cardiovascular medicine medical knowledge self-assessment program.* Philadelphia: American College of Physicians, 1998.

Marelli AJ, Moodie DS. Adult congenital heart disease. In: Topel E, ed. *Textbook of Cardiovascular Medicine*, 2nd ed. Philadelphia: Lippincott Williams & Wilkins, 2002.

Moss AJ, Adams FH, Emmanouilides GC, eds. *Heart disease in infants, children and adolescents*, 2nd ed. Baltimore: Williams & Wilkins, 1977.

Murphy JG, Gersh BJ, Mair DD, et al. Long-term outcome in patients undergoing surgical repair of tetralogy of Fallot. *N Engl J Med* 1993;329:593–599.

CHAPTER 9

Physiology/Biochemistry

Marc S. Penn

QUESTIONS

1. At the completion of a cycle of excitation-contraction coupling, cytosolic Ca^{2+} is sequestered in the sarcoplasmic reticulum by what adenosine triphosphatase?

   A. glyceraldehyde phosphate dehydrogenase
   B. sarcoplasmic-endoplasmic reticulum calcium ATPase type 2 (SERCA2)
   C. adenylyl cyclase
   D. V-adenosine triphosphatase
   E. L-type calcium channels

2. In myocardium from patients with CHF, the SERCA2 to phospholamban ratio has been shown to be

   A. increased
   B. unchanged
   C. decreased

3. Downregulation of signaling along the adrenergic pathway in failing myocardium is due to all the below *except*

   A. overexpression of beta-adrenoreceptor (β-AR) kinase
   B. downregulation of the β_2-receptor
   C. phosphodiesterase inhibitors
   D. beta-blocker therapy
   E. ACE inhibitors

4. The most efficient methodology for the delivery of cDNA for gene therapy presently being used in clinical trials is

   A. adeno-associated virus
   B. bacteriophage
   C. adenovirus
   D. plasmid DNA
   E. liposomes

265

5. All of the delivery vectors listed below allow for the possibility of stable integration of genetic material into chromosomal DNA *except*

   A. adeno-associated virus
   B. adenovirus
   C. plasmid DNA
   D. liposomes

6. Arterial thrombosis after plaque rupture is initiated by

   A. tissue plasminogen activator
   B. factor XIII
   C. protein C
   D. activated protein C
   E. tissue factor

7. Blood-borne markers of inflammation that have been shown to predict the presence of CAD or acute coronary syndrome include the following *except*

   A. high-sensitivity C-reactive protein
   B. interleukin-6
   C. myeloperoxidase
   D. interferon alpha
   E. serum amyloid A

8. Potential mediators of lipid oxidation *in vivo* include all of the following *except*

   A. myeloperoxidase
   B. lipoxygenase
   C. ceruloplasmin
   D. catalase
   E. ischemia

9. Low levels of gene expression can be detected by

   A. Northern blot
   B. Western blot
   C. reverse transcriptase-polymerase chain reaction (RT-PCR)
   D. Southern blot
   E. gene transfer

10. DNA can be cut at sites of specific sequences using

    A. hybridization
    B. restriction enzymes
    C. RT-PCR
    D. pepsin
    E. desalting column

11. Oxidized LDL can be characterized by the following *except*

    A. positive charge
    B. cytotoxicity
    C. high malondialdehyde levels
    D. recognition by the scavenger receptor
    E. low vitamin E

12. The final common pathway of platelet aggregation is mediated through

    A. adenosine diphosphate binding
    B. collagen
    C. thrombin
    D. $\alpha_v\beta_3$ receptor
    E. glycoprotein (GP)IIb/IIIa receptor

13. Inducers of smooth muscle cell proliferation include

    A. platelet-derived growth factor β
    B. basic fibroblast growth factor (bFGF)
    C. transforming growth factor β
    D. thrombin
    E. oxidized LDL

14. Apoptosis of a cell is indicated by all of the following *except*

    A. phosphatidylserine in the outer leaflet
    B. high caspase 3 activity
    C. low annexin-V binding
    D. DNA laddering
    E. low cytoplasmic cytochrome C levels

15. Inhibitors of cardiac myocyte apoptosis include

    A. insulin-like growth factor-1β
    B. dobutamine
    C. ischemia
    D. caspase 3
    E. Bid cleavage

ANSWERS

1. B. SERCA2.

2. C. Decreased.

3. D. Intracellular calcium (Ca^{2+}) plays an integral role in contraction and relaxation in cardiac myocytes, a process tightly controlled by mechanisms that regulate its rise and fall. During depolarization, Ca^{2+} entry through the L-type Ca^{2+} channels triggers an exponential release of Ca^{2+} from the sarcoplasmic reticulum through ryanodine receptors, resulting in activation of contractile proteins. At the completion of a cycle of excitation-contraction coupling, cytosolic Ca^{2+} is sequestered in the SR by the SR-Ca^{2+} adenosine triphosphatase (SERCA2a) pump (~75%) or exported extracellularly via the Na/Ca exchanger (~25%) located on the sarcolemmal membrane. Cardiomyocytes isolated from humans with CHF are characterized by contractile dysfunction as evidenced by decreased systolic force generation, prolonged relaxation, and elevated diastolic force. Abnormalities in Ca^{2+} homeostasis, including reduced SR Ca^{2+} release, elevated diastolic Ca^{2+} levels, and a reduced rate of Ca^{2+} removal, parallel the contractile dysfunction seen in the failing myocardium. Furthermore, a reduction in frequency-dependent systolic force and Ca^{2+} can be witnessed in failing human myocytes. Key components in the development of the derangements in contraction and

relaxation observed in CHF have been shown to be SERCA2a and its regulatory protein, phospholamban. SERCA2a controls function of Ca^{2+} re-uptake after myocytes contraction and serves to regulate Ca^{2+} transients initiating diastolic relaxation. Phospholamban exerts an inhibitory effect on SERCA2a functioning, reducing its ability to assist in removal of cytosolic Ca^{2+} after contraction, a mechanism believed to result in the diastolic dysfunction seen in CHF patients. The ratio of SERCA2a:phospholamban has been demonstrated to be decreased in patients with CHF, resulting in the derangements described previously. With this improved understanding of calcium homeostasis in failing hearts, interests have pointed toward methods of ameliorating these dysfunctional mechanisms.

Heart failure results in dramatic changes in certain neurotransmitter and hormone receptors. The majority of the changes occur in the heart and generally can be classified as regulatory phenomena that withdraw the failing heart from adrenergic stimulation. However, these changes also can result in alterations of excitation-contraction coupling and, ultimately, contribute to CHF. Derangements in β-adrenergic signaling, including β-AR receptor downregulation, β-AR uncoupling from second messenger systems, and upregulation of β-AR kinase, have been demonstrated as significant components of heart failure. Phosphodiesterase inhibitors, such as milrinone, are used to increase β-adrenergic signaling by bypassing the β-AR. ACE-Is have no effect on β-adrenergic signaling. Beta-blockers increase β-adrenergic signaling by increasing the density of β-AR on the cardiomyocyte cell surface.

4. C. Adenovirus.

5. B. Adenovirus does not allow for the possibility of stable integration. Replication-defective adenoviral vectors have emerged as the primary modality for gene transfer in a variety of preclinical and clinical studies of gene therapy. A number of properties have resulted in the popularity of these vectors for cardiovascular gene therapy. Adenoviral vectors are rendered replication incompetent by deleting the early (E1A and E1B) genes responsible for viral gene expression from the genome and are stably integrated into the host cells in an extrachromosomal form. This decreases the risk of integration into the host cell genome and mutagenesis. Adenoviral vectors have been shown to result in transient expression of therapeutic genes *in vivo*, peaking at 7 days and lasting approximately 4 weeks.

Unlike replication-defective adenoviral vectors, adeno-associated virus vectors do not express any viral gene products, rendering them significantly less immunogenic. This vector demonstrated efficient and stable integration of its transgene with a minimal inflammatory response.

Multiple studies have demonstrated the feasibility of *in vivo* gene transfer into myocardial cells by direct injection of plasmid DNA. These vectors have the enticing qualities of being relatively nonimmunogenic and nonpathogenic, with the potential to stably integrate in the cellular genome, resulting in long-term gene expression in postmitotic cells *in vivo*. Furthermore, plasmid DNA is rapidly degraded in the blood stream; therefore, the chance of transgene expression in distant organ systems is negligible. The use of bacteriophage for gene transfer is presently theoretical and not under consideration for clinical use at this time.

6. E. Tissue factor. Tissue factor binding to factor VII is the initiating event for the extrinsic blood coagulation cascade. The complex can also cleave factor

IX and contribute to activation of the intrinsic cascade as well. Tissue factor is normally not expressed in the vasculature, but, in atherosclerotic vessels, tissue factor is expressed by macrophages and smooth muscle cells. Tissue factor expression is increased in the lesions of patients who present with unstable angina. On plaque rupture, the exposure of tissue factor to blood-borne coagulation factors leads to thrombus formation.

7. D. Interferon alpha has not been shown to predict the presence of CAD or acute coronary syndrome. Increased levels of each of these circulating markers have been found in patients with CAD compared to the levels found in control populations.

8. D. Lipoxygenase, myeloperoxidase, and ceruloplasmin are all expressed by activated macrophages and lead to lipid oxidation. Ischemia, in particular ischemia-reperfusion, leads to generation of free radicals and lipid peroxidation. Catalase is an antioxidant by reacting with hydrogen peroxide and releasing water.

9. C. RT-PCR. RT-PCR is capable of finding a single copy of RNA. Northern blot analysis requires at least 5 to 10 µg of total RNA. Western blot analysis is for determining protein levels. Southern blot analysis is for genotyping and requires multiple copies of DNA. Gene transfer is not a detection method.

10. B. Restriction enzymes. Restriction enzymes cleave DNA at sites of specific DNA sequences. Pepsin cleaves protein at specific sites. RT-PCR is discussed in the answer to question 9, and hybridization refers to the process of annealing DNA to RNA or DNA.

11. A. Oxidized LDL has a higher electrophoretic mobility compared to native LDL due to its negative charge. LDL does not oxidize until its vitamin E content is reduced. It is highly cytotoxic to cells in culture. Oxidized LDL is not recognized by the LDL receptor; rather, it is recognized by the scavenger receptor. The level of LDL oxidation is quantified by its ability to generate high malondialdehyde levels.

12. E. GPIIb/IIIa receptor. Adenosine diphosphate, collagen, and thrombin bind independently, leading to platelet activation and, ultimately, to expression of the GPIIb/IIIa receptor. GPIIb/IIIa receptor expression leads to platelet clumping by binding to surrounding activated platelets. The $\alpha_v\beta_3$ receptor does not lead to platelet aggregation.

13. C. Transforming growth factor β. Platelet-derived growth factor β, bFGF, and thrombin are all smooth muscle mitogens. Oxidized LDL causes smooth muscle cell proliferation through the autocrine release of bFGF. Transforming growth factor β alters the smooth muscle cell phenotype from a proliferative to a synthetic state and, thus, is antiproliferative.

14. C. Low annexin-V binding does not indicate apoptosis of a cell. Cellular apoptosis is characterized by increased phosphatidylserine expression in the outer leaflet of the plasma membrane that leads to increased annexin-V binding. Intracellular markers of apoptosis include increased caspase 3, decreased cytochrome C levels, and evidence of DNA laddering.

15. A. Insulin-like growth factor-1β. Insulin-like growth factor-1β overexpression has been shown to be cardioprotective due to decreased apoptosis in the setting of myocardial ischemia. Dobutamine has been shown to induce cardiomyocyte apoptosis. Caspase 3 and Bid cleavage are cytoplasmic markers of apoptosis.

SUGGESTED READING

Akhter SA, Skaer CA, Kypson AP, et al. Restoration of beta-adrenergic signaling in failing cardiac ventricular myocytes via adenoviral-mediated gene transfer. *Proc Natl Acad Sci U S A* 1997;94(22):12100–12105.

Annex BH. Differential expression of TF protein in directional atherectomy specimens from patients with stable and unstable coronary syndromes. *Circulation* 1995;91:619–622.

Askari AT, Penn MS. Targeted gene therapy for the treatment of cardiac dysfunction. *Semin Thorac Cardiovasc Surg* 2002;14:167–177.

Bristow MR, Ginsburg R, Minobe W, et al. Decreased catecholamine sensitivity and beta-adrenergic-receptor density in failing human hearts. *N Engl J Med* 1982;307(4):205–211.

Chai YC, Howe PH, DiCorleto PE, et al. Oxidized low density lipoprotein and lysophosphatidylcholine stimulate cell cycle entry in vascular smooth muscle cells. Evidence for release of fibroblast growth factor-2. *J Biol Chem* 1996;27:17791–17797.

Chisolm GM 3rd, Hazen SL, Fox PL, et al. The oxidation of lipoproteins by monocytes-macrophages. Biochemical and biological mechanisms. *J Biol Chem* 1999;274:25959–25962.

del Monte F, Williams E, Lebeche D, et al. Improvement in survival and cardiac metabolism after gene transfer of sarcoplasmic reticulum Ca(2+)-ATPase in a rat model of heart failure. *Circulation* 2001;104(12):1424–1429.

French B, Mazur W, Geske RS, et al. Direct in vivo gene transfer into porcine myocardium using replication-deficient adenoviral vectors. *Circulation* 1994;90(5):2414–2424.

Guzman RJ, Lemarchand P, Crystal RG, et al. Efficient gene transfer into myocardium by direct injection of adenovirus vectors. *Circ Res* 1993;73(6):1202–1207.

Gwathmey JK, Copelas L, MacKinnon R, et al. Abnormal intracellular calcium handling in myocardium from patient with end-stage heart failure. *Circ Res* 1987;61(1):70–76.

Gwathmey JK, Slawsky MT, Hajjar RJ, et al. Role of intracellular calcium handling in force-interval relationships of human ventricular myocardium. *J Clin Invest* 1990;85(5):1599–1613.

Hajjar RJ, Schmidt U, Kang JX, et al. Adenoviral gene transfer of phospholamban in isolated rat cardiomyocytes. Rescue effects by concomitant gene transfer of sarcoplasmic reticulum Ca(2+)-ATPase. *Circ Res* 1997;81(2):145–153.

Hessler JR, Morel DW, Lewis LJ, et al. Lipoprotein oxidation and lipoprotein-induced cytotoxicity. *Arteriosclerosis* 1983;3(3):215–222.

Kadambi VJ, Ponniah S, Harrer JM, et al. Cardiac-specific overexpression of phospholamban alters calcium kinetics and resultant cardiomyocyte mechanics in transgenic mice. *J Clin Invest* 1996;97(2):533–539.

Kessler PD, Podsakoff GM, Chen X, et al. Gene delivery to skeletal muscle results in sustained expression and systemic delivery of a therapeutic protein. *Proc Natl Acad Sci U S A* 1996;93:14082–14087.

Kitsis RN, Buttrick PM, McNally EM, et al. Hormonal modulation of a gene injected into rat heart in vivo. *Proc Natl Acad Sci U S A* 1991;88(10):4138–4142.

Kohler C. Evaluation of caspase activity in apoptotic cells. *J Immunol Methods* 2002;265:97–110.

Li Q, Li B, Wang X, et al. Overexpression of insulin-like growth factor-1 in mice protects from myocyte death after infarction, attenuating ventricular dilation, wall stress, and cardiac hypertrophy. *J Clin Invest* 1997;100:1991–1999.

Lin H, Parmacek MS, Morle G, et al. Expression of recombinant genes in myocardium in vivo after direct injection of DNA. *Circulation* 1990;82(6):2217–2221.

Losordo DW, Vale PR, Symes JF, et al. Gene therapy for myocardial angiogenesis: initial clinical results with direct myocardial injection of phVEGF$_{165}$ as sole therapy for myocardial ischemia. *Circulation* 1998;98:2800–2804.

Lowes BD, Gilbert EM, Abraham WT, et al. Myocardial gene expression in dilated cardiomyopathy treated with beta-blocking agents. *N Engl J Med* 2002;346(18):1357–1365.

Mercadier JJ, Lompre AM, Duc P, et al. Altered sarcoplasmic reticulum Ca2(+)-ATPase gene expression in the human ventricle during end-stage heart failure. *J Clin Invest* 1990;85(1):305–309.

Morel DW, Hessler JR, Chisolm GM. Low density lipoprotein cytotoxicity induced by free radical peroxidation of lipid. *J Lipid Res* 1983;24:1070–1076.

Moreno PR, Bernardi VH, Lopez-Cuellar J, et al. Macrophages, smooth muscle cells, and tissue factor in unstable angina. Implications for cell-mediated thrombogenicity in acute coronary syndromes. *Circulation* 1996;94:3090–3097.

Morgan JP. Abnormal intracellular modulation of calcium as a major cause of cardiac contractile dysfunction. *N Engl J Med* 1991;325:625.

Nilsson J. Cytokines and smooth muscle cells in atherosclerosis. *Cardiovasc Res* 1993;27:1184–1190.

Reidy MA, Fingerle J, Lindner V. Factors controlling the development of arterial lesions after injury. *Circulation* 1992;86[6 Suppl]:III43–46.

Reutlingsperger CP. Visualization of cell death in vivo with the annexin V imaging protocol. *J Immunol Methods* 2002;265:123–132.

Rifai N, Ridker PM. Inflammatory markers and coronary heart disease. *Curr Opin Lipidol* 2002;13(4):383–389.

Robbins M, Topol EJ. Inflammation in acute coronary syndromes. *Cleve Clin J Med* 2002;69[Suppl 2]:SII130–SII142.

Rosenberg RD, Aird WC. Vascular-bed-specific hemostasis and hyper-coagulable states. *N Engl J Med* 1999;340(20):1555–1564.

Schmidt U, Hajjar RJ, Helm PA, et al. Contribution of abnormal sarcoplasmic reticulum ATPase activity to systolic and diastolic dysfunction in human heart failure. *J Mol Cell Cardiol* 1998;30(10):1929–1937.

Schwinger RH, Munch G, Bolck B, et al. Reduced Ca(2+)-sensitivity of SERCA 2a in failing human myocardium due to reduced serin-16 phospholamban phosphorylation. *J Mol Cell Cardiol* 1999;31(3):479–491.

Svensson EC, Marshall DJ, Woodard K, et al. Efficient and stable transduction of cardiomyocytes after intramyocardial injection or intracoronary perfusion with recombinant adeno-associated virus vectors. *Circulation* 1999;99(2):201–205.

Topol EJ, Byzova TV, Plow EF. Platelet GPIIb-IIIa blockers. *Lancet* 1999;353:227–231.

Toschi V, Gallo R, Lettino M, et al. Tissue factor modulates the thrombogenicity of human atherosclerotic plaques. *Circulation* 1997;95:594–599.

Vale PR, Losordo DW, Milliken CE, et al. Randomized, single-blind, placebo-controlled pilot study of catheter-based myocardial gene transfer for therapeutic angiogenesis using left ventricular electromechanical mapping in patients with chronic myocardial ischemia. *Circulation* 2001(103):2138–2143.

Whitmer JT, Kumar P, Solaro RJ. Calcium transport properties of cardiac sarcoplasmic reticulum from cardiomyopathic Syrian hamsters (BIO 53.58 and 14.6): evidence for a quantitative defect in dilated myopathic hearts not evident in hypertrophic hearts. *Circ Res* 1988;62(1):81–85.

Wolff JA, Malone RW, Williams P, et al. Direct gene transfer into mouse muscle in vivo. *Science* 1990;247(4949 Pt 1):1465–1468.

Zhang R, Brennan ML, Fu X, et al. Association between myeloperoxidase levels and risk of coronary artery disease. *JAMA* 2001;286(17):2136–2142.

CHAPTER 10

Hypertension

Matthew G. Deedy

QUESTIONS

1. A 55-year-old man presents to the emergency department with severe, progressive shortness of breath at rest over the last 12 hours. He denies any cardiac history, including MI, CHF, and known valvular heart disease. He denies any history of hypertension, hyperlipidemia, diabetes, or a family history of premature CAD, although he smokes two packs of cigarettes daily. He denies any history of chest, back, or abdominal discomfort. A recent treadmill ECG was normal, according to the patient.

The patient appears dyspneic after moving to the examination table.
Pulse is 120 bpm.
BP is 250/120 mm Hg.
Respiratory rate is 45 breaths per minute.
There is an elevated jugular venous pulse to the angle of his jaw.
Inspiratory crackles are noted in all lung fields.
His heart is tachycardic and regular, an S_4 is present, and no murmurs are audible.
His abdomen is thin and soft; systolic and diastolic bruits are noted.
His extremities are warm, bilateral femoral artery bruits are noted, and the femoral pulses are palpable but diminished.
ECG shows sinus tachycardia and borderline LV hypertrophy (LVH) by voltage criteria. No acute ST segment or T-wave changes are present.
Chest radiograph reveals a normal mediastinum with bilateral perihilar alveolar infiltrates.

Which of the following is included in the most appropriate initial management of this patient?

A. O_2, IV diltiazem bolus and continuous infusion, and IV furosemide
B. O_2, IV morphine, and sublingual nifedipine
C. O_2, IV furosemide, and PO metoprolol
D. IV furosemide, sodium nitroprusside IV infusion, and O_2
E. immediate spiral CT scan to rule out aortic dissection

2. The same patient is admitted to the hospital for management of his hypertension. Acute MI is ruled out with three normal troponin-T values. A TTE reveals normal LV size and function with mild LVH and structurally normal valves. After 3 days, he has been converted to a PO regimen, including metoprolol, 100 mg twice daily; amlodipine, 10 mg daily; and hydrochlorothiazide (HCTZ), 50 mg daily. He is discharged home to follow-up with you in 2 weeks.

At the follow-up appointment, the patient feels well and denies any shortness of breath or chest pain with exertion. He has stopped smoking and is walking for 15 min daily, limited mainly by lower extremity cramping while walking. His BP is 160/90 mm Hg; his heart rate at rest is 50 bpm. The laboratory evaluation is shown below:

Sodium, 137 mmol per L
Creatinine, 1.7 mg per dL
Potassium, 4.5 mmol per L
Glucose, 90 mg per dL
Hemoglobin, 13.5 g per dL
Cholesterol, 210 mg per dL
LDL, 129 mg per dL
HDL, 33 mg per dL
Triglyceride, 240 mg per dL
Urinalysis normal, no active sediment

Based on the above, what is the most appropriate management at this time?

A. continue the current drug regimen plus simvastatin, 40 mg nightly
B. schedule captopril-enhanced radionuclide renal scan
C. increase metoprolol to 200 mg twice daily and observe
D. schedule lower extremity pulse volume recordings
E. add clonidine, 0.1 mg twice daily, and observe

3. All of the following statements regarding therapy with enalapril are true *except*

A. Plasma renin and angiotensin-II levels increase with therapy.
B. Its antihypertensive effect is reduced by nonsteroidal antiinflammatory drugs.
C. Its use is contraindicated in patients with bilateral renal artery stenosis.
D. All-cause mortality is reduced by approximately 40% in patients with New York Heart Association (NYHA) class IV CHF.
E. Circulating bradykinin levels increase as a result of reduced degradation.

4. A 72-year-old obese woman presents for evaluation of exertional dyspnea and lightheadedness. The patient describes a history of hypertension for the past 5 years that her primary physician has been managing with triamterene/HCTZ, 37.5/25.0 mg, one-half tablet daily. She denies exertional chest discomfort and a history of MI or CHF. The patient describes breathlessness climbing stairs and occasional lightheadedness with activity or after standing up from a seated position.

BP is 166/80 mm Hg.
Pulse is regular and 88 bpm.
Body mass index is 35 kg per m^2.

The jugular venous pulse is not elevated.

Carotid upstrokes are brisk.

Her lungs are clear bilaterally.

Her heart is regular, with a 3/6 systolic ejection murmur at the left upper sternal border. The murmur peaks in midsystole and radiates to the carotids. S_1 and S_2 are normal, and an S_4 is present. The murmur increases slightly when the patient stands and decreases with the patient supine.

The abdomen is obese and otherwise unremarkable. Lower extremities are warm, with mild pitting edema to the mid-calf.

What is the most appropriate management option?

A. Increase triamterene/HCTZ, 37.5/25.0 mg, to a whole tablet daily, and arrange for consultation with a nutritionist for weight loss and instructions on a low-sodium diet.

B. Discontinue triamterene/HCTZ, order a TTE, and initiate therapy with long-acting verapamil, 240 mg daily.

C. Initiate therapy with lisinopril, 10 mg daily; continue triamterene/HCTZ; and order a TTE.

D. Initiate therapy with atenolol, 50 mg daily; discontinue triamterene/HCTZ; and order a TTE.

E. Refer the patient for aortic valve replacement for symptomatic aortic stenosis.

5. Which of the following methods can improve patient adherence to antihypertensive therapy?

A. encouraging home BP monitoring

B. patient education about the disease and reinforcement of appropriate lifestyle modifications

C. use of inexpensive and simple regimens with long-acting medications

D. early follow-up after initiation of therapy for a BP check and assessment for the presence of side effects

E. all of the above

6. ACE-inhibitor use is indicated in all of the following patients *except*

A. a 37-year-old woman with type 1 diabetes mellitus and proteinuria

B. an asymptomatic 55-year-old man with a history of inferior MI, an ejection fraction of 35%, and no ischemia on a treadmill TTE at 11.5 METS

C. a 63-year-old woman with an idiopathic dilated cardiomyopathy, NYHA class II CHF symptoms, and a resting BP of 110/50 mm Hg

D. a 34-year-old woman with eclampsia who is 36 weeks pregnant

E. a 57-year-old man with hypertension and a serum creatinine level of 2.2 mg per dL

7. All of the following statements regarding hypertension in heart transplant recipients are true *except*
   A. Hypertension occurs in approximately two-thirds of patients after heart transplantation.
   B. Hypertension related to cyclosporine therapy is mediated through vasoconstriction.
   C. Cyclosporine doses should be increased when diltiazem therapy is initiated to maintain adequate immunosuppression.
   D. Hypertension typically responds to treatment with vasodilators.
   E. Monotherapy with diuretics for hypertension should be avoided.

Questions 8–12

Match the antihypertensive medication with its associated side effect. Each answer should be used only once.

8. Clonidine   A. gynecomastia

9. Losartan   B. bronchospasm

10. Spironolactone   C. lupus-like syndrome

11. Hydralazine   D. dry mouth

12. Atenolol   E. angioedema

13. A 60-year-old man with a history of type 2 diabetes presents to your office for a cardiovascular evaluation. He denies any history of smoking, hyperlipidemia, MI, stroke, or TIA.

    Body mass index is 25 kg per m^2.
    BP is 160/95 mm Hg.
    Pulse is regular at 76 bpm.
    There are normal carotid upstrokes without bruits.
    The jugular venous pulse is normal.
    His lungs are clear to auscultation bilaterally.
    His heart is regular, with a normal S_1 and S_2; an S_4 is present.
    The abdominal aorta is not palpable, and there are no abdominal bruits.
    The peripheral pulses are normal.

    All of the following are true statements regarding the management of this patient *except*

    A. Initial treatment with doxazosin would be associated with a twofold increase in risk for developing CHF compared to initial treatment with chlorthalidone.
    B. Regression of LVH would be more likely with atenolol than with losartan.
    C. Treatment with ramipril would be expected to lower his risk of death by nearly 25% over the next 4.5 years.
    D. Initial treatment with losartan would be expected to reduce his combined risk for death, MI, and stroke by 13% over the next 5.5 years, compared to treatment with atenolol.
    E. Treatment with ramipril would be expected to lower his risk for overt nephropathy by nearly 25% over the next 4.5 years.

14. A 37-year-old man is brought to the emergency department with crushing substernal chest discomfort for the last 90 min. He denies any history of chest pain in the past. He smokes cigarettes but denies a history of hypertension, hyperlipidemia, diabetes, or a family history of premature CAD. He describes a crushing substernal chest pressure that radiates to his left arm.

He is short of breath, appears agitated and combative, and smells of alcohol. BP on arrival is 175/95 mm Hg.
Pulse is 100 bpm and regular.
The head and neck examination is remarkable for dilated pupils, brisk carotid upstrokes, and no jugular venous distention.
His lungs are clear.
His heart is tachycardic and regular, with a normal S_1 and S_2; an S_4 is present. His extremities are warm with palpable, symmetric pulses.
ECG reveals sinus tachycardia at 102 bpm and 2-mm ST segment elevation in leads II, III, and aVF. There are ST segment depressions in leads I, aVL, V_1, and V_2.

Appropriate initial therapy includes all of the following *except*

A. aspirin, 325 mg PO
B. sublingual nitroglycerin, followed by an IV nitroglycerin infusion
C. supplemental O_2 by nasal cannula
D. metoprolol, 5 mg IV every 5 min up to 15 mg, followed by 50 mg PO
E. diltiazem, 30 mg PO

Questions 15–19

Match each patient below with his or her recommended target BP according to the recommendations outlined in the Sixth Report of the Joint National Committee on Prevention, Detection, Evaluation, and Treatment of High Blood Pressure (JNC VI). Individual answers can be used more than once.

15. A 55-year-old man with type 2 diabetes mellitus

16. A 70-year-old woman with NYHA class II CHF

17. A 70-year-old woman with uncomplicated hypertension

18. A 36-year-old man with type 1 diabetes mellitus and proteinuria greater than 1 g per 24 hours

19. A 65-year-old woman with a serum creatinine of 2.0 g per dL

    A. less than 140/90 mm Hg
    B. less than 160/90 mm Hg
    C. less than 130/85 mm Hg
    D. less than 125/75 mm Hg
    E. less than 135/85 mm Hg

20. A 40-year-old woman presents to your office for a cardiovascular evaluation. She has no significant past medical history and is taking no medications at this time. She denies any chest discomfort or breathlessness with exertion, but she does not exercise regularly. Her father experienced an MI when he was 52 years old, and both parents are treated for hypertension. She does not smoke cigarettes or drink alcohol. She does not know if her cholesterol has ever been checked.

Her physical examination is unremarkable.
BP is 138/88 mm Hg.
Pulse is regular at 76 bpm.
Body mass index is 29 kg per m^2.
An ECG shows sinus rhythm and is normal.

All of the following are appropriate recommendations for this patient *except*

A. She should perform 30 to 45 min of aerobic activity every day, if possible.
B. A fasting lipid profile should be checked.
C. She should initiate therapy with HCTZ, 12.5 mg daily, and follow-up in 6 months for a BP check.
D. She should reduce her salt intake to less than 6 g per day.
E. She should set a goal weight that corresponds to a body mass index of 25 kg per m^2.

21. All of the following statements regarding hypertension in older patients are true *except*

A. Very high BP measurements can be due to pseudohypertension.
B. Treatment of isolated systolic hypertension with thiazide diuretics or long-acting dihydropyridine calcium channel blockers reduces the risk of fatal and nonfatal stroke.
C. Target BP for patients older than 60 years with isolated systolic hypertension is below 160/90 mm Hg.
D. Amiloride and HCTZ reduce stroke and coronary event rates more than atenolol.
E. Treatment benefits for patients with stage 1 isolated systolic hypertension (systolic BP 140 to 159 mm Hg) have not been demonstrated in randomized controlled trials.

22. A 55-year-old man presents to your office for a preoperative evaluation before planned shoulder surgery. He denies any cardiac history, including MI and CHF. He reports a history of borderline hypertension and states that his usual BP is approximately 150/90 mm Hg. He is active and played singles tennis regularly until his shoulder injury. He denies any chest pain, dyspnea with exertion, or change in his activity tolerance. He has never had an ECG or stress test.

The cardiovascular examination is unremarkable.
BP is 162/92 mm Hg.
ECG shows sinus rhythm at 68 bpm and is normal.

What is the most appropriate recommendation at this point?

A. Proceed with surgery only if a stress ECG is normal.
B. Proceed immediately to surgery with a low risk for perioperative events.
C. Initiate therapy with amlodipine, 5 mg daily, and proceed with surgery.
D. Initiate therapy with atenolol, 25 mg daily, and proceed with surgery only if a stress ECG is normal.
E. Initiate therapy with atenolol, 25 mg daily, and proceed with surgery.

23. You are seeing a 73-year-old woman in the recovery area after a cardiac catheterization. The procedure was performed to evaluate recent symptoms, including exertional breathlessness and lightheadedness and a loud systolic ejection murmur best heard at the upper left sternal border.

Angiography did not reveal significant obstructive CAD.

LV systolic function is normal.

A pressure tracing from the cardiac catheterization is shown (Fig. 1).

BP is 175/90 mm Hg.

Heart rate is 100 bpm.

The patient is reporting mild shortness of breath.

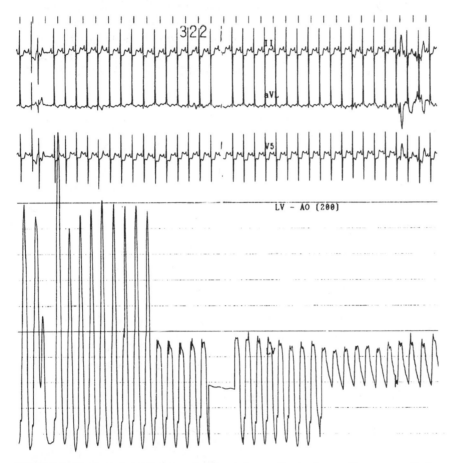

FIGURE 1 Continuous pressure recording during pullback of a multipurpose catheter from the apex of the LV to the ascending aorta (Ao).

What is the most appropriate next step in the management of this patient?

A. Administer nitroglycerin, 0.4 mg sublingually, and initiate a continuous, IV nitroglycerin infusion with close monitoring of the BP.

B. Administer hydralazine, 10 mg IV; monitor the patient closely; and repeat if there is no response.

C. Administer furosemide, 40 mg IV, and assess the urine output in 1 hour.

D. Observe the patient with supplemental O_2.

E. Administer metoprolol, 5 mg IV; monitor the patient closely; and repeat if needed.

24. A 57-year-old woman presents to the emergency department for evaluation of severe chest pain. The patient is a smoker and has a history of hypertension and hyperlipidemia. She describes the abrupt onset of severe, tearing pain in the midsternal area that radiates to the midscapular area.

The patient appears uncomfortable.
Her BP is 190/110 mm Hg in both upper extremities.
Pulse is regular at 110 bpm.
The head and neck examination reveals brisk carotid upstrokes without audible bruit, and there is no jugular venous distention.
Her lungs are clear bilaterally.
Her heart is tachycardic and regular, with an S_4, S_1, and S_2 present. A II/VI systolic ejection murmur is present at the second right intercostal space.
Her abdomen is soft, with normal bowel sounds, and is not tender.
The upper and lower extremity pulses are palpable and symmetric.
An ECG reveals sinus tachycardia and LVH with secondary repolarization abnormality.

Which of the following is included in the most appropriate initial management of this patient?

A. metoprolol, 5 mg IV, repeated every 5 min, titrated to a mean arterial pressure below 70 mm Hg and a pulse below 60 bpm
B. immediate sodium nitroprusside infusion titrated to a systolic BP less than 110 mm Hg
C. nitroglycerin, 0.4 mg sublingually, followed by a continuous infusion, up to 200 µg per minute
D. nifedipine, 10 mg sublingually
E. hydralazine, 10 mg IV, repeated in 30 min if the systolic BP remains approximately 110 mm Hg

25. A 33-year-old woman presents to your clinic for evaluation of hypertension. She is referred after a BP of 146/100 mm Hg was detected during a routine examination. She denies any history of elevated BP. There is no family history of hypertension at a young age. She does not exercise regularly and has only noticed mild fatigue and occasional headaches over the last 6 months. She is not taking any medications.

Physical Examination

BP is 152/102 mm Hg.
Pulse is 76 bpm and regular.
Body mass index is 28 kg per m².
Her head and neck examination is unremarkable.
Her lungs are clear bilaterally.
Her heart is regular, with a normal S_1 and S_2 without an S_3, S_4, or murmur.
Her abdomen is soft and mildly obese, with normal bowel sounds. No abdominal bruits are noted.
Her peripheral pulses are normal, and there is no lower extremity edema.
ECG reveals sinus rhythm with borderline LVH by voltage criteria.

Laboratory Studies

Complete blood cell count is normal.
Urinalysis is normal.
Sodium, 138 mEq per L.
Potassium, 3.1 mEq per L.

Creatinine, 0.9 mg per dL.
Glucose, 90 mg per dL.
Cholesterol, 196 mg per dL.
HDL-C, 60 mg per dL.

Which of the following is included in the most appropriate management at this time?

A. Instruct the patient regarding regular exercise and weight loss and repeat BP in 3 months.
B. Initiate treatment with triamterene/HCTZ, 37.5/25 mg daily, and repeat BP in 3 months.
C. Initiate therapy with atenolol, 25 mg daily.
D. Instruct the patient regarding strict sodium restriction, and check the plasma renin activity.
E. Initiate therapy with HCTZ, 25 mg daily.

ANSWERS

1. D. IV furosemide, sodium nitroprusside IV infusion, and O_2. This presentation is most consistent with a hypertensive emergency with acute LV failure and pulmonary edema. Aortic dissection is unlikely in the absence of chest or back pain; however, it is appropriate to consider aortic dissection in this patient. Over 90% of patients with aortic dissection present with severe pain, and this patient describes no pain. IV vasodilators and adrenergic inhibitors are the mainstay of therapy for hypertensive emergencies, based on their ability to rapidly lower BP. The goal of therapy is to rapidly lower the mean arterial BP by no more than 25% within minutes to 2 hours. This will prevent or limit target organ damage, including intracranial hemorrhage, MI, aortic dissection, and pulmonary edema. Excessive falls in pressure may precipitate renal, cerebral, or myocardial ischemia. A more normal BP should be approached after several hours.

   IV diltiazem is contraindicated in the setting of pulmonary edema. IV furosemide is appropriate for the management of pulmonary edema and frank fluid overload. Morphine may be helpful in this setting; however, it may result in sedation or changes in mental status that can confuse the clinical situation when hypertensive encephalopathy is a concern. Sublingual nifedipine should be avoided, as it can cause excessive falls in BP and has been associated with adverse outcomes. The longer onset of action of PO metoprolol makes it less useful in this situation. In general, beta-adrenergic blockers should be used cautiously in the patient with pulmonary edema. Sodium nitroprusside is a potent arterial vasodilator and is very effective for the management of hypertensive emergencies. It is most safely used in an ICU setting with invasive arterial BP monitoring.

2. B. Schedule captopril-enhanced radionuclide renal scan. This patient has persistently elevated BP over 140/90 mm Hg with triple drug therapy, consistent with resistant hypertension. This should prompt the clinician to consider causes of secondary hypertension. The clinical presentation and examination in this patient suggest renovascular hypertension. This diagnosis should be considered with (a) the abrupt onset of hypertension after the

patient is 50 years old; (b) systolic or diastolic abdominal bruits; (c) a history of smoking, particularly in the patient with evidence of peripheral vascular disease; (d) normal urinalysis; and (e) a history of flash pulmonary edema. Renovascular hypertension is important to identify, because appropriate treatment can lower the risk of renal failure and improve BP control. The addition of a statin is reasonable; however, the patient will likely derive greater benefit from the identification of renal artery stenosis. The resting heart rate is 50 bpm on the current dose of metoprolol. Although a higher dose may lower the BP more, it will likely result in undesired side effects that may cause the patient to discontinue the metoprolol altogether. Lower-extremity pulse volume recordings are helpful for localizing the level of obstruction in patients with intermittent claudication. This patient does not have limb-threatening ischemia; therefore, management of hypertension is most important for the long run. Clonidine may be helpful for additional BP control; however, evaluation for renovascular hypertension is appropriate at this point.

3. A. Enalapril is an ACE inhibitor that blocks the conversion of angiotensin I to angiotensin II. Plasma renin and angiotensin-I levels increase with ACE-inhibitor treatment, whereas angiotensin-II and aldosterone levels decrease acutely with treatment. With long-term ACE-inhibitor use, aldosterone levels can return to pretreatment levels. ACE inhibitors also inhibit the degradation of the vasodilator, bradykinin. Increased bradykinin levels are thought to be the cause of the dry cough that some patients experience with ACE-inhibitor therapy.

ACE inhibitors have effects on the renal vasculature. They reduce both preglomerular (afferent) and postglomerular (efferent) arteriolar resistance, thereby reducing glomerular capillary hydraulic pressure. For this reason, their use is contraindicated in patients with bilateral renal artery stenosis who are particularly dependent on high efferent arteriolar resistance to maintain glomerular capillary hydraulic pressure. Patients with CHF maintain renal blood flow partly through an increase in renal vasodilating prostaglandins. Inhibition of prostaglandin synthesis by nonsteroidal antiinflammatory drugs can result in reduced renal blood flow, glomerular filtration, and oliguric renal failure. Nonsteroidal antiinflammatory drugs increase sodium retention and thereby reduce the BP-lowering effects of ACE inhibitors.

ACE inhibitors improve survival in CHF patients. The Cooperative North Scandinavian Enalapril Survival Study (CONSENSUS) studied hospitalized patients with NYHA class IV CHF symptoms and found over 40% reduction in mortality with 6 months of therapy with enalapril. Subsequent studies have demonstrated improved survival in all patients with CHF symptoms and LV systolic dysfunction and reduced hospitalizations in those with asymptomatic reductions in LV systolic function.

4. D. Initiate therapy with atenolol, 50 mg daily; discontinue triamterene/HCTZ; and order a TTE. This patient has poorly controlled systolic hypertension and physical examination findings suggestive of hypertrophic cardiomyopathy (HCM). The murmur of aortic stenosis usually decreases with standing and does not change in the supine position, whereas the murmur of HCM increases with standing and decreases in the supine position. TTE is the method of choice for diagnosing HCM. HCM typically presents with

exertional dyspnea, chest pain, syncope, arrhythmia, or sudden death. HCM is a heterogeneous disease both genetically and phenotypically. A variation occurs in elderly patients with proximal septal hypertrophy and a decrease in the angle between the LVOT and the ascending aorta. This morphology change can result in a narrowed LVOT and a propensity to develop systolic anterior motion of the mitral valve with resulting obstruction to LV outflow. LVOT obstruction is exacerbated by conditions or medications that reduce preload and afterload or increase inotropy. This patient's lightheadedness and exertional dyspnea may be multifactorial, with contributions from LVOT obstruction, diastolic dysfunction, obesity, and, perhaps, ischemia. However, LVOT obstruction exacerbated by diuretic use is likely the major contributor. By reducing preload, diuretics increase LVOT obstruction and can exacerbate symptoms in HCM. The mainstay of therapy for HCM is beta-blockade. Nondihydropyridine calcium channel blockers can be used in this condition; however, verapamil in this patient is less desirable, as it may exacerbate the patient's lower extremity edema, and beta-blockers have strong data supporting their use in systolic hypertension. ACE inhibitors, like lisinopril, can exacerbate symptoms related to LVOT obstruction by decreasing afterload.

5. E. All of the above. All of the above methods can help improve adherence to therapy. Noncompliance with antihypertensive therapy contributes to inadequate BP control in more than two-thirds of patients with hypertension. Patients should understand the goals of therapy along with the consequences of inadequate control. It is the responsibility of the health care professional to educate patients such that they are informed participants in their care. Appropriate follow-up and encouragement to reach treatment goals should be provided to increase the likelihood of adherence to therapy.

6. D. ACE inhibitors delay the development of end-stage renal disease in patients with type 1 diabetes mellitus and proteinuria (greater than 1 g/24 hours) and patients with renal insufficiency. The use of ACE inhibitors is *absolutely contraindicated* in pregnancy. Hydralazine has a long safety record in the treatment of hypertension in pregnancy. ACE inhibitors improve functional capacity, reduce hospitalizations due to CHF, and improve survival for patients with symptomatic CHF. ACE inhibitors reduce reinfarction rates and improve survival for patients with a history of MI and LV dysfunction.

7. C. Approximately two-thirds of patients develop hypertension after heart transplantation. Cyclosporine and tacrolimus both increase BP, and sodium retention related to chronic steroid use can also increase BP. The BP elevation related to cyclosporine is related to vasoconstriction and usually responds to vasodilators. Calcium channel blockers and ACE inhibitors are frequently used for BP control. Diltiazem and verapamil decrease the metabolism of cyclosporin and tacrolimus, so doses of these immunosuppressive agents should be *decreased* when diltiazem or verapamil are initiated. Diuretics should not be used as monotherapy, because they can exaggerate prerenal azotemia and induce gout.

8. D. Dry mouth.

9. E. Angioedema.

10. A. Gynecomastia.

11. C. Lupus-like syndrome.

12. B. Bronchospasm.

All antihypertensive medications can cause dizziness and hypotension. Clonidine is a centrally acting alpha-agonist that can be associated with severe rebound hypertension, sedation, dry mouth, sexual dysfunction, bradycardia, and nausea. Losartan is an angiotensin receptor blocker that can be associated with hyperkalemia, hepatotoxicity, leukopenia, agranulocytosis, and angioedema. The incidence of angioedema with angiotensin receptor blockers is less than that which occurs with ACE inhibitors. Spironolactone is a potassium-sparing diuretic that can be associated with hyperkalemia, gynecomastia, and, rarely, anaphylaxis and agranulocytosis. Hydralazine is a direct arterial vasodilator that can be associated with the development of a lupus-like syndrome and, rarely, neutropenia and agranulocytosis. Atenolol is a beta$_1$-selective beta-blocker that can cause bronchospasm, although the frequency is less than that associated with nonselective beta-blockers.

13. B. The Antihypertensive and Lipid-Lowering Treatment to Prevent Heart Attack Trial (ALLHAT) is a multicenter, randomized, placebo-controlled trial designed to determine whether the incidence of fatal coronary heart disease and nonfatal MI differs between different antihypertensive medications. The medications under study in the trial include doxazosin, chlorthalidone, amlodipine, and lisinopril. The doxazosin arm of the trial was stopped prematurely due to a significantly increased incidence of cardiovascular disease events, particularly CHF. The incidence of CHF in the doxazosin arm was twice that observed in the chlorthalidone arm.

The Losartan Intervention For Endpoint Reduction in Hypertension study (LIFE) is a multicenter, randomized, placebo-controlled trial assessing therapy with losartan compared to atenolol in a group of patients with hypertension and LVH. Compared to patients treated with atenolol, patients treated with losartan experienced a 13% reduction in the primary end points of death, MI, and stroke in the 5.5-year follow-up period. Patients treated with losartan also experienced a greater reduction in LVH compared to those treated with atenolol.

The Heart Outcomes Prevention Evaluation study (HOPE) evaluated ramipril in a group of patients older than 55 years at high risk for cardiovascular events. In the prespecified subgroup of patients with diabetes, ramipril therapy resulted in a 24% reduction in total mortality after 4.5 years of follow-up compared to patients treated with placebo. Overt nephropathy was also reduced by 24%.

14. D. Metoprolol, 5 mg IV every 5 min up to 15 mg, followed by 50 mg PO is not appropriate initial therapy. This patient presents with a history and ECG consistent with an acute inferior MI. He has evidence of adrenergic stimulation with tachycardia, hypertension, and dilated pupils. This com-

bination of findings along with agitation suggests cocaine intoxication. Hypertension in this setting is related to cocaine's sympathomimetic effects and alpha-adrenergic stimulation. MI can be related to vasospasm, thrombus formation in the absence of CAD, or intense myocardial O_2 demand in the presence of a fixed atherosclerotic plaque. Plaque rupture is not the typical etiology of cocaine-related MI. Appropriate therapy includes aspirin, supplemental O_2, and heparin, as well as the aggressive use of nitrates for relief of vasospasm. Calcium channel blockers are also indicated for the treatment of vasospasm and hypertension in this group of patients. The use of beta-blockers in this setting has been associated with an *increase* in mortality, most likely due to unopposed alpha-adrenergic stimulation with resulting hypertension. Labetalol, a combined alpha- and beta-blocker, may not result in the hypertensive response associated with beta-blockers; however, its use has not been studied in randomized controlled trials.

15. C. Less than 130/85 mm Hg.

16. C. Less than 130/85 mm Hg.

17. A. Less than 140/90 mm Hg.

18. D. Less than 125/75 mm Hg.

19. C. Less than 130/85 mm Hg.

JNC VI recommends different target BPs for different patients, depending on comorbid conditions and risk for adverse events. A target BP below 140/90 mm Hg is recommended for patients with uncomplicated hypertension. Patients with diabetes, renal failure, and heart failure are at increased risk for events, including MI, stroke, CHF exacerbations, and progression of renal failure; the recommended target BP is below 130/85 mm Hg for these patients. Patients with renal failure and more than 1 g of proteinuria in 24 hours are at particularly high risk for developing end-stage renal disease; the recommended target BP for these patients is below 125/75 mm Hg. The American Diabetes Association and the American College of Cardiology recommend a target BP below 130/80 mm Hg for all patients with diabetes.

20. C. This patient has high-normal BP according to the JNC VI guidelines. She falls in risk group B because of her family history of CAD. The most appropriate intervention for this patient includes lifestyle modifications, including regular exercise, weight reduction, and salt restriction. She does not require drug therapy at this time, but she should have a repeat BP check in 1 year. A fasting lipid profile is appropriate in this patient given her age and family history of premature CAD.

21. C. Hypertension in older patients is very common. Pseudohypertension can be seen when an older patient has noncompliant, incompressible vessels, resulting in falsely high sphygmomanometer readings. Treatment of isolated systolic hypertension reduces the risk for both fatal and nonfatal stroke. The Systolic Hypertension in the Elderly Program (SHEP) trial evaluated a stepped-care approach to the management of isolated systolic hypertension in patients older than 60 years. Patients were randomized to

placebo or chlorthalidone for initial therapy; atenolol was added to patients in the treatment arm if target BP was not reached. Major cardiovascular events were reduced 32% in the treatment arm after 4.5 years of follow-up; there was a trend to reduced mortality in the treatment arm [relative risk = 0.87 (0.73–1.05)]. Stroke risk was reduced by 36% in the treatment arm. The Systolic Hypertension-Europe (Syst-Eur) trial was a randomized, placebo-controlled trial of the long-acting dihydropyridine calcium channel blocker, nitrendipine. Patients older than 60 years were included if they had a resting systolic BP of 160 to 219 mm Hg and a diastolic BP below 95 mm Hg. Therapy with enalapril or HCTZ was added for those patients in the treatment arm who did not reach target BP values. There was a trend to decreased mortality in the treatment group after 2 years of follow-up. The stroke rate was reduced by 42%, and the cumulative rate of fatal and nonfatal cardiovascular end points was reduced by 31% in the active treatment arm. Randomized trials evaluating isolated systolic hypertension have not included patients with resting systolic BPs in the 140 to 159 mm Hg range; however, observational studies have shown that BPs in this range are associated with increased rates of cardiovascular events compared to patients with normal BP.

According to the JNC VI guidelines, the BP target for patients with isolated systolic hypertension is the same as for patients with uncomplicated hypertension—below 140/90 mm Hg. The Medical Research Council Trial of Treatment of Hypertension in Older Adults randomized patients 65 to 74 years old with systolic BPs of 160 to 209 mm Hg and diastolic BPs below 115 mm Hg to treatment with either atenolol or placebo or amiloride/HCTZ or placebo. After adjusting for baseline characteristics, the diuretic group had significant reductions in the risk for stroke, coronary events, and all cardiovascular events compared to placebo, whereas the atenolol group did not.

22. E. Initiate therapy with atenolol, 25 mg daily, and proceed with surgery. This patient is at low risk for cardiovascular events at the time of his intermediate-risk shoulder surgery, based on his functional capacity, lack of ischemic symptoms, and normal ECG. No functional study is necessary. However, the patient has untreated stage 2 hypertension. Treatment with a cardioselective beta-blocker before and after surgery is appropriate and may lower his risk for perioperative cardiovascular events. Calcium antagonists have not been shown to reduce perioperative event rates. The target BP is below 140/90 mm Hg for this patient with uncomplicated hypertension.

23. E. Administer metoprolol, 5 mg IV; monitor closely; and repeat if needed. The tracing is a continuous pullback from the LV apex to the ascending aorta and is consistent with HCM. The patient has elevated systolic pressures at the LV apex. As the catheter is withdrawn across the LVOT obstruction, the peak systolic pressure drops, and the diastolic pressure remains unchanged because the catheter remains in the LV cavity. The diastolic pressure increases as the catheter is withdrawn across the aortic valve, and the systolic pressure remains stable because there is no pressure gradient across the aortic valve. Patients with HCM often present with exertional chest discomfort, breathlessness, and lightheadedness. Conditions that reduce LV filling, or preload, tend to exacerbate symptoms, as the LVOT obstruction occurs earlier in systole. Examples include dehydration, over diuresis, and bleeding. Conditions that reduce afterload tend to result in an

increase in heart rate and myocardial contractility, thereby increasing LVOT obstruction. This usually occurs with medications, including vasodilators such as amyl nitrite, hydralazine, and sodium nitroprusside.

In this case, the patient has HCM, is hypertensive, and is short of breath at rest. The goal of therapy is to reduce BP without significantly decreasing LV preload or afterload. Beta-blockade is ideal for this patient, as it will reduce heart rate and contractility, resulting in increased preload and decreased myocardial O_2 demand. Nitrates significantly reduce preload and modestly reduce afterload and could exacerbate the patient's symptoms. Hydralazine is a potent arterial vasodilator that decreases afterload and often causes tachycardia, both of which would exacerbate LVOT obstruction in this patient. Furosemide is a loop-diuretic that decreases LV preload and would increase in LVOT obstruction. Finally, this patient has severe HCM, with a resting LVOT gradient of 100 mm Hg, and is short of breath. With a measured systolic BP of 174 mm Hg, the estimated pressure at the LV apex would be nearly 275 mm Hg. Observation alone at this point would not be appropriate.

24. A. Metoprolol, 5 mg IV, repeated every 5 min, titrated to a mean arterial pressure below 70 mm Hg and a pulse below 60 bpm. This patient has a history and presentation suggestive of aortic dissection with the abrupt onset of severe, tearing chest pain. Radiation to the midscapular area suggests type B dissection of the descending thoracic aorta. The goal of therapy in this situation is to control BP and pain and reduce the rate of change of pressure development in the aorta (dP/dT). This will reduce the likelihood of extension of the dissection. Beta-blockers are ideal because they reduce heart rate and BP and exert a negative inotropic effect, thereby reducing the dP/dT. Sodium nitroprusside can be used in combination with beta-blockers if needed for additional BP control, but only after the institution of adequate beta-blockade. Nitroglycerin is not likely to be effective for this patient's chest pain and does not have a potent antihypertensive effect. Sublingual nifedipine is not recommended in any clinical situation and would be particularly dangerous in this situation due to its potent vasodilator properties and propensity to increase dP/dT. Likewise, hydralazine is a direct arterial vasodilator, increases dP/dT, and would not be recommended in this situation.

25. D. Instruct the patient regarding strict sodium restriction, and check the plasma renin activity. This patient has many features suggestive of primary aldosteronism, the cause of hypertension in approximately 1% of patients. Primary aldosteronism is more common in women, with the peak incidence from 30 to 50 years of age. Patients typically present with diastolic hypertension, fatigue, and headache. Unprovoked hypokalemia is a clue to its presence. When hypokalemia is noted in a patient with hypertension, plasma renin activity should be checked. Low plasma renin activity suggests a primary mineralocorticoid excess syndrome. Elevated plasma aldosterone levels after saline loading confirm the diagnosis and should be followed up with an abdominal CT scan to rule out adrenal adenoma. BP control can usually be achieved with strict sodium restriction and spironolactone. HCTZ could result in severe hypokalemia and should be avoided unless used with potassium supplementation. Atenolol may lower the BP but should not be the first choice of therapy in this situation. Although important, weight loss and exercise are unlikely to control BP in this patient.

NOTES

SUGGESTED READING

Bhalla H. Hypertensive crisis. In: Marso SP, Griffin BP, Topol EJ, eds. *Manual of cardiovascular medicine.* Philadelphia: Lippincott Williams & Wilkins, 2000:434–445.

Foody J. Cardiovascular risk factors. In: Marso SP, Griffin BP, Topol EJ, eds. *Manual of cardiovascular medicine.* Philadelphia: Lippincott Williams & Wilkins, 2000:455–481.

Gerber JG, Nies AS. Antihypertensive agents and the drug therapy of hypertension. In: Gilman AG, ed. *Goodman and Gilman's the pharmacological basis of therapeutics*, 8th ed. New York: Pergamon Press, Inc., 1990:784–813.

Joint National Committee on Prevention, Detection, Evaluation, and Treatment of High Blood Pressure. The sixth report of the Joint National Committee on Prevention, Detection, Evaluation, and Treatment of High Blood Pressure (JNC VI). *Arch Intern Med* 1997;157:2413–2446.

Renlund DG, Taylor DO. Cardiac transplantation. In: Topol EJ, ed. *Textbook of cardiovascular medicine*, 2nd ed. Philadelphia: Lippincott Williams & Wilkins, 2002:1915–1934.

Rudd P, Osterberg. Hypertension: context, pathophysiology, and management. In: Topol EJ, ed. *Textbook of cardiovascular medicine*, 2nd ed. Philadelphia: Lippincott Williams & Wilkins, 2002:91–122.

CHAPTER 11

Pericardial Disease

Monvadi B. Srichai and Wael A. Jaber

QUESTIONS

1. A 45-year-old woman with a history of treated carcinoma of the breast presents to the local emergency department with a few days of severe chest pain. In the emergency department, she appears ill and pale and in moderate discomfort. Her BP is 135/60 mm Hg, her respiratory rate is 24 breaths per minute, her heart rate is 82 bpm, and her temperature is 100.8°F. The resident on call reads her CXR as unremarkable. Her ECG is shown in Figure 1.

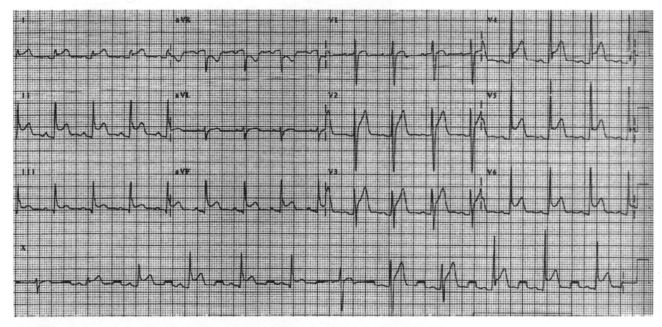

FIGURE 1 (From Wagner GS, ed. *Marriott's practical electrocardiography*, 9th ed. Baltimore: Williams & Wilkins, 1994, with permission.)

What is the most reasonable next step?

A. Give aspirin and nitroglycerin and prepare to administer thrombolytics.
B. Call the cardiac intervention team and rush to the catheterization laboratory for emergency coronary intervention.
C. Give a nonsteroidal antiinflammatory medication.
D. Discharge the patient and refer her for a gastroenterology follow-up as an outpatient.

2. You are called to see a 21-year-old female immigrant from Russia who presents to the emergency department with worsening left-sided chest pain of 6 months' duration. She also reports marked shortness of breath while walking to her daily job in a local supermarket. In addition, she has noticed "puffiness" in her lower extremities. However, she has attributed most of her symptoms to long hours of standing and dust in the warehouse. In addition to normal vital signs, her physical examination reveals quiet heart sounds. The rest of her examination is significant for distended neck veins, marked hepatosplenomegaly, and 3+ lower extremities edema. Her CXR is shown in Figure 2.

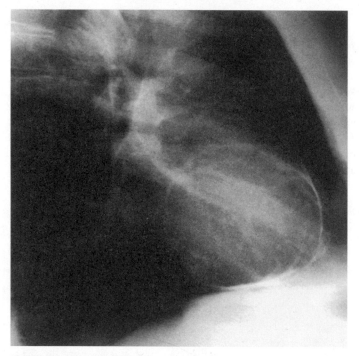

FIGURE 2 (From Pohost GM, O'Rourke GA, Berman DS, et al., eds. *Imaging in cardiovascular disease.* Philadelphia: Lippincott Williams & Wilkins, 2000, with permission.)

All of the following are appropriate diagnostic tests *except*

A. right and left cardiac catheterization
B. TEE
C. blood samples for liver function testing and hepatitis
D. cardiac CT
E. MRI

3. A 59-year-old man with a history of CAD and remote coronary bypass surgery presents with progressive dyspnea and vague chest pain. He had a stress echocardiogram for these symptoms that demonstrated normal LV function with no stress-induced wall motion abnormalities. However, he

returned to the emergency department a few days later with recurrent symptoms. This time the house officer examining the patient notes 3+ pedal edema. The patient is admitted and started on diuretics. His blood tests are as follows:

White blood cell count = 11,000
Hemoglobin = 14.2
Platelets = 172,000
Albumin = 4.6
Urea = 11
Creatinine = 0.9

Owing to the recurrent symptoms, his cardiologist decides to refer him for a right and left heart catheterization. The coronary grafts are all patent. The tracings from the study are shown in Figure 3.

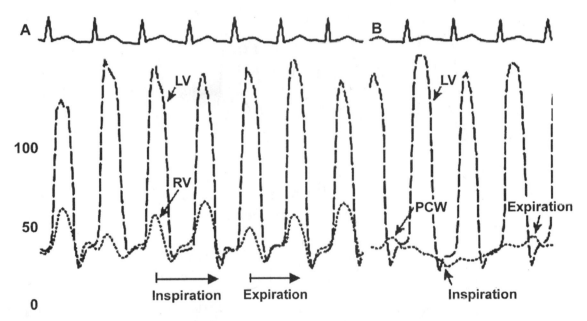

FIGURE 3 PCW, pulmonary capillary wedge.

What is the most logical explanation of this patient's symptoms?

A. constrictive pericardial disease
B. small vessel CAD
C. diastolic dysfunction related to his chronic CAD
D. cardiac amyloid
E. cardiac tamponade

4. A 73-year-old man with no cardiac history presents with chronic lower extremities edema. His primary care physician attributed his symptoms to old age. He was treated with hydrochlorothiazide. Initially, he reported a good response to the therapy, but, over the past few months, his edema recurred, and doubling the diuretic dose did not alleviate his symptoms. On his initial examination, you notice distended neck veins and a quiet precordium. He has mild hepatomegaly and 4+ pedal edema. A TTE is suboptimal due to the patient's inability to lie flat and obstructive lung disease. His blood work is as follows:

White blood cell count = 6,000
Hemoglobin = 12.7
Platelets = 225,000
Urea = 43
Creatinine = 2.4
Albumin = 3.6

A cardiac catheterization is performed. He has normal coronary arteries with mild impairment in LV systolic function. The tracings from the study are shown in Figure 4.

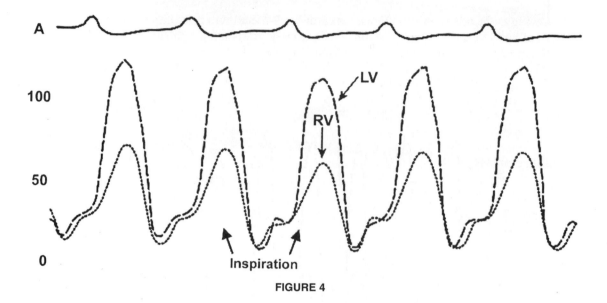

FIGURE 4

What is your explanation of his symptoms?

A. You agree with his primary care physician. You tell the patient that he probably has peripheral venous insufficiency.

B. This patient has significant diastolic dysfunction, and his prognosis is guarded.

C. This patient's symptoms are due to the LV systolic dysfunction and volume overload.

D. This patient should be referred for surgical evaluation for possible pericardial stripping.

5. A 56-year-old male smoker with a family history significant for CAD is presenting with dyspnea on exertion and nonexertional vague chest pain. His physical examination and his initial ECG are unremarkable. His CXR demonstrates an increased cardiac silhouette. There is also a small nodule seen in his right upper lobe. The radiologist is not certain about its significance. Given his risk factors and symptoms, he is referred for a perfusion stress test. The images from the stress test are shown in Figure 5.

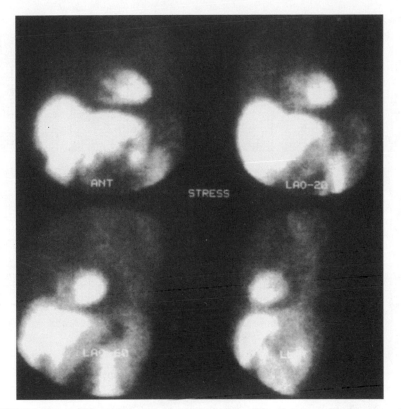

FIGURE 5 (From Pohost GM, O'Rourke GA, Berman DS, et al., eds. *Imaging in cardiovascular disease*. Philadelphia: Lippincott Williams & Wilkins, 2000, with permission.)

Which of the following does the patient clearly have?

A. He has coronary ischemia and should be referred for coronary angiography.
B. There is no evidence of pathology to justify his symptoms.
C. His symptoms are related to impairment of RV filling and pericardial disease.
D. He has mild ischemia and can be treated medically.

6. A 58-year-old man, with cardiac risk factors of tobacco use, hypertension, and hypercholesterolemia, presented to the emergency department a few days ago with an acute onset of left-sided chest pain. His evaluation revealed a diaphoretic man in moderate discomfort. An ECG was performed and showed a pattern consistent with an inferior wall acute MI. The patient was treated with thrombolytics. Forty-five minutes after the initial dose of the thrombolytics, he felt better and had complete resolution of his symptoms and normalization of the ECG. On the third day after the event, he reports midsternal chest pain, vague in nature, with mild diaphoresis and shortness of breath. An ECG is performed, as shown in Figure 6.

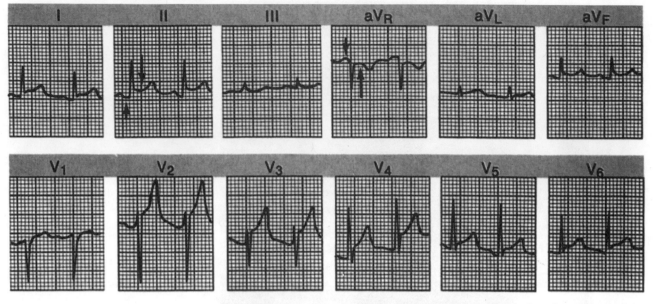

FIGURE 6 (From Braunwald E, ed. *Heart disease: a textbook of cardiovascular medicine*, 5th ed. Philadelphia: WB Saunders, 1997, with permission.)

Which of the following should you tell the patient is the next step in managing his condition?

A. There is evidence of reocclusion of the infarct-related artery, and a percutaneous intervention is needed.

B. There is evidence of reocclusion of the infarct-related artery, and re-bolus with thrombolytics and heparin is indicated.

C. He is showing signs of early postinfarction pericarditis, and a nonsteroidal antiinflammatory medication should be started.

D. An LV aneurysm has developed, and a TTE is needed to evaluate the extent of the aneurysm.

7. A 19-year-old male college student presents to his local physician for evaluation of a dry cough. His symptoms started 3 days ago but now appear to be resolving. He had planned a trip overseas but was concerned and is now seeking advice. His physical examination is unremarkable. A CXR is performed and is read as showing an enlarged right cardiac silhouette. A TTE is ordered, which is shown in Figure 7.

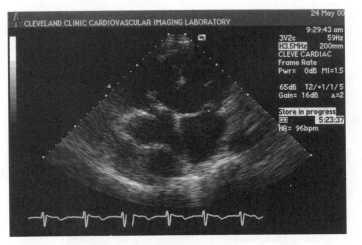

FIGURE 7

The patient most likely has which of the following conditions?

A. He has a pericardial cyst that is benign; no further treatment should be offered.
B. He has cardiac tamponade requiring a pericardial tap.
C. He has a pleural effusion.
D. There is no pathology. The CXR was misread.
E. He has mesothelioma.

8. An 82-year-old man, who has a history of CAD with two surgical coronary revascularizations, is presenting with a few months' history of dyspnea on exertion, increased abdominal girth, and pedal edema. An evaluation performed in the office of his local cardiologist showed a slightly depressed LV EF of 45%. His cardiologist refers him to your center with the differential diagnosis of constrictive versus restrictive heart disease. All of the following echocardiographic markers support constrictive physiology *except*

A. dissociation between intracardiac and intrathoracic pressures
B. exaggerated ventricular interdependence in diastolic filling
C. respiratory difference greater than 20 cm per second in superior vena cava flow velocities
D. increased atrial pressures and equalization of end-diastolic pressures

9. You are called to the emergency department to see a 74-year-old man. He has a history of heavy smoking and hypertension. The patient cannot remember his medications, but he reports not taking them on a routine basis. In the past few hours before presentation, he experienced a sudden onset of severe left-sided chest pain with radiation to the left scapula. Approximately half an hour later, he noted some difficulty breathing. In the emergency department, he is noted to be diaphoretic and in significant respiratory distress. His physical examination reveals a BP of 160/90 mm Hg, elevated jugular venous pressures, and a quiet precordium. His ECG is reported as sinus tachycardia with no acute ST-T changes. After initial pain and BP management, a TEE is performed to rule out aortic dissection. The findings of the TTE are shown in Figure 8.

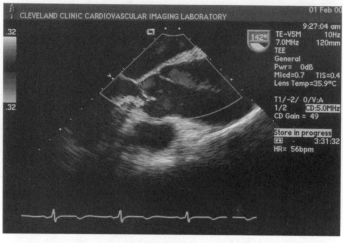

FIGURE 8

What is your recommendation?

A. The patient should have immediate surgical intervention.

B. The patient needs BP control and surgical evaluation once he is medically stabilized.

C. The patient should have percutaneous pericardial drainage to manage the cardiac tamponade and then a surgical evaluation.

D. The diagnosis is unclear; a CT scan or an aortic angiogram is needed.

10. A 42-year-old man was referred for evaluation of symptomatic MR. He was diagnosed with mitral valve prolapse that was not suitable for repair. Given his family history of CAD and tobacco use, he underwent a coronary angiogram, which revealed no evidence of obstructive coronary disease. He underwent an uneventful mitral valve replacement. He was extubated and transferred from the ICU 48 hours after the operation. On postoperation day 3, you note the patient to be pale and lethargic and in mild respiratory distress. His BP is 100/60 mm Hg. His cardiac and lung examination is compromised by the presence of rapid breathing and chest tubes. His ECG reveals NSR at 97 bpm with no acute ST-T changes. A TTE is performed. Selected views are shown in Figure 9A.

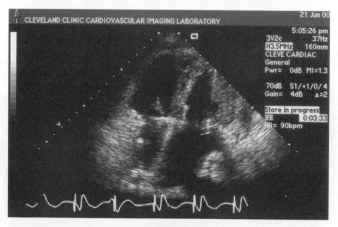

FIGURE 9A

As the patient continues to deteriorate and becomes hypotensive, a TEE is performed next, as shown in Figure 9B.

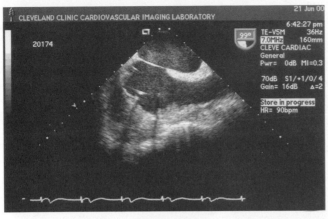

FIGURE 9B

What should you recommend?

A. Immediate surgical exploration of the pericardium.
B. Percutaneous aspiration of the fluid present in the pericardium.
C. Immediate surgical intervention for malfunction of the prosthetic mitral valve.
D. A 500-cc bolus of IV normal saline solution should be started because the patient is dehydrated, and no further intervention is needed.

11. A 49-year-old black man with hypertension and chronic renal insufficiency presents with dyspnea and fluid overload with decreased urine output. He is treated in the hospital with diuretics, and his symptoms improve. However, his renal function continues to deteriorate with an increasing BUN of 90 and a creatinine of 5.4. In addition, the patient is noted to have several bruises on his arms from needlestick blood draws and IV lines. On hospital day 4, the patient is noted to be hypotensive and tachycardic: BP, 80/40 mm Hg; heart rate, 110 bpm. No jugular venous distention is noted, but heart sounds are diminished, and a loud pericardial rub is heard. His TTE is shown in Figure 10.

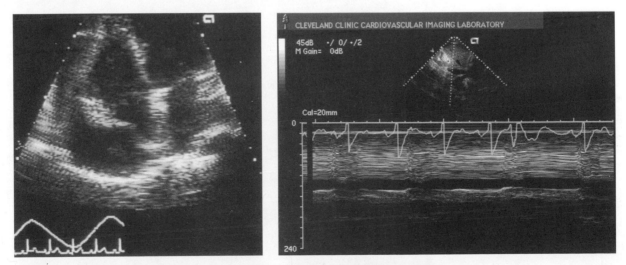

FIGURE 10 (From Otto CM, Pearlman AS. *Textbook of clinical echocardiography*. Philadelphia: WB Saunders, 1995, with permission.)

What is the next step in management?

A. urgent pericardiocentesis
B. IV hydration
C. immediate dialysis
D. the continuation of diuretics with serial TTE

12. A 42-year-old white male chef is brought into the emergency department after a motor vehicle accident in which he fell asleep at the wheel and ran into a tree. He is reporting anterior chest discomfort and shortness of breath. He relates no prior medical conditions and takes no medications. Vitals are stable with a BP of 120/60 mm Hg and a heart rate of 90 bpm. His ECG is shown in Figure 11A.

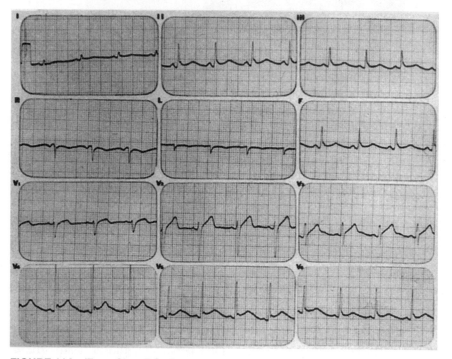

FIGURE 11A (From Chou T-C. *Electrocardiography in clinical practice*, 4th ed. Philadelphia: WB Saunders, 1996, with permission.)

A TTE is performed. Diastolic images are shown in Figure 11B.

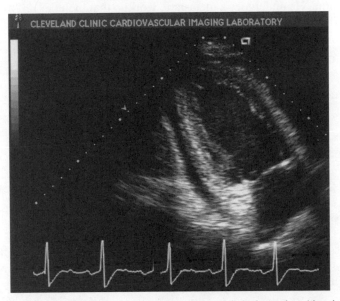

FIGURE 11B (From Chou T-C. *Electrocardiography in clinical practice*, 4th ed. Philadelphia: WB Saunders, 1996, with permission.)

Laboratory tests show modest elevation of creatinine phosphokinase at 240. Which of the following is the most reasonable next step in managing this patient?

A. Start the patient on a nonsteroidal antiinflammatory agent with follow-up as an outpatient in 1 week.
B. Admit the patient for observation on telemetry with a follow-up TTE.
C. The patient needs immediate percutaneous revascularization.
D. Send the patient for surgical treatment of pericardial rupture.

13. A 22-year-old white man is newly diagnosed with non-Hodgkin's lymphoma. He undergoes a metastatic workup that includes an MRI of the chest and abdomen, which is shown in Figure 12.

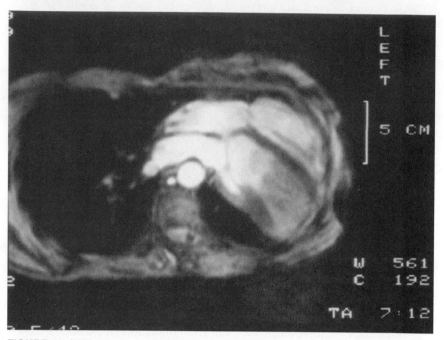

FIGURE 12 (MRI image was provided by Dr. Richard White, Head, Section of Cardiovascular Imaging, Departments of Radiology and Cardiovascular Medicine, The Cleveland Clinic Foundation.)

The plan is for chemotherapy, but you are consulted for cardiac assessment before beginning chemotherapy. Radionuclide ventriculography shows a normal LV EF of 65%. What should you recommend?

A. ordering a TTE to delineate the abnormality
B. cardiothoracic surgical consultation before starting chemotherapy
C. exercise stress testing
D. proceeding with chemotherapy without further cardiac evaluation

14. A 32-year-old white man presented initially with low-grade fever, cough, and pleuritic chest pain. He was found on ECG to have diffuse ST segment elevation. A TTE revealed a large pericardial effusion, and serologies were positive for Coxsackievirus B infection. He was diagnosed with acute viral pericarditis and treated with indomethacin. He returns 4 weeks later for follow-up and states that he no longer has any pain, but he notes some mild ankle swelling. His ECG is normal. A repeat TTE shows resolution of the effusion but new findings consistent with mild constriction. What is the next step in managing this patient?

A. Obtain cardiac MRI to better assess the pericardium.
B. Have a cardiothoracic surgical consultation for pericardectomy.
C. Reassure the patient and observe him over the next 3 months for worsening of symptoms.
D. Start a course of steroids.

15. All of the following statements concerning pericarditis post-MI are true *except*

    A. Thrombolytic therapy has reduced the incidence by 50%.
    B. It occurs most commonly after inferior infarctions.
    C. Typical diagnostic electrocardiographic changes of acute pericarditis are rare.
    D. Atrial tachyarrhythmias are common.

16. A 56-year-old Asian man, who recently emigrated from Thailand, presents to the emergency department with cough, fever, and chills. He is noted to have a BP of 80/50 mm Hg and a regular pulse at a rate of 135 bpm. CXR shows cardiomegaly. A two-dimensional echocardiography is shown in Figure 13A, and Doppler interrogation of the mitral inflow is shown in Figure 13B.

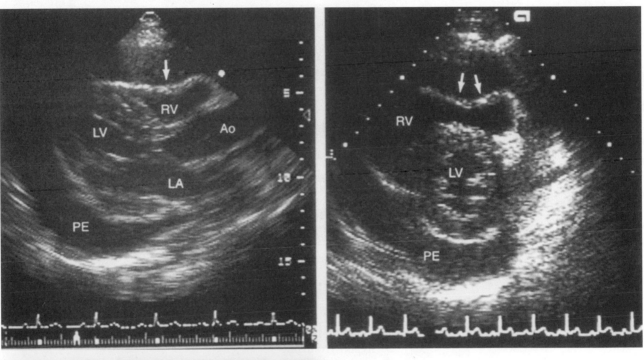

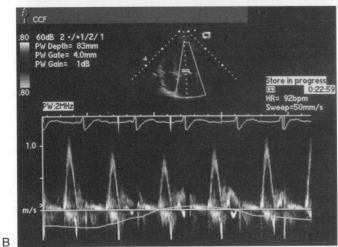

FIGURE 13

All of the following are expected on physical examination *except*

A. Kussmaul's sign
B. Ewart's sign
C. pulsus paradoxus
D. absent Y descent on jugular venous waveforms

17. A 64-year-old white woman, with a history of breast carcinoma in her 20s treated with mastectomy and radiation, is undergoing preoperative evaluation for knee surgery. She has not had a recurrence of breast cancer since her initial treatment, and she has no other medical problems. Her preoperative CXR demonstrates cardiomegaly. TTE is performed and is shown in Figure 14.

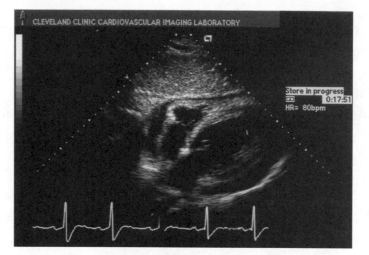

FIGURE 14

Which of the following is the least likely cause of this patient's effusion?

A. radiation pericarditis
B. hypothyroidism
C. viral pericarditis
D. recurrent malignant pericarditis

18. A 63-year-old white woman with a history of left-sided breast cancer, which was treated with lumpectomy and radiation therapy 30 years ago, presents with new-onset lower extremity edema, hepatomegaly, and ascites. The CT scan of the chest is shown in Figure 15.

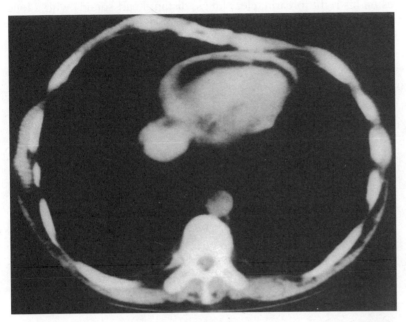

FIGURE 15

All of the following features may be present on TTE *except*

A. septal bounce
B. diastolic septal shudder
C. no respiratory variation of mitral inflow
D. myocardial tethering

19. For constrictive pericarditis, factors associated with a worse prognosis after pericardiectomy include all of the following *except*

A. older age
B. arrhythmia
C. history of irradiation
D. presence of pericardial effusion on preoperative TTE

20. A 66-year-old woman with diabetes mellitus, hypertension, and a 50-pack-per-year tobacco history is seen in the emergency department for shortness of breath. She is noted on examination to have distended neck veins (16 cm), tachycardia with distant heart sounds, clear lungs, and pulsus para-doxus of 20 mm Hg. A CXR shows normal heart size. All of the following should be included on the differential *except*

A. hypertrophic obstructive cardiomyopathy
B. partial obstruction of the superior vena cava
C. cardiac tamponade
D. chronic obstructive pulmonary disease

21. A 44-year-old white man with rheumatoid arthritis is referred to your office for evaluation after his rheumatologist heard a loud heart sound. On questioning, the patient mainly reports joint pains in his fingers. He denies any chest discomfort or shortness of breath. He has been on methotrexate and prednisone for the past year. His examination is significant for mild erythema and swelling of his distal interphalangeal joints, rheumatoid nod-

ules on his right forearm, clear lungs, distant heart sounds with a loud friction rub, and moderate peripheral edema. You order a TTE to further assess his heart. Selective images are shown in Figure 16.

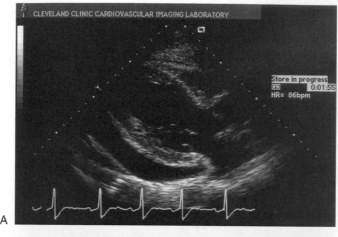

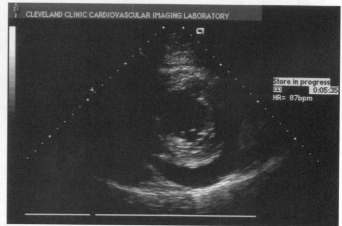

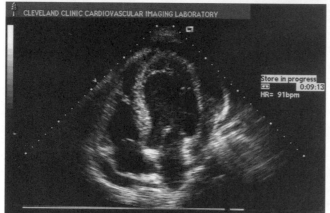

FIGURE 16

What is your recommendation?

A. Because he currently has no cardiac symptoms, no further treatment is needed except to continue methotrexate and prednisone.

B. You want the patient to start indomethacin, continue methotrexate and prednisone, and follow up in 4 weeks.

C. The best treatment at this time for his pericardial effusion is drainage with the instillation of steroids to prevent recurrence.

D. A surgical evaluation for pericardiectomy is necessary because the findings on his TTE indicate that he will develop problems in the future if this is not taken care of soon.

22. A 55-year-old white man presents for evaluation of chest pain. He has no prior medical problems, but he has noted burning epigastric and chest discomfort for the past few months for which he was taking antacids with some relief of his symptoms. However, because the symptoms persisted, he sought medical attention and was referred for an esophagogastroduodenoscopy, which was performed earlier today. He was found to have a fundal hiatal her-

nia with a gastric ulcer that was cauterized, and he was started on omeprazole. On returning home, he noted a new sharp anterior chest pain, somewhat positional related, that was not relieved with antacids or omeprazole. This pain progressively worsened over the next few hours, and he came to the emergency department. Examination in the emergency department revealed a temperature of 38.1°C, a heart rate of 110 bpm, and a BP of 120/70 mm Hg. Lung sounds were clear. Heart sounds appeared normal with the patient sitting upright, but they were diminished with the patient lying in the supine position. An ECG did not show any acute ST-T wave abnormalities to suggest infarction. A CXR was performed, as shown in Figure 17.

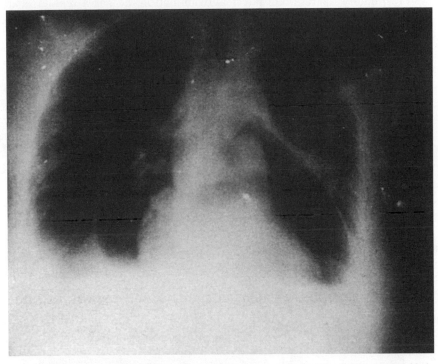

FIGURE 17 (From Spodick DS. *The pericardium: a comprehensive textbook.* New York: Marcel Dekker, 1997, with permission.)

You are called to further assess the patient. After reviewing the available data, which of the following is your next step?

A. Immediate surgical consultation.
B. Immediate pericardiocentesis.
C. Start a nonsteroidal antiinflammatory medication and admit him for observation.
D. No further treatment is needed, because his symptoms are due to the hiatal hernia.

23. In patients who have congenital absence of the pericardium, which of the following is a common finding?

A. cardiac displacement to the left on CXR
B. sinus bradycardia on ECG
C. cardiac hypermobility with postural changes on TTE
D. absence of preaortic pericardial recess on CT
E. all of the above

24. A 71-year-old man presents to the hospital with palpitations of 2 to 3 days' duration. He has no known medical history, and he is not on any medications. Initial evaluation is unremarkable except for a BP of 160/90 mm Hg and an ECG showing AFib with a ventricular rate of 120 to 130 bpm. Given the duration of his symptoms, he is treated with beta-blockers for rate control and heparin for anticoagulation. On hospital day 2, he is referred for early transesophageal guided cardioversion. The TEE reveals normal LV and RV function. There are no echocardiographic contraindications for cardioversion. An uneventful cardioversion is performed, and the patient converts to NSR. On hospital day 3, the patient is found in marked respiratory distress. On physical examination, he has a regular heart rate with a loud audible click over the precordium. A CXR is performed, as shown in Figure 18.

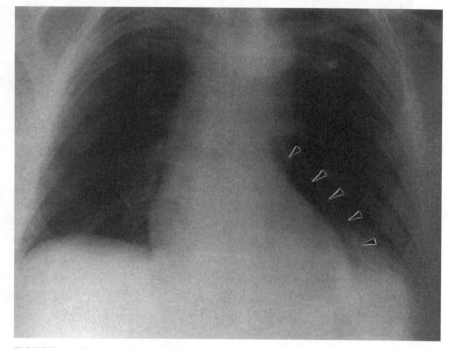

FIGURE 18 (From Spodick DS. *The pericardium: a comprehensive textbook.* New York: Marcel Dekker, 1997, with permission.)

What does this patient have?

A. He has a pulmonary embolism and should be treated with thrombolytics.
B. He has a hiatal/diaphragmatic hernia with compression of the heart by the fundus of stomach.
C. He has an iatrogenic pneumohydropericardium; immediate drainage and surgical attention are needed.
D. He has a recurrence of AFib.

25. Among the causes of pulsus paradoxus are all of the following *except*

A. large pericardial effusion
B. chronic obstructive lung disease
C. morbid obesity
D. constrictive pericardial disease

26. The etiologies of granulomatous pericarditis (Fig. 19) include which of the following?

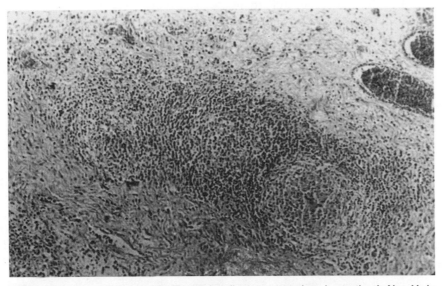

FIGURE 19 (From Spodick DS. *The pericardium: a comprehensive textbook*. New York: Marcel Dekker, 1997, with permission.)

A. infections: tuberculosis, histoplasmosis
B. connective tissue diseases and rheumatoid arthritis
C. environmental exposures: silicosis, asbestosis
D. idiopathic pericarditis
E. all of the above

27. A 59-year-old woman with a history of chronic renal insufficiency presents to the emergency department with anterior left-sided chest pain. She reports that the chest pain started after her last dialysis 7 days ago. She appears lethargic and in mild respiratory distress. The physical examination demonstrates a BP of 160/90 mm Hg and a heart rate of 100 bpm. On cardiac auscultation, a loud friction rub is heard. An ECG is obtained (Fig. 20).

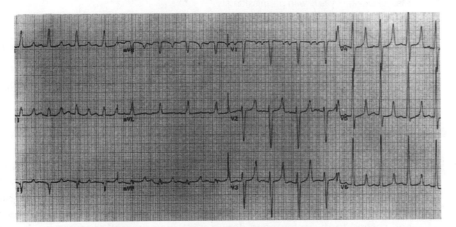

FIGURE 20 (From Spodick DS. *The pericardium: a comprehensive textbook*. New York: Marcel Dekker, 1997, with permission.)

What is the most important next step in this case?

A. Perform emergency dialysis.

B. Obtain an echocardiogram.

C. Prepare for pericardiocentesis.

D. Admit the patient to the cardiac care unit to rule out MI.

28. An 82-year-old woman with no history of cardiac disease or malignancy is seen at your office for weakness, fatigue, constipation, and lower extremities swelling. Her daughter reports that she was in very good health until 6 months ago when she was admitted to the hospital with pneumonia. Her daughter noticed that she was discharged from the hospital on no medications. Her concern was that her mother had been on a pill for a long time for her "glands." On physical examination, the patient is an elderly woman who appears her age. She is pale, lethargic, and somewhat confused. Her skin is dry, and she has a BP of 100/60 mm Hg and a heart rate of 52 bpm. The chest examination reveals marked reduction in air entry in the lower third of her lung fields. She has normal heart sounds. Marked edema of the lower extremities is also noted. An ECG is obtained and is shown in Figure 21.

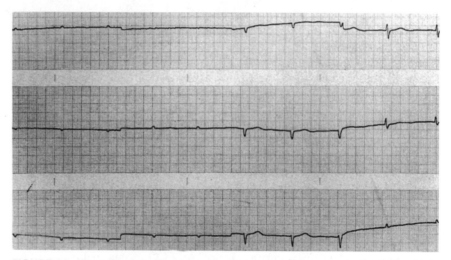

FIGURE 21 (From Spodick DS. *The pericardium: a comprehensive textbook.* New York: Marcel Dekker, 1997, with permission.)

The initial concern and management of this patient involves all of the following *except*

A. She is in cardiac tamponade and needs an immediate pericardial tap.

B. She is in a hypothyroid state and needs her medications restarted.

C. She is in CHB, and a pacemaker should be inserted.

D. She is in cardiogenic shock, and an IABP should be inserted.

29. A 29-year-old woman with known insulin-dependent diabetes mellitus was found unconscious 1 hour after an office party. Initial assessment by the emergency medical service team showed a BP of 90/60 mm Hg. Her pulse was 120, and her blood sugar was 870 mg per dL. She was given SC insulin and rushed to the emergency department. You are called to see her because of her abnormal ECG (Fig. 22).

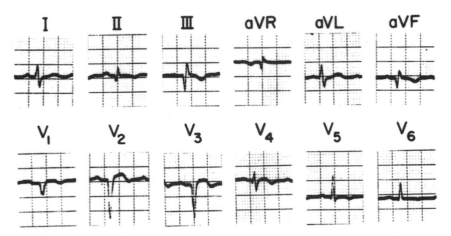

FIGURE 22 (From Spodick DS. *The pericardium: a comprehensive textbook*. New York: Marcel Dekker, 1997, with permission.)

She is noted to be semiconscious. The emergency physician has already started her on IV insulin drip and hydration. What is your recommendation at this juncture?

A. She is having an acute MI, and immediate restoration of coronary flow is essential.
B. She has ECG evidence of hyperkalemia, and she needs IV calcium and, possibly, dialysis.
C. Continue the current management; the ECG will improve with the resolution of ketoacidosis.
D. Her ECG predicts high-degree AV block; a standby external pacemaker should be available.

30. Which of the following is the most common neoplastic pericardial tumor in adults?

A. neuroma
B. hemangioma
C. mesothelioma
D. teratoma

ANSWERS

1. C. Give a nonsteroidal antiinflammatory medication. The clinical presentation of few days of severe chest pain does not favor an acute MI. Furthermore, the ECG tracing supports the diagnosis of pericarditis. Therefore, cardiac catheterization or thrombolytics are not appropriate. The only reasonable answer is to start the patient on antiinflammatory medications and obtain a TTE to rule out pericardial effusion.

2. C. Blood samples for liver function testing and hepatitis are not appropriate diagnostic tests. The patient is a young adult immigrant. Her chronic symptoms mainly suggest RV and LV failure. The CXR shows typical changes of calcific pericardial disease. All of the listed tests except those in choice C would be appropriate to help confirm the diagnosis. A right and left heart

catheterization could probably confirm the diagnosis, although assessing the coronary arteries is not indicated. TEE could have been used before obtaining the CXR to evaluate the etiology of the biventricular failure. Passive congestion of the liver is common in patients with constrictive pericarditis.

3. A. Constrictive pericardial disease. This patient did not have evidence of ischemia on a recent stress test. Furthermore, there is no evidence of obstructive disease in his coronaries or grafts. His tracings mostly support the diagnosis of constriction, given the diastolic equalization of pressures in the cardiac chambers and the typical square root sign. Amyloidosis would typically show signs of restrictive hemodynamics with no respiratory variation. Echocardiography typically shows increased LV wall thickness. Additionally, a diagnosis of tamponade should have been evident by echocardiography, which the patient had before heart catheterization. Otherwise, hemodynamic tracings of cardiac tamponade would look exactly the same as for constriction.

4. B. This patient has significant diastolic dysfunction, and his prognosis is guarded. He has evidence of restrictive LV filling (advanced diastolic dysfunction) in the absence of CAD. The differential diagnosis in his age group includes amyloidosis (especially considering concomitant renal dysfunction), hemochromatosis, and other infiltrative processes.

5. C. His symptoms are related to impairment of RV filling and pericardial disease. This patient with the main presentation of dyspnea has an increased cardiac silhouette. The nuclear image provided shows a circumferential echolucency surrounding the heart. This is consistent with a large pericardial effusion, and he most likely has right atrial and RV diastolic compromise. There is no evidence of a perfusion defect to suggest ischemia.

6. C. He is showing signs of early postinfarction pericarditis, and a nonsteroidal antiinflammatory medication should be started. This patient had an MI 72 hours ago that was successfully treated with thrombolytics. The ECG shows diffuse ST elevation with PR depression. These findings support the diagnosis of post-MI pericarditis. The ECG changes are new and nonlocalizing. Most patients improve with nonsteroidal antiinflammatory medications.

7. A. He has a pericardial cyst that is benign; no further treatment should be offered. The TTE and CXR show a pericardial cyst. Pericardial cysts are usually smooth structures containing transudative fluid. They are frequently only 2 or 3 cm in diameter, often located at the right cardiodiaphragmatic angle, and clinically silent. However, cysts can be associated with chest pain, dyspnea, cough, and arrhythmias likely due to compression of adjacent tissues. They can also become secondarily infected. In this patient, whose nonspecific symptoms appear to be resolving, no further treatment is needed.

8. C. Respiratory difference greater than 20 cm per second in superior vena cava flow velocities does not support constrictive physiology. The limitation on ventricular expansion imposed by the constricting pericardial sac will lead to ventricular "competition" for volume during the filling phase. The respiratory variations in the superior vena cava are typically less than 20 cm per second in constriction.

9. A. The patient should have immediate surgical intervention. This patient has evidence of acute type A aortic dissection with extension to the pericar-

dium, as evidenced by the pericardial effusion on the TEE. He should be immediately referred for surgical repair. If the diagnosis were not certain based on the TEE, then CT, MRI, or aortic angiography would be needed to better define the anatomy. The safest and most efficient management of patients with aortic dissection is to carry out all diagnostic procedures in the operating room. Pericardial drainage often gives only temporary relief or no relief of the tamponade, and the subsequent increase in BP disrupts sealing clots, accelerating intrapericardial leakage.

10. A. Immediate surgical exploration of the pericardium. The TTE and TEE demonstrate a pericardial hematoma compromising right atrial and RV filling. This is an indication for surgical exploration and evacuation of the hematoma.

11. B. IV hydration. This patient has evidence of pericarditis likely related to uremia, as he is close to requiring dialysis. Although his TTE shows signs of tamponade (right atrial collapse, moderate-sized effusion, and respiratory variation across the mitral inflow), there is no jugular venous distention, and the inferior vena cava is small sized, indicating that this patient has been overdiuresed. His hypotension and tachycardia are related to dehydration. He should, therefore, be treated with IV hydration.

12. B. Admit the patient for observation on telemetry with a follow-up TTE. The ECG shows findings consistent with an anterior wall injury, and the TTE shows a small pericardial effusion. Given this patient's history, he most likely has a cardiac contusion. Although the prognosis for recovery is generally excellent, these patients require careful monitoring and follow-up for late complications, which range from ventricular arrhythmias to cardiac rupture. Hence, the most logical answer to this question is to admit the patient to a telemetry bed with follow-up TTE.

13. D. Proceeding with chemotherapy without further cardiac evaluation. This patient's MRI shows congenital absence of the pericardium. This is a benign condition usually found incidentally. No specific cardiac treatment is needed unless there is entrapment of one of the cardiac chambers.

14. C. Reassure the patient and observe him over the next 3 months for worsening of symptoms. The natural history of acute viral or idiopathic pericarditis is usually short and self-limited. Occasionally, mild forms of constriction may develop weeks after the initial event, but they usually resolve without any specific treatment. No further treatment is indicated unless he becomes more symptomatic or develops signs of cardiac tamponade.

15. B. All of the answers except for B are true. Pericarditis after acute MI is usually associated with larger infarcts, as indicated by their more common presentation with anterior Q-wave infarctions.

16. A. Kussmaul's sign is not expected on physical examination. This patient has findings of cardiac tamponade on his TTE with large pericardial effusion and respiratory variation of mitral inflow pattern. In constrictive pericarditis or restrictive cardiomyopathy, the jugular venous pressure may not fall appropriately or may even increase with inspiration, a finding known as *Kussmaul's sign*. This finding may also be seen with RV infarction, but it is very uncommon and seldom noted in cardiac tamponade in which intratho-

racic pressures are transmitted through the pericardial sac. Ewart's sign—dullness to percussion of the left lung base—can be seen in any syndrome with a large pericardial effusion resulting in compression of the left lower lobe. Pulsus paradoxus, which is an exaggeration of the normal inspiratory drop in systolic arterial pressure exceeding 12 to 15 mm Hg, commonly occurs in cardiac tamponade. In addition, there is often a lack of a sharp X and Y descent with sometimes absent Y descent reflecting poor RV filling during diastolic due to high intrapericardial pressures causing RV collapse.

17. D. Recurrent malignant pericarditis. It would be extremely unusual for a patient to develop recurrence of breast carcinoma 20 years after successful treatment, especially without other signs of recurrence. More often, these patients have pericardial effusions related to cardiac disease, hypothyroidism, radiation pericarditis, or idiopathic pericarditis.

18. C. This patient has evidence of pericardial calcifications and symptoms consistent with constrictive pericarditis. All of the above findings except for choice C are seen with constrictive pericarditis. The heart and pulmonary vessels are intrathoracic, and, normally, both are simultaneously affected by respiratory pressure changes. In constrictive pericarditis, transthoracic pressures are not transmitted to the cardiac chambers. Hence, when inspiration decreases intrathoracic and pulmonary pressures, cardiac pressures remain high. Consequently, total pulmonary venous flow is decreased during inspiration, decreasing LV filling. Thus, respiratory variation is observed on Doppler interrogation of mitral inflow.

19. D. Presence of pericardial effusion on preoperative TTE is not included. Poorer results after surgical pericardiectomy are seen (a) with inadequate resection; (b) in uncorrected coronary disease; (c) with higher New York Heart Association classifications for "congestive failure"; (d) in older age; (e) after radiation pericarditis; (f) with chronicity—including peripheral organ failure (especially renal and hepatic) and ascites or edema, or both, which are ominous; (g) with severe myocardial atrophy and fibrosis (detectable by CT and MRI); and (h) with significant arrhythmias reflecting myocardial impairment.

20. A. Hypertrophic obstructive cardiomyopathy should not be included on the differential. The physical findings described in this case are seen in superior vena cava syndrome, obstructive lung disease, and tamponade. The presence of pulsus paradoxus is not observed in hypertrophic obstructive cardiomyopathy because the less compliant LV resists the phasically changing pericardial pressure.

21. D. A surgical evaluation for pericardiectomy is necessary because the findings on his TTE indicate that he will develop problems in the future if this is not taken care of soon. The patient is currently symptomatic with edema of the lower extremities. Furthermore, he has a pericardial friction rub suggestive of an active pericardial process likely related to his rheumatologic disease process. He is already on methotrexate and prednisone as antiinflammatory medications. Pericardial effusions related to rheumatoid arthritis often progress to constriction despite antiinflammatory therapy, and early management consisting of pericardial stripping is recommended.

22. B. The next step is an immediate pericardiocentesis. This patient has signs of early sepsis. Furthermore, the CXR shows pneumopericardium that likely developed secondary to gastric perforation from the esophagogas-

troduodenoscopy and cauterization of the ulcer. This patient needs immediate referral to surgery for repair.

23. E. All of the above. All are common findings in congenital absence of the pericardium.

24. C. He has an iatrogenic pneumohydropericardium; immediate drainage and surgical attention are needed. This patient had a TEE that most likely resulted in an esophageal tear with communication to the pericardial sac. On the CXR, there is a lucent triangle outlining the pericardium with pericardial passage over the aortic arch.

25. D. Constrictive pericardial disease is not a cause of pulsus paradoxus. Pulsus paradoxus depends on increased RV filling volume with inspiration. In constriction, although the RV filling velocity increases with inspiration, there is minimal change in the RV volume.

26. E. All of the above. Granulomas are focal nodules or masses made of granulation tissue and fibrous tissue with a variable degree of leukocytic infiltration. All the above entities have been linked to formation of granulomas.

27. A. Perform emergency dialysis. This patient has missed her dialysis session and is now presenting with hyperkalemia (note peaked T waves on ECG) and uremic pericarditis. The most essential step is to start dialysis to treat the hyperkalemia.

28. B. This patient has myxedema due to untreated hypothyroidism. The ECG shows sinus bradycardia, low QRS voltage, and nonspecific T-wave changes. The treatment is thyroid hormone replacement, which is almost always followed by steady regression of the effusion. Drainage is rarely needed in these situations, and if medical treatment is initiated early, one can avoid the precipitation of cholesterol in the pericardium and cholesterol pericarditis.

29. C. Continue the current management; the ECG will improve with the resolution of ketoacidosis. Patients presenting with diabetic ketoacidosis can have ECG features that are typical of stage I pericarditis and hypokalemia. The treatment is usually that of ketoacidosis. The ECG returns to normal after resolution of the acidosis.

30. C. Mesothelioma. Teratoma is the most common pericardial tumor in infancy and childhood. Neuroma and hemangioma are uncommon enough to be considered curiosities.

SUGGESTED READING

Buck M, Ingle JN, Giuliani ER, et al. Pericardial effusion in women with breast cancer. *Cancer* 1987;60(2):263–269.

Hoit BD. Management of effusive and constrictive pericardial heart disease. *Circulation* 2002;105(25):2939–2942.

Klein AL, Asher CR. Diseases of the pericardium, restrictive cardiomyopathy, and diastolic dysfunction. In: Topol EJ, ed. *Textbook of cardiovascular medicine*, 2nd ed. Philadelphia: Lippincott Williams & Wilkins, 2002.

Spodick DS. *The pericardium: a comprehensive textbook*. New York: Marcel Dekker, 1997.

CHAPTER 12

Common Echocardiographic Images in Cardiovascular Medicine

Brian P. Griffin

QUESTIONS

1. A 47-year-old diabetic is admitted with fever and shortness of breath. The patient has had poorly controlled diabetes and frequent urinary tract infections. A TTE is technically difficult. A TEE is performed. A long-axis image of the aortic valve is shown. Based on the TEE image of the valve, what is the most likely cause of the fever (Fig. 1)?

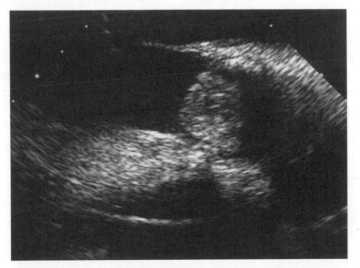

FIGURE 1 A transesophageal long-axis view of the aortic valve.

A. staphylococcal endocarditis
B. streptococcal endocarditis
C. fungal endocarditis
D. valve myxoma
E. none of the above

2. A 70-year-old woman recently underwent coronary artery bypass grafting. She is seen back in the emergency room with shortness of breath. A TTE is performed on her. Based on the accompanying apical four-chamber view (diastolic frame), what would the best course of action be now (Fig. 2)?

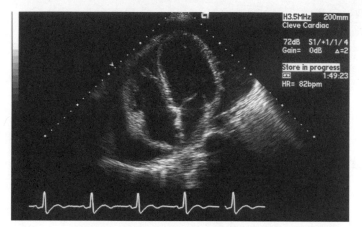

FIGURE 2 An apical four-chamber transthoracic image of the heart.

A. thoracentesis
B. pericardiocentesis
C. assessment of respiratory variation on mitral and tricuspid inflow Doppler velocities
D. arterial blood gas measurement
E. exploratory thoracotomy

3. A 55-year-old man is seen in the emergency room. He is cyanotic, with pulse oximetry O_2 saturation of 85%; pulse, 102 bpm; BP, 85/40; temperature, 38°C. His ECG shows LBBB. His wife says he had chest pain a few days ago but thought it was indigestion. His wife, when questioned, thinks he may have had a heart murmur before but is not sure. He is intubated due to declining oxygenation. TTE is unrevealing due to inadequate images. A TEE is performed to assess the cause of his hemodynamic compromise. Based on the accompanying multiplane TEE images, what is the most likely cause of his compromise (Fig. 3)?

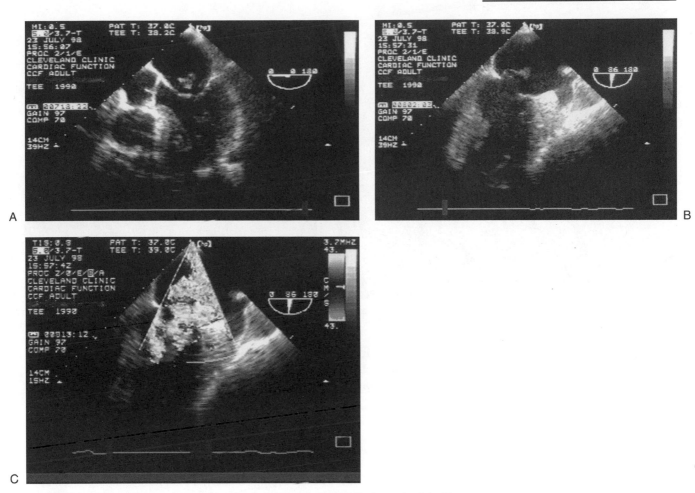

FIGURE 3 TEE multiplane views In systole. **A:** 0-Degree view. **B, C:** Approximately 90-degree vicw.

A. mitral valve prolapse
B. endocarditis of the mitral valve
C. acute aortic dissection
D. VSD
E. papillary muscle rupture

4. You are asked to consult on a 45-year-old man who has had staphylococcal endocarditis of the aortic valve that has been treated for 6 weeks with appropriate antibiotics and who is being followed by an internist in a rural area. A TEE was performed 3 days ago to assess the status of his infection and the hemodynamic severity of the aortic regurgitation. Based on the accompanying TEE images of the aortic valve, which of the following should you recommend (Fig. 4)?

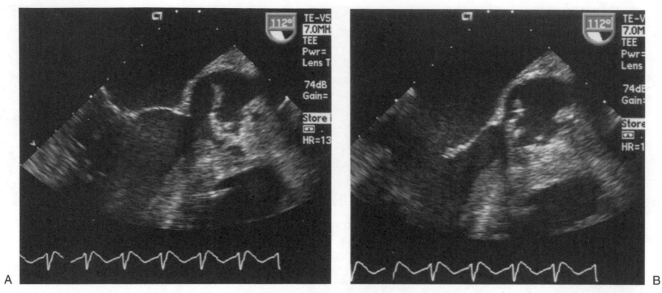

FIGURE 4 TEE long-axis view of the aortic valve and aorta in systole **(A)** and diastole **(B)**.

A. serial follow-up every 6 months after discontinuation of antibiotics
B. antibiotic treatment and urgent surgery
C. additional antibiotic treatment for 4 weeks
D. MRI to define aortic pathology
E. none of the above

5. A 25-year-old woman presents with acute chest pain that has been present frequently over the last year but is considerably worse over the last week. She describes it as a squeezing substernal pain not reliably provoked by any specific activity. Her examination findings are unremarkable. You request an ECG and a two-dimensional TTE. The technician calls you to review the TTE before you have seen the ECG. Based on the accompanying TTE image, which of the following will her ECG most likely show (Fig. 5)?

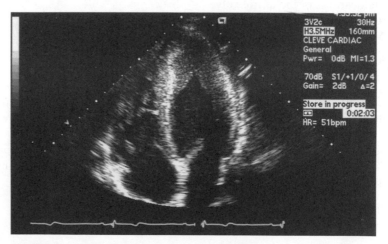

FIGURE 5 Transthoracic apical four-chamber view.

A. normal findings, except for early repolarization
B. ST elevation anteriorly
C. normal findings
D. anterior symmetric T-wave inversion
E. RBBB pattern

6. A 70-year-old man is admitted with a cerebrovascular accident. He has no prior cardiac history and is on no medication. He is in new-onset AFib. A head CT scan shows a nonhemorrhagic infarct. His TTE suggests a mass in the left atrium. A TEE is performed. Based on the associated TEE image, what is the best form of treatment now (Fig. 6)?

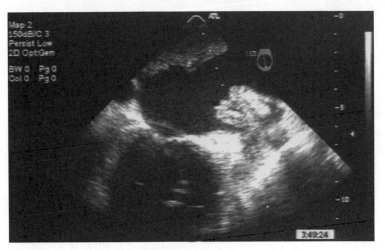

FIGURE 6 TEE two-chamber view of the left atrium and LV.

A. thrombolysis
B. heparinization followed by warfarin treatment
C. urgent surgical exploration of the heart
D. rehabilitation
E. slow anticoagulation with warfarin

7. A 37-year-old woman is seen in the clinic for vague chest discomfort. This occurs infrequently, but when it occurs, it is a burning feeling associated with diaphoresis. She has had to sit down with the pain. There is no significant family history of CAD. She has never smoked. Her grandmother has diabetes. Her BP is 100/60 mm Hg. Her heart rate is 65 bpm. Her LDL-C is 132 mg per dL, and her HDL is 52 mg per dL. An ECG shows diffuse T-wave flattening but no other changes. She undergoes a stress TTE. This shows no evidence of wall motion abnormalities at rest or on exercise. She achieves 10.2 METS and 90% maximum predicted heart rate. She stops because of fatigue. On the TTE, a concern is raised about the possibility of an abnormality on the aortic valve leaflets. There is no stenosis or regurgitation. A TEE is performed to define the possible aortic valve abnormality more clearly. Based on the TEE images of the aortic valve, what is the most likely diagnosis (Fig. 7)?

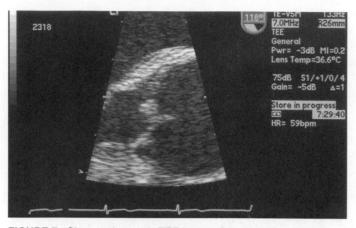

FIGURE 7 Close-up long-axis TEE image of the aortic valve.

A. Lambl's excrescences
B. vegetation on an abnormal valve
C. myxoma of the aortic valve
D. unicuspid aortic valve
E. papillary fibroelastoma

8. A 42-year-old man presents with new-onset dyspnea. He has been seen in a satellite office, where a TTE has been performed. Unfortunately, the only portion of the study available for your review is an M-mode recording. Based on the accompanying tracing (Fig. 8), what is the most likely diagnosis?

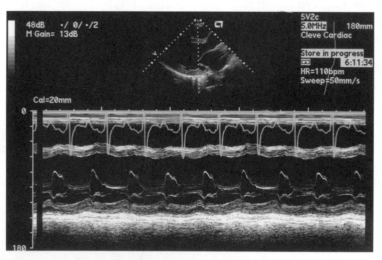

FIGURE 8 Parasternal long-axis M-mode image.

A. dilated cardiomyopathy
B. mitral stenosis
C. severe aortic regurgitation
D. left atrial myxoma
E. tamponade from pericardial effusion

9. A 59-year-old woman presents with new-onset AFib. Based on the accompanying TTE image, what is the most appropriate advice to give her (Fig. 9)?

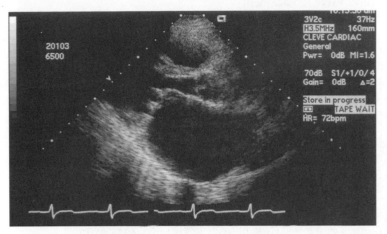

FIGURE 9 Parasternal long-axis transthoracic diastolic frame.

A. She is unlikely to return to NSR with cardioversion.
B. She is likely to need long-term warfarin.
C. She needs urgent surgery.
D. She has had AFib frequently.
E. Cardioversion is contraindicated.

10. A 70-year-old woman is admitted to a local hospital with an acute MI with a modest rise in her cardiac enzymes. As she had presented 12 hours after the onset of pain and there was no significant ST elevation on arrival, no thrombolytic was given. She had no further chest pain but developed sudden onset of shortness of breath 72 hours after admission. Her oxygenation has progressively declined, so that now she needs to be ventilated. She is transferred to you for further management. Because her TTE images are difficult to interpret due to the poor imaging windows, a TEE is performed. Meanwhile, her BP is 90/60 mm Hg, and her heart rate is 100 bpm. Her PA catheter has become dislodged in transit. Based on the accompanying TEE image, what is the best immediate course of action (Fig. 10)?

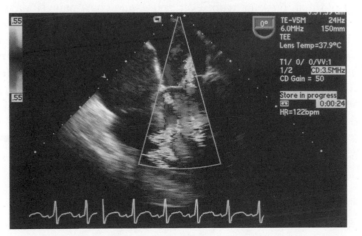

FIGURE 10 Transesophageal four-chamber image (systole).

A. pericardiocentesis
B. IABP insertion
C. IV nitroglycerin
D. mitral valve replacement
E. pulmonary angiogram

11. You are asked to see a 19-year-old college basketball star with a newly recognized murmur. He has been asymptomatic, but all of the team has undergone a physical examination recently. To help screen players, a local hospital has donated an old M-mode TTE machine. The accompanying tracing has been acquired on this player (Fig. 11).

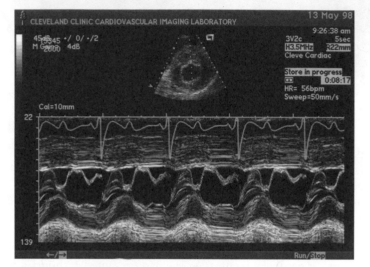

FIGURE 11 Parasternal M-mode image.

What is the most likely diagnosis?

A. physiologic LV hypertrophy
B. mitral valve prolapse
C. aortic stenosis
D. normal heart
E. hypertrophic cardiomyopathy

12. A 67-year-old man presents with fever and vague chest pain 10 days post coronary artery bypass graft. He has had a nonproductive cough. When you see him, he has a fever of 38.2°C. His BP is 141/76 mm Hg. His pulse is 89 bpm and regular. His incisions appear well healed. His venous pressure is 5 cm above the sternal angle. He has no murmurs but has an S_4. He has decreased air entry bilaterally on examination of the lungs, but no rub is heard anywhere. He has been taking a baby aspirin and a statin. An ECG is unremarkable. His hematocrit is 35%, and his white blood count is 11.3, with a leftward shift. A TTE is performed. Based on the accompanying image, what is the best course of treatment (Fig. 12)?

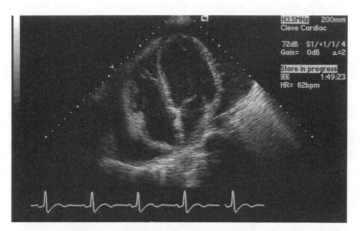

FIGURE 12 Apical four-chamber transthoracic image.

A. IV antibiotics after surveillance blood cultures
B. a course of nonsteroidal antiinflammatory drugs
C. diagnostic and therapeutic pericardiocentesis
D. IV diuretics
E. PO antibiotics for community-acquired pneumonia

13. A previously healthy young man presents with severe dyspnea. He is seen in the emergency room. The technician has just acquired this M-mode image when he desaturates and needs urgent ventilation (Fig. 13).

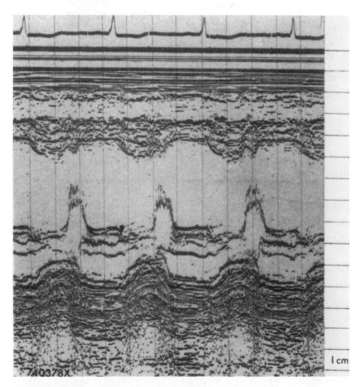

FIGURE 13 Parasternal M-mode image.

You are called to see him. Based on his M-mode image, the cause of his dyspnea is apparent. What is the most likely cause of his dyspnea?

A. severe MR with flail mitral valve
B. endocarditis of the mitral valve
C. severe acute aortic insufficiency
D. intracardiac tumor
E. dilated cardiomyopathy

14. An internist sees a 28-year-old woman for the first time. He hears an apical systolic murmur. She is asymptomatic but has recently lost weight on an over-the-counter medication recommended by her fitness consultant. The internist refers her for a consultation. You request a TTE. The parasternal short-axis image of the mitral valve is shown (Fig. 14).

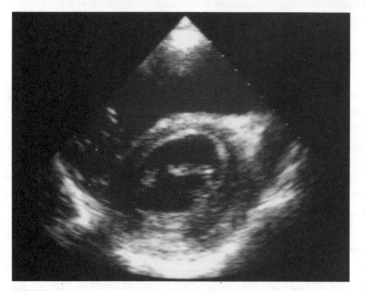

FIGURE 14 Parasternal short-axis transthoracic image.

Based on this image, what is the most likely cause of the apical systolic murmur?

A. congenital cleft mitral valve
B. mitral valve prolapse
C. rheumatic disease
D. anorexiant valvulopathy
E. lupus valvulopathy

15. A 65-year-old man comes to see you for a routine consultation. He is currently having intermittent rapid palpitations that he is aware of but that do not cause him to stop activity. He had an MI 1 year ago but has had no angina since. He has not seen a cardiologist since. He is currently taking an aspirin; a low-dose beta-blocker; furosemide, 20 mg daily; and a statin. His physical examination reveals that he has an S_4, and a soft systolic and questionable diastolic murmur are heard at the apex. His BP is 105/80 mm Hg. You refer him for a TTE to assess his LV function. The echocardiographer calls you to review the accompanying TTE images. Based on the image, what is the most appropriate immediate step (Fig. 15)?

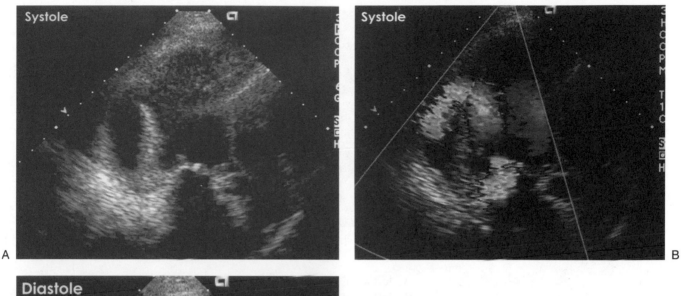

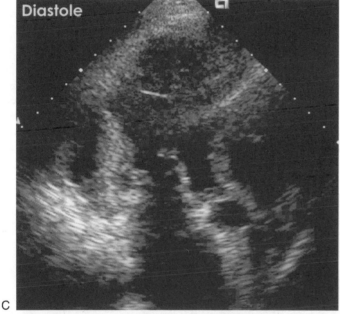

FIGURE 15 Long-axis apical images in systole **(A,B)** and diastole **(C)**.

A. no additional testing or treatment
B. afterload reduction; schedule a nuclear stress test
C. referral to EP for possible ablation
D. consider anticoagulation
E. cardiac catheterization, with consideration for possible open-heart surgery

16. A 65-year-old woman has a murmur on physical examination. She has been losing weight and has a cough and has had some blood streaking of her sputum. She is in NSR on examination and has an apical diastolic murmur and a loud P_2. A TTE indicates a mass in the left atrium. A TEE is performed to solidify the diagnosis. Based on the accompanying TEE image, what is the most likely diagnosis (Fig. 16)?

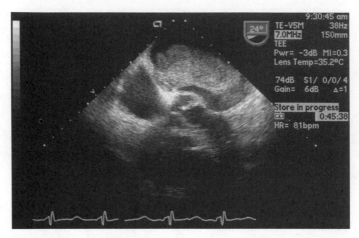

FIGURE 16 TEE image.

A. left atrial myxoma
B. left atrial thrombus
C. cardiac sarcoma
D. metastatic melanoma
E. secondary cardiac involvement with bronchogenic carcinoma

17. A 70-year-old South American man presents with ankle edema and pleural effusions. He has lived in the United States most of his adult life. He has no cardiac history. He has been fatigued but not unduly short of breath. He has trace proteinuria on urinalysis. Based on the accompanying M-mode tracings, which of the following is most likely to be diagnostic (Fig. 17)?

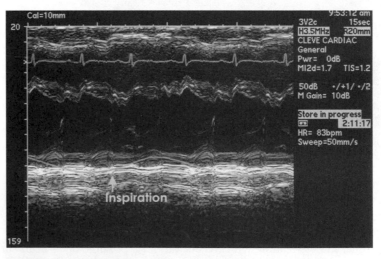

FIGURE 17 Parasternal M-mode and respirometer.

A. myocardial biopsy
B. left-heart catheterization
C. MRI of the heart
D. fat pad biopsy
E. Doppler tracings with respirometer

18. A 45-year-old man presents with acute chest pain. His ECG shows T-wave inversion throughout. His BP is 150/90 mm Hg. An emergency TTE is performed, but the images are suboptimal. A TEE is performed. Based on the accompanying TEE image, what is the best approach to the patient now (Fig. 18)?

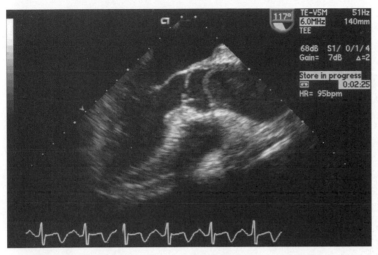

FIGURE 18 TEE long-axis image of the ascending aorta and aorta.

A. intraaortic balloon placement
B. thrombolysis and possible percutaneous transluminal coronary angioplasty
C. immediate consultation of cardiothoracic surgery
D. BP control with possible elective cardiovascular surgery
E. spiral CT to confirm diagnosis

19. A young man presents with fatigue and paroxysmal rapid heartbeats. Based on the accompanying image, what is the most likely diagnosis (Fig. 19)?

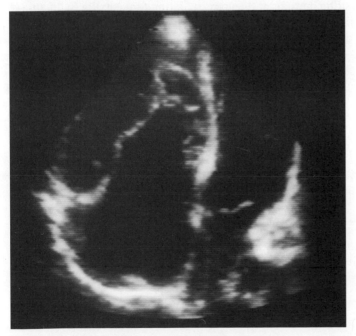

FIGURE 19 Transthoracic apical four-chamber image.

A. RV dysplasia
B. chronic pulmonary embolism
C. Eisenmenger's atrial septal defect (ASD)
D. primary pulmonary hypertension
E. Ebstein's anomaly

20. Based on the accompanying image, which of the following physical signs is this patient likely to have (Fig. 20)?

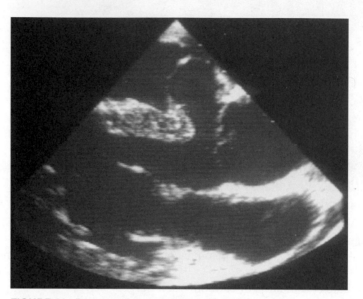

FIGURE 20 Parasternal transthoracic long-axis image.

A. a harsh pansystolic murmur heard at left sternal border
B. fixed splitting of the S_2, a diastolic rumble at left fourth intercostal space, and a systolic murmur at second left intercostal space
C. pansystolic murmur at the apex, radiating to the axilla, with an S_3
D. a continuous murmur heard at the left sternal border
E. none of the above

Match the following CXRs with their respective valve lesion (Figs. 21 through 24).

21.

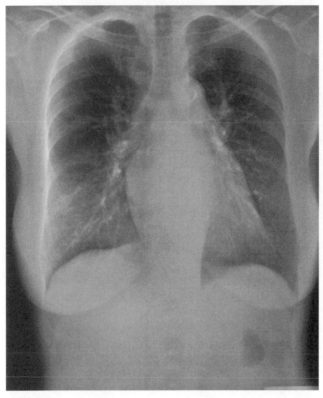

FIGURE 21 PA CXR.

22.

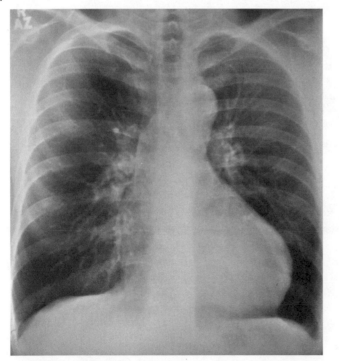

FIGURE 22 PA CXR.

23.

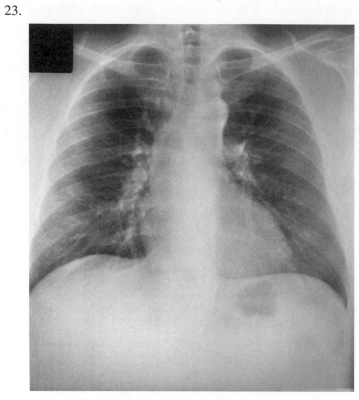

FIGURE 23 PA CXR.

24.

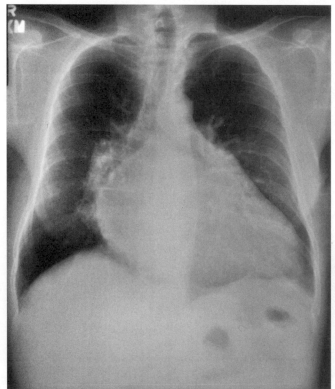

FIGURE 24 PA CXR.

A. aortic stenosis
B. aortic regurgitation
C. mitral stenosis
D. MR

25. The condition displayed in the accompanying images (Fig. 25) may be associated with all of the following *except*

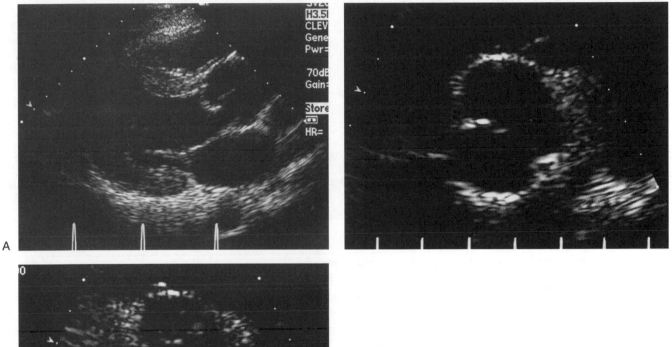

FIGURE 25 Transthoracic image: parasternal long-axis image **(A)** and short-axis images of the aortic valve in diastole **(B)** and systole **(C)**.

A. aortic stenosis
B. Williams syndrome
C. aortic dissection
D. aortic regurgitation
E. coarctation of the aorta

26. The accompanying images are most consistent with which of the following (Fig. 26)?

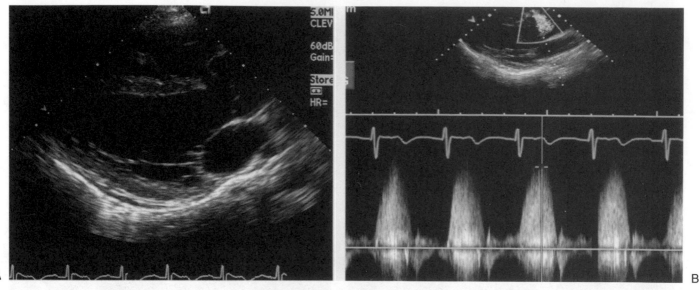

FIGURE 26 Parasternal long-axis transthoracic image **(A)** and a continuous-wave Doppler image **(B)**.

A. tetralogy of Fallot
B. Gerbode defect
C. endocardial cushion defect
D. ischemic VSD
E. Ebstein's anomaly

ANSWERS

1. C. Fungal endocarditis. The image shows a vegetation of the aortic valve. It is of large size, suggesting a fungal infection. This is more common in diabetics. Valve myxoma is rare, although it could present with fever. Both staphylococcal and streptococcal infections of the aortic valve can lead to large vegetations, but the bulky nature of this example is very suggestive of a fungal infection.

2. C. Assessment of respiratory variation on mitral and tricuspid inflow Doppler velocities. The image shows a moderate-sized pericardial effusion but is not diagnostic of tamponade. The best course of action is to assess for hemodynamic findings consistent with tamponade physiology to determine if the pericardial effusion is hemodynamically significant and is contributing to the shortness of breath. These findings include respiratory variation of the inflow velocities. In tamponade physiology, the mitral inflow velocity is reduced on inspiration and increases on expiration, whereas the tricuspid velocity decreases on expiration and increases on inspiration. The woman was mildly hypoxic and had a respiratory tract infection that responded to antibiotic therapy. The pericardial effusion diminished spontaneously, without the need for pericardiocentesis.

3. E. Papillary muscle rupture. The images show severe MR and a flail mitral valve with an attached mass. Papillary muscle rupture is the most likely cause, as he had chest pain a few days before, and the appearance of the mass is suggestive of the head of a papillary muscle. Papillary muscle rupture occurs usually between day 2 and day 7 after an MI. It occurs in approximately 1% of all myocardial infarcts and is most common with an inferior wall infarction, as the posterior descending artery supplies the posteromedial papillary muscle. The anterolateral papillary muscle is usually supplied jointly by the left anterior descending artery and the circumflex artery. Papillary muscle rupture requires emergency cardiac surgery.

4. B. Antibiotic treatment and urgent surgery. The patient has an abscess at the aortic valve, as indicated by the presence of echolucent areas and thickening of the aortic wall around the aortic valve. TEE is highly sensitive and specific in the detection of aortic valve abscess and is much more accurate than TTE in diagnosis. No other test is usually necessary to confirm the diagnosis. Abscess of the aortic valve is frequently seen with staphylococcal infections and requires urgent surgical treatment. A homograft is frequently used in this situation as a valve replacement, as it reduces the likelihood of residual infection postoperatively.

5. D. Anterior symmetric T-wave inversion. The patient has apical hypertrophic cardiomyopathy (Yamaguchi syndrome). This is uncommon in Western countries but relatively frequent in Japan. It is associated with chest pain. The hypertrophy of the LV is most marked apically, as illustrated on the TTE, and it is not associated with dynamic outflow obstruction. The ECG shows characteristic giant symmetric T-wave inversion over the precordial leads. The prognosis is more favorable than for other hypertrophic cardiomyopathies presenting at a young age. Chest pain may respond to a beta-blocker or a calcium blocker.

6. B. Heparinization followed by warfarin treatment. The patient has a large thrombus involving the body and appendage of the left atrium. The most important consideration now is to prevent further embolization. A CT scan has shown no evidence of hemorrhage. Therefore, anticoagulation is indicated. This is best achieved quickly by heparinization followed by warfarin. There is no indication for thrombolysis. This has potential risks of bleeding and embolization, and in the setting of sessile thrombus attached to the walls will have little benefit. Similarly, surgical exploration is not indicated. An uncommon indication for surgical exploration might be a mobile large thrombus present in any of the cardiac chambers. Rehabilitation, of course, is indicated in all stroke patients but does not of itself address the need to prevent further embolization.

7. E. Papillary fibroelastoma. The woman has no evidence of CAD. She has a small mass attached to the aortic valve leaflet. There is no evidence of any hemodynamic effect associated with this mass. This excludes unicuspid aortic valve. This is always associated with severe aortic stenosis. Vegetation on a hemodynamically normal valve is also very unlikely. Lambl's excrescences are seen as a degenerative process in elderly patients and usually are strand-like in nature rather than discrete masses, as in this case. A myxoma of the aortic valve is very rare. Papillary fibroelastomas, on the other hand, are more common but often not detected due to their small size. In a series from the Cleveland Clinic, almost one-half of them involved the aortic

valve. They can occur on either side of the valve, but the aortic side is the more common presentation. They frequently have a stalk and highly mobile elements and often have a shimmering stippled appearance. They have a predilection for embolization. For this reason, surgical excision should be considered when there is a history of possible embolism, a left-sided lesion with a stalk, or a tumor of a size larger than 1 cm, even in the absence of symptoms. This woman had the fibroelastoma surgically removed through a small incision, with no residual regurgitation or stenosis. Her symptoms disappeared, and it seems likely that she was embolizing to her coronary vessels from the tumor. Her coronary angiogram, performed before surgery, was normal.

8. A. Dilated cardiomyopathy. The patient has a dilated LV. The excursion of the septum and the posterior wall is reduced in systole, suggesting global reduction in contractility. The distance of the anterior mitral valve leaflet from the septum (E point–septal separation) is larger than 2 cm, supporting reduced contractile function. The anterior and posterior leaflets of the mitral valve move fully and in opposite directions, which makes either mitral stenosis or left atrial myxoma unlikely. There is no diastolic flutter of the anterior mitral valve leaflet or of the septum and no premature closure of the mitral valve to suggest aortic regurgitation, although, of course, aortic regurgitation may cause LV enlargement and global dysfunction. No pericardial effusion is evident to suggest that tamponade is a possibility.

9. B. She is likely to need long-term warfarin. The TTE shows the typical diastolic doming of mitral stenosis. It is likely that once AFib occurs in mitral stenosis, it will recur or become chronic. Once AFib occurs in mitral stenosis, consideration should be given to the use of long-term anticoagulation, because the combination of AFib and mitral stenosis is associated with a very high embolic risk in the absence of anticoagulation. Although the left atrium is enlarged in this patient, this is likely as a consequence of the mitral stenosis and does not necessarily imply prior episodes of AFib. The onset of AFib of itself is not an indication for surgical intervention in mitral stenosis. The symptomatology, exercise capacity, and pulmonary pressures, in addition to the valve area, are paramount in this decision process. Cardioversion is neither contraindicated nor likely to be unsuccessful in somebody with both AFib and mitral stenosis. Obviously, because of the increased embolic risk, meticulous attention to anticoagulation algorithms must be given before embarking on cardioversion in this situation.

10. B. IABP insertion. The image shows a VSD with flow from the LV to the RV. Some MR is also seen. In this scenario, in a patient with hemodynamic compromise, an IABP will help support the BP and reduce the shunt. Early surgical closure is the treatment of choice. Acquired VSD may occur with either an anterior or an inferior infarction. An anterior MI is usually associated with an apical septal defect, whereas with an inferior MI, the defect is typically in the posterobasal region.

11. E. Hypertrophic cardiomyopathy. The tracing shows classical features of hypertrophic cardiomyopathy. The septum is almost 3 cm thick and is thicker than the posterior wall (asymmetric septal hypertrophy). Systolic anterior motion of the mitral valve is seen, with the valve leaflet touching the septum in systole.

12. B. A course of nonsteroidal antiinflammatory drugs. The patient has evidence of both a pericardial and a pleural effusion on the TTE. These findings, in addition to the fever and mildly elevated white count, are suggestive of the postpericardiotomy syndrome. This syndrome is seen typically in the first few weeks post–open-heart surgery and is thought to be immune-mediated. It usually responds to nonsteroidal antiinflammatory medication. Rarely, steroids are necessary. Careful monitoring of the pericardial fluid is needed, especially in those requiring anticoagulation, as a rapid increase in fluid volume may lead to cardiac tamponade. There are no findings in this presentation to suggest tamponade either clinically or on TTE. Thoracentesis may also be required if a pleural fluid collection is increasing in size or contributing to dyspnea.

13. C. Severe acute aortic insufficiency. The M-mode tracing shows a number of features of severe aortic insufficiency. The most important is early closure of the mitral valve. This occurs before the QRS complex. This is indicative of a very high diastolic LV pressure that shuts the mitral valve early. On color Doppler, diastolic MR is seen in this instance for the same reason. Additionally, there is fine fluttering of the mitral valve leaflets, suggestive of aortic insufficiency. Furthermore, the LV septum and posterior walls show increased amplitude of motion, indicative of a volume overload on the LV. Early closure of the mitral valve can also be seen with prolonged first-degree block.

14. A. Congenital cleft mitral valve. The patient has the typical appearance of a cleft in the anterior leaflet of the mitral valve. This is often associated with septum primum ASD and other endocardial cushion defects. Mitral valve prolapse is difficult to diagnose, except in the long-axis views, and is not reliably diagnosed in this view. Rheumatic disease causes thickening of the mitral leaflets, often with concomitant mitral stenosis. Anorexiant valvulopathy produces an appearance similar to rheumatic disease in terms of thickening, but without significant stenosis or doming of the valve. Lupus valvulopathy may produce thickening and calcification of the leaflets in addition to the noninfective vegetations of Libman-Sacks endocarditis.

15. E. Cardiac catheterization, with consideration for possible open-heart surgery. The accompanying image shows a pseudoaneurysm of the LV. The appearance here is characteristic, with an abrupt outpouching seen in both systole and diastole. Flow is seen to enter the aneurysm through a narrow neck (less than 50% of the body of the aneurysm). As there is a risk of further rupture, consideration is given to surgical patching of the pseudoaneurysm and possible revascularization. A true aneurysm is associated with a more gradual onset and a wide neck (greater than 50%) compared to the body of the aneurysm. Pseudoaneurysm formation is due to contained rupture of the heart by pericardium and thrombus. It is often clinically silent, although occasionally to-and-fro murmurs are heard because of blood entering and leaving the aneurysm.

16. A. Left atrial myxoma. The TEE image shows a characteristic appearance of a left atrial myxoma arising by a stalk from the interatrial septum. All of the other conditions could cause an atrial mass but are unlikely to arise in this fashion. The loud P_2 and hemoptysis are due to pulmonary hypertension. Bronchogenic carcinoma may infiltrate the atrium directly or, more commonly, via a pulmonary vein.

17. C. MRI of the heart. The patient has constrictive pericarditis, as indicated by ventricular interdependence and diastolic septal bounce. The RV fills at the expense of the LV with inspiration, and the septum moves toward the left. The opposite effect is seen with expiration, in which LV filling is augmented. These findings are most consistent with constrictive rather than restrictive physiology. MRI is likely to show thickening of the pericardium, encasement of the heart, and impaired diastolic filling of the ventricles. Left-heart catheterization without right-heart catheterization is unlikely to be diagnostic of constrictive pericarditis. Although Doppler tracings with respirometry are helpful in distinguishing constriction from restriction, they are unlikely to be definitive. Both myocardial biopsy and fat pad biopsy are useful in the diagnosis of infiltrative disorders that cause restrictive cardiomyopathy. They would be indicated if a restrictive pathology were considered most likely.

18. C. Immediate consultation of cardiothoracic surgery. The TEE shows a dissection flap in the ascending aorta. This is an indication for urgent surgical intervention. Intraaortic balloon placement is potentially hazardous, as by augmenting diastolic pressure, it may increase aortic regurgitation and if placed in the false lumen may extend the intimal tear. BP control is important while surgery is being arranged, but this image depicts a type A dissection for which urgent surgery is indicated. In a type B dissection confined to the descending aorta, watchful waiting with BP control and a beta-blocker are indicated, with possible elective surgery if the aortic dilatation is severe, if symptoms persist, or if there is evidence of substantial impaired perfusion of major organs. Spiral CT scan is a useful test to diagnose aortic dissection, but the TEE image is diagnostic, and another confirmatory test is not necessary and is potentially hazardous, as it will possibly delay surgical treatment.

19. E. Ebstein's anomaly. The image shows the typical appearance of Ebstein's anomaly, in which the septal leaflet of the tricuspid valve is apically displaced. This is associated with an accessory pathway and arrhythmia in many patients. RV dysplasia is also associated with ventricular arrhythmias but not with tricuspid abnormalities. The RV wall is often thin and parchment-like, with infiltration of lipid and fibrous tissue elements. The diagnosis may be difficult to define by TTE, and MRI is the technique of choice in diagnosis. Both primary pulmonary hypertension and Eisenmenger's ASD cause RV enlargement and dysfunction. Both may be associated with secondary tricuspid regurgitation but do not affect the septal leaflet of the tricuspid valve.

20. E. None of the above. The image shows a membranous septal aneurysm. No flow crosses from the LV to the RV. This patient started out life with a VSD. However, tissue (usually a portion of the tricuspid valve) has become attached to the defect causing closure of the VSD and leaving a residual aneurysm. Occasional flow can be heard going in and out of this area, and tricuspid regurgitation due to impaired coaptation of the leaflets is often heard. However, none of the murmurs listed would be expected. A is the murmur of a VSD with left-to-right shunting. B is the murmur consistent with ASD. C is the murmur of severe MR. D is the murmur heard with a fistula or patent ductus arteriosus.

21. C. Mitral stenosis. The x-ray shows the double shadow along the right heart border, consistent with left atrial enlargement. Additionally, the pulmonary

vessels are prominent. The overall cardiac silhouette is not markedly enlarged, as the LV is not enlarged in isolated mitral stenosis.

22. B. Aortic regurgitation. There is marked cardiac enlargement—the so-called cor bovinum or cow's heart. The ascending aorta is unfolded and dilated.

23. A. Aortic stenosis. The cardiothoracic silhouette is not significantly enlarged. The apex of the LV is lifted off the left hemidiaphragm, consistent with ventricular hypertrophy rather than dilatation. The ascending aorta is prominent.

24. D. MR. There is marked LV enlargement. There is a double density along the right heart border, consistent with left atrial enlargement. There is marked splaying of the main bronchi, consistent with marked atrial enlargement.

25. B. The images show a bicuspid aortic valve. This is associated with aortic dissection, aortic stenosis and regurgitation, and coarctation of the aorta. Williams syndrome is associated with supravalvular aortic stenosis but not with valvar aortic stenosis.

26. A. Tetralogy of Fallot. The images show a VSD and an aorta that is malaligned with regard to the ventricular septum, such that it overrides the septum. Normally, the ventricular septum merges smoothly with the anterior wall of the ascending aorta at the aortic valve. Additionally, there is a VSD. These are two features seen in tetralogy of Fallot. The others are severe infundibular or valvular pulmonic stenosis and RV hypertrophy. A Gerbode defect is communication between the LV and right atrium. This is possible, as the tricuspid valve is usually placed somewhat apically as compared to the mitral valve. Gerbode defects are usually acquired, often in the setting of prosthetic mitral endocarditis. None of the other conditions are typically associated with an overriding aorta.

SUGGESTED READING

Otto CM, ed. *The practice of clinical echocardiography,* 2nd ed. Philadelphia: W.B. Saunders Company, 2002.
Topol EJ, ed. *A textbook of cardiology*, 2nd ed. Philadelphia: Lippincott Williams & Wilkins, 2002.

Index

Page numbers followed by *f* refer to figures; those followed by *t* refer to tables.

Abciximab, 113, 145
    contraindications for, 167, 179–180
    half-life of, 167, 180
    thrombocytopenia from, 167, 179–180
Abdominal aortic aneurysm
    diagnosis of, 191, 208
    management of, 191, 208
ACE inhibitors. *See* Angiotensin-converting enzyme
        inhibitors
ACIP, 108, 135
Action potential, 17, 29
Acute coronary syndrome
    angioplasty in, 76, 95
    blood-borne markers of inflammation predictive of, 266,
        269
    revascularization with PCI and CABG in, 110, 138
    severe stenosis with thrombus in, 76f, 95
    stenting in, 76, 95
    ticlopidine in, 75–76, 95
Adenosine
    in cardiac transplant patients, 3, 19
    reduction of, 1, 18
Adenosine diphosphate inhibitor, 166–167, 178. *See also*
        Clopidogrel, Ticlopidine
Air Force/Texas Coronary Atherosclerosis Prevention Study
        (AFCAPS/TexCAPS), 112, 142
Aldosteronism, primary, hypertension in, 280–281, 287
Alpha$_1$-blockers, survival improvement with, 163, 176
Alteplase, dosage of, 169, 182
American College of Cardiology/American Heart Association
        (ACC/AHA) Class I guidelines
    regarding early risk management for unstable angina and
        NSTMI, 108, 135
    regarding management of diabetes mellitus and UA/non–Q-
        wave myocardial infarction, 110, 139
    regarding management of unstable angina and NSTMI,
        109–110, 135, 136, 137f
    regarding revascularization in acute coronary syndrome,
        110, 138
    regarding risk stratification in chronic stable angina, 111,
        139–140

Amiodarone, 15, 28–29
    drug effect of, 3, 19
    elimination of, 1, 18
    indications for, 170–171, 183
    properties of, 170, 182
    side effects of, 171, 183
Amitriptyline, overdose of, 9, 25
Amlodipine, chronic use of, 221, 235
Amyloidosis, treatment of, 229, 238
Angina
    effect of smoking on, 112, 143–144
    stable. *See* Stable angina
    unstable. *See* Unstable angina
Angiography
    in acute myocardial infarction, 83, 98
    indications for, 105, 109, 131, 135, 193
Angioplasty
    in acute coronary syndrome, 76, 95
    in acute myocardial infarction, 80, 96
    placement of stents during, 93, 101
Angiotensin-converting enzyme inhibitors, 161, 174, 282. *See*
        also specific drugs
    benefits on systolic dysfunction of, 161, 174
    contraindications for, 161, 175
    indications for, 275, 283–284
    side effects of, 162, 175–176
    sodium depletion and, 161, 174–175
Angiotensin II-receptor blockers, 162, 175–176
    indications for, 162, 175
    side effects of, 162, 175–176
Ankle-brachial index, 198–199, 200, 213–214, 214, 215
Anorectic agents, 46–47, 64
Anterior symmetric T-wave inversion, echocardiographic
        images of, 318–319, 318f, 333
Antiarrhythmic drugs, 170, 182
    with active metabolites, 1, 18
    in atrial fibrillation, 1, 18
    inotropic effects of, 2, 18
    reverse use dependence of, 2, 18
    as sodium channel blockers, 3, 19
    use, dependence of, 2, 18

Antiarrhythmic drugs—*continued*
    Vaughan Williams class III, 3, 19
Antibiotic prophylaxis
    after aortic valve replacement, 41, 62
    in dental extraction, 56, 68
Anticoagulation. *See also* Warfarin
    long-term systemic, 169, 181
    in pregnancy, 56–57, 68
Antihypertensive therapy. *See also specific therapies*
    adherence to, 275, 283
    side effects of, 276, 284
Antithrombotic therapy, for atrial fibrillation, 166, 179
Aortic aneurysm
    abdominal. *See* Abdominal aortic aneurysm
    ascending
        diagnosis of, 195–196, 210–211
        treatment of, 196, 211, 211f
    diagnosis of, 187, 204
Aortic coarctation, 35, 59
    blood pressure control in, 243, 257
    cardiac catheterization image of, 250f, 262
    characteristic chest radiography findings in, 253, 263
    common coexisting congenital anomaly in, 241, 255
    complications of unrecognized, 241, 255–256
    gender preponderance of, 249, 261
    physical findings in, 252, 262
    surgical repair in, 245, 258
Aortic dissection
    blood pressure reduction in, 280, 287
    diagnosis of, 191, 208
    imaging of, 195–196, 206f, 207f, 210–211
    type A
        echocardiographic images of, 327, 327f, 336
        with extension to pericardium, 295–296, 296f, 310–311
Aortic homograft valve, incidence of endocarditis with, 54, 67
Aortic insufficiency, 37, 59
    emergent cardiac surgery for, 40, 61
    severe, 39–40, 43, 61, 62
    severe acute, 323–324, 323f, 335
Aortic regurgitation, 39, 51–52, 60–61, 66
    echocardiographic images of, 329f, 337
    evaluation of, 187, 188
Aortic replacement surgery
    elective, 189, 205
    emergent, 196, 211, 211f
Aortic stenosis, 37, 59
    asymptomatic, 38–39, 60
    echocardiographic images of, 330f, 337
    pregnancy and, 247, 260
    severe, 44–45, 64
        prognosis of, 45, 64
        sudden death from, 45, 64
    supravalvular, associated disease conditions of, 252, 263
    surgical procedures for, 248, 261
    symptomatic, 51, 65–66
    valvular and subvalvar compared, 243, 257

valve recommendations for, 51, 66
Aortic ulcer, penetrating, diagnosis of, 192–193, 192f, 208–209, 209f
Aortic valve
    bicuspid. *See* Bicuspid aortic valve
    echocardiographic images of abscess at, 317–318, 318f, 333
    quadricuspid, 255f, 263
    replacement of, 37, 38–39, 40, 41, 59, 60, 61, 62
Apoptosis, 267, 269
    inhibitors of cardiac myocyte, 267, 270
Argatroban, 168, 181
Arrhythmia, 1–30
    secondary to accessory pathway, 53, 53f, 66–67
    treatment of, 1. *See also* Antiarrhythmic drugs
    ventricular, 229, 238
Arterial occlusion, 74, 75f, 94–95, 200, 215
Arterial Revascularization Therapies Study (ARTS), 129, 153
Arterial switch procedure, 248, 261
Arterial thrombosis, after plaque rupture, 266, 269
Arteriovenous fistula, 119f, 152
Aspirin, 166
    versus clopidogrel, 116, 151
    and ramipril, 228, 237
    versus warfarin, 116, 151
Aspirin therapy, indications for, 71, 73–74, 73f, 94
Asymptomatic Cardiac Ischemia Pilot (ACIP), 108, 135
Asystole, prognosis for, 6, 22
Atenolol
    effects of renal function on, 226–227, 237
    side effects of, 276, 284
Atheroma
    aortic arch, 196, 212, 212f
    in ascending aorta, 192f
    diagnosis of, 196, 211
Atherosclerotic lesions, 106, 132–133
Atorvastatin
    complications of, 166, 178
    lipid-lowering ability of, 111, 141, 165, 178
Atorvastatin Versus Revascularization Treatment (AVERT) trial, 111, 141
Atrial fibrillation
    acute pharmacologic conversion to sinus rhythm of, 3, 19
    anticoagulation for, 17, 29
    chronic, pacing modality for, 8, 24
    external cardioversion of, 15, 28
    flecainide for, 16, 29
    new-onset, echocardiographic images of, 321, 321f, 334
    and renal insufficiency, 1, 18
    use of digoxin in, 16, 29
Atrial implantable cardioverter-defibrillator (AICD), 224–225, 236. *See also* Implantable cardioverter defibrillator (ICD)
Atrial septal defect
    gender preponderance of, 249, 261
    indications for surgical closure of, 247, 260

natural history of, 246, 259–260
ostium primum, 241, 254f, 255, 263
ostium secundum, 247, 260
Atrial undersensing, after dual-chamber pacemaker placement, 10, 10f, 25
Atrioventricular block
second degree, at infra-Hisian level, 13, 13f, 27
treatment for, 9, 25
Atrioventricular nodal reentrant tachycardia, 3–4, 17, 17f, 20, 29–30
diagnosis of, 7, 23
orthodromic, 4, 20
Azotemia, prerenal, treatment of, 225–226, 236

Ball-and-cage valve, sounds from, 44, 63
Beta-blockers, 160f, 162, 173, 175, 221, 234
in acute myocardial infarction, 80, 83, 96, 98
contraindications for, 160, 162, 173–174, 176
effects of renal function on, 226–227, 237
mechanism of benefit of, 162, 176
in new-onset congestive heart failure, 225, 236
in prevention of sudden cardiac death, 6, 22–23
properties of, 163, 176
in vasovagal syncope, 6, 22
Bicuspid aortic valve, 36, 59, 241–242, 255, 256
characteristic echocardiography findings in, 254f, 263
echocardiographic images of, 331f, 337
gender preponderance of, 249, 261
Bioprosthetic valve, in mitral valve replacement, 35, 59
Bisoprolol, properties of, 163, 176
Blalock-Taussig procedure, 248, 261
Blood pressure. See also Hypertension
intraarterial, 194, 210
lower extremity, 36, 59
management of, 199–200, 214
target, 277, 285
Bradycardia, treatment of, 8, 24
Breast cancer, pericarditis and, 302, 302f, 312
Brockenbrough response, 116, 117f, 152
Brugada's syndrome, 14, 27
Bupropion
contraindications for, 80, 96
for smoking cessation, 79, 96
Bypass Angioplasty Revascularization Investigation (BARI), 112, 143

CABG. See Coronary artery bypass graft (CABG)
Calcium channel blockers
in new-onset congestive heart failure, 225, 236
properties of, 164, 177
Captopril
in acute myocardial infarction, 81, 97
indications for, 161, 175
Carcinoid, 32–33, 58
Cardiac arrest, out-of-hospital, 6, 22
Cardiac Arrhythmia Suppression Trial I (CAST I), 2, 18–19

Cardiac Arrhythmia Suppression Trial II (CAST II), 2, 18–19
Cardiac necrosis, 107, 133
Cardiac tamponade, 301–302, 301f, 311
diagnosis of, 190, 206, 206f, 234, 239
differential diagnosis of, 303, 312
treatment of, 190, 207
Cardiogenic shock
acute myocardial infarction and, 82, 97
LV assist device for, 224, 236
treatment of, 223–224, 235
Cardiomegaly, etiology of, 302, 302f, 312
Cardiomyopathy
constrictive, 234, 239
dilated, 228, 237
echocardiographic images of, 320, 320f, 334
treatment of, 228, 237
hypertrophic, 71–72, 72f, 94, 229, 238
blood pressure reduction in, 279–280, 279f
cardiac catheterization image of, 251f, 262
differential diagnosis of, 303, 312
dual-chamber pacing in, 8, 24–25
echocardiographic images of, 322, 334
management of, 275, 283
ischemic, pharmacologic therapy for, 15, 28–29
peripartum
prognosis of, 222, 235
recurrent, 228, 237
treatment of, 162, 175
well-compensated, 225, 236
Cardioversion, 166, 178. See also Implantable cardioverter defibrillator (ICD)
indications for, 230, 238
for mitral stenosis, 46, 64
Carotid artery stenosis, audible bruits in, 202, 217
Carotid endarterectomy
indications for, 202, 217
risk of stroke and death associated with, 201, 216–217
Carotid pulse, diagnosis of, 232f–234f, 239
CASS, 108, 134–135
CAST I, 2, 18–19
CAST II, 2, 18–19
Catheterization, cardiac. See also Angiography
in aortic regurgitation, 39
for constrictive pericardial disease, 290–291, 291f, 310
indications for, 50–51, 65–66, 192, 208
Cerebral aneurysm, rupture of, 190, 207–208
Cholestyramine
lipid-lowering ability of, 165, 178
and warfarin, 168, 181
Chronic obstructive pulmonary disease (COPD)
differential diagnosis of, 303, 312
palpitations associated with, 10, 25
Cigarette smoking. See Smoking
Cilostazol, 202, 217
Claudication, 198, 213
severe intermittent, 200, 215

Claudication—*continued*
  treatment of, 202, 217
  warfarin and, 193, 209
Click-murmur complex, 42–43, 62
Clonidine
  hypertensive emergency and, 163, 176–177
  side effects of, 276, 284
Clopidogrel
  antiplatelet effects of, 166–167, 179
  versus aspirin, 116, 151
  mechanism of action of, 79, 95–96
  side effects of, 166, 179
Clopidogrel versus Aspirin in Patients at Risk of Ischemic
      Events (CAPRIE) trial, 116, 151
Cluster shocks, 6, 22
Coarctation of aorta. *See* Aortic coarctation
Cocaine intoxication
  management of, 277, 285
  myocardial infarction due to, 84
Complete heart block
  catheter-induced, 9, 25
  corrective action for, 10, 26
  at infra-Hisian level, 13, 13f, 26
  at level of atrioventricular node, 12, 12f, 26
  pacemaker placement for, 10, 26
Conduction system, electrophysiologic testing of, 14, 27, 28
Congenital heart disease, 241–263, 261t. *See also specific
      disorders*
Congestive heart failure, 221–239
  acute, 33, 58
  characteristics of, 221, 234
  prognosis correlation of, 226, 236
  recurrent, 36–37
  SERCA2 to phospholamban ratio in, 265, 267
  symptomatic exercise limitation in, 226, 236
  treatment of, 224, 225, 236
Contusion, cardiac, diagnosis of, 298–299, 298f, 299f, 311
COPD. *See* Chronic obstructive pulmonary disease (COPD)
Coronary arteriovenous fistula, 244, 257
Coronary artery. *See also* Coronary artery disease
  left anterior descending. *See* Left anterior descending
      coronary artery
  left main. *See* Left main coronary artery
  most common anomaly of, 243, 257
  right. *See* Right coronary artery (RCA)
Coronary artery bypass graft (CABG)
  in diabetic patients, 112, 143
  indications for, 110, 111, 138, 140, 227–228, 237
Coronary artery disease, 105–155. *See also specific disorders*
  blood-borne markers of inflammation predictive of, 266,
      269
  homocysteine as risk factor for, 130, 155
  incidence of nonsignificant, 114, 148
  risk factors for, 113, 144–145
  sudden cardiac death and, 7, 23
Coronary Artery Surgery Study (CASS), 108, 134–135

Coronary heart disease, risk factors for, 106, 131
Coronary perforation, 89f, 101
Cor triatriatum, 243, 253f, 256–257, 263
C-reactive protein
  decrease of, 79, 96
  and risk of myocardial infarction, 79, 96

Dental extraction, prophylactic antibiotics for, 56, 68
Diabetes mellitus
  in coronary artery disease, 110, 139
  myocardial infarction and
    mortality of, 83, 98
    risk of, 93, 102
  type 2, 165–166, 276, 284
Dialysis, in refractory heart failure, 54, 67
Diastolic dysfunction, prognosis of, 291–292, 292f, 310
Diastolic filling pattern, 230t, 238
Digoxin
  in atrial fibrillation, 16, 29
  dosage of, 159, 173
  effects on concentrations of, 161, 174
  increased serum levels of, 2, 18
  mechanisms of, 171, 183
  reduction of hospitalization and, 222, 235
Diltiazem, 163, 177
Diuretics, 77, 95
  contraindications for, 6, 22
  effects of on left ventricular volume loop, 232f, 239
  loop, 170, 182
DNA cutting, 266, 269
Dobutamine, 172, 184
  chronic use of, 221, 235
Dofetilide
  in acute myocardial infarction, 83, 98
  contraindications for, 2, 18, 171, 183
  indications for, 229, 238
  inotropic effects of, 2, 18
Dressler's syndrome, 85, 99
Drug use, chronic, mortality of, 221, 235
Dyspnea, exertional, 34–35, 42, 58–59

Ebstein's anomaly, 53–54, 67, 245, 258–259
  characteristic chest radiography findings in, 252, 263
  echocardiographic images of, 246f, 259, 327–328, 327f,
      336
  management of, 248, 260
  physical findings in, 252, 262
Echocardiography
  with amyl nitrate, 43–44, 62
  dobutamine, 37, 59
  Doppler, 54, 67
  stress, 38, 60
Edema, pedal, 291
Eisenmenger's syndrome, 197, 213
  characteristic chest radiography findings in, 252, 263
  contraindications for, 245, 259

physical findings in, 252, 262
pregnancy and, 247, 248, 260
Ejection fraction, improvement of, 221, 222, 234, 235
Enalapril, 274, 282
Endocarditis
  enterococcal, 173, 185
  fungal, 315–316, 315f, 332
  native valve
    etiology of, 55, 68
    indications for surgery in, 56, 68
  prophylaxis, 43, 62, 172, 184, 247, 260
  prosthetic valve, 56, 68
  risk factors for, 56, 68
End-stage renal failure, coronary atherosclerotic lesions in, 130, 154–155
Enoxaparin, 168, 180
Esophageal spasm, 71, 94
Ethacrynic acid, 170, 182
Ethanol, and warfarin, 160–161, 174
Excitation-contraction coupling, 265, 267
Exercise stress testing, 88, 100, 108, 134
Exercise tolerance, improvement of, 226, 236

Fenofibrate, 165, 178
Fibrillin, 198, 213
Fibrinolytic therapy
  mortality in acute myocardial infarction and, 80, 96
  and pericarditis in myocardial infarction, 85, 99
Flecainide, 2, 18, 170, 182–183
  as sodium channel blocker, 3, 19
  as treatment for atrial fibrillation, 16, 29
  use dependence of, 2, 18
Fontan procedure, 248, 261
Free radicals, depletion of, 164, 177
Furosemide, complications of, 169–170, 182

Gemfibrozil
  complications of, 166, 178
  lipid-lowering ability of, 165, 178
Gene expression, low levels of, 266, 269
Gene therapy, delivery of cDNA for, 265, 268
Gene transfer, adenovirus and, 266, 268
Giant cell arteritis, diagnosis of, 188, 205
Global Utilization of Streptokinase and t-PA for Occluded Coronary Arteries (GUSTO)-I trial, 85, 99, 107
Global Utilization of Streptokinase and t-PA for Occluded Coronary Arteries (GUSTO)-III trial, 81, 96
Glucagon
  indications for, 226, 236
  intravenous, 9, 25
Glycoprotein IIb/IIIa inhibitors, 167, 179, 180

Half-life, parameters of, 159, 173
Heart failure. See also Congestive heart failure
  acute decompensated, 231, 238
  class III, 162, 176

diastolic, 228, 237
refractory, 54, 67
Heart rate recovery, abnormal, mortality of, 227, 237
Heart transplantation
  hypertension and, 276, 283
  indications for, 227, 237
Heparin
  binding of, 167, 180
  after transient ischemic attack, 45, 64
Hirudin, bleeding due to, 114, 148–149
HOPE (Heart Outcomes Prevention Evaluation) trial, 106, 132
Hydralazine, 164, 177–178
  side effects of, 276, 284
Hydration, intravenous, indications for, 298, 311
Hydrochlorothiazide, 278, 286
Hyperkalemia, treatment of, 307–308, 307f, 313
Hypertension, 273–288
  with acute LV failure and pulmonary edema, 274, 281–282
  diagnosis of, 36, 59
  in heart transplant recipients, 276, 283
  management of, 163, 164, 176, 177, 278–279, 286–287
  in older patients, 278, 286
  resistant, 274, 282
  systolic, 275, 283
Hyperviscosity syndrome, 247, 260
Hypocalcemia, 170, 182
Hypotension
  etiology of, 89, 89f, 100, 101
  from right ventricular infarction, 76, 95
Hypothyroidism, treatment of, 308, 313

Ibutilide, 3, 19
Implantable cardioverter defibrillator (ICD), 5, 21
  atrial, 224–225, 236
  implantation procedure for, 5, 21
  inappropriate shocks from, 5, 21
  indications for, 4–5, 21
  multiple shocks from, 6, 22
  prior myocardial infarction and, 82, 97
Infrapopliteal arterial disease, revascularization in, 201, 216
Inotropic agents, 171–172, 183–184
  effects of on left ventricular volume loop, 232f, 239
  long-term intravenous, 172, 184
Intraaortic balloon pump, 86, 100
Intraatrial reentry, in atrial flutter, 9, 25
Intracerebral bleed, etiology of, 190, 207–208
Intracranial hemorrhage, risk factors for, 85, 86, 99, 100, 169
Ischemia, 86–87, 87f, 100

Kawasaki disease, 129, 153–154
Ketoacidosis, diabetic, abnormal ECG in, 308–309, 308f, 313
Kussmaul's sign, 301–302, 311–312

Labetalol, properties of, 163, 176
Left anterior descending coronary artery
  anomalous origin of, 124f, 153

Left anterior descending coronary artery—*continued*
  occlusion of, 74, 75f, 94–95
  severe stenosis of, 126f, 153
  stenosis of, 87–88, 87f, 100
Left atrial myxoma, echocardiographic images of, 325–326, 326f
Left atrial thrombus, echocardiographic images of, 319, 319f, 333
Left circumflex artery
  anomalous origin of, 121f, 152
  occlusion of, 77–78, 77f, 95
  ostial stenosis of, 120f, 152
  severe stenosis of, 127f, 129f, 153
Left main coronary artery
  anomalous origin of, 123f, 152
  stenosis of, 118f, 152
Left subclavian artery, diagnosis of stenosis of, 201, 216
Left ventricle
  echocardiographic images of pseudoaneurysm of, 324–325, 325f, 335
  function of, 92, 92f, 101
    assessment of, 227, 237
    improvement of, 221, 235
    reduced compliance, 227, 237
  regression of hypertrophy of, 276, 284–285
  rupture of, 204, 219
  shift of volume loop, 231, 238
Lepirudin, 168, 181
Lidocaine, intravenous, in acute myocardial infarction, 83, 98
Lipid-lowering therapy, 165–166, 178–179
  compared to percutaneous coronary revascularization, 111, 141
  indications for, 114, 147t
Lipid oxidation, mediators of, 266, 269
Long-QT syndrome, 14, 27
Loop diuretics, 170, 182
Losartan, 164, 177–178
  indications for, 229, 238
  side effects of, 276, 284
Lovastatin, 112, 142
Low-density lipoprotein
  characteristics of, 266, 269
  levels indicating lipid-lowering therapy, 114, 147t
Low-molecular-weight heparin, 168, 180–181, 181t. *See also* Heparin
Lymphedema
  etiology of, 204, 219
  evaluation of, 203–204, 218

Magnesium, intravenous, 83, 98
Magnetic resonance angiography, in aortic dilation, 188, 204
Marfan's syndrome
  with aortic dilation, aortic replacement surgery for, 189, 205
  diagnosis of, 188, 189f, 205
  genetic defect associated with, 198, 213
  pregnancy and, 247, 260

Membranous septal aneurysm, echocardiographic images of, 328, 328f, 336
Metoprolol, contraindications for, 160, 173–174
Mexiletine, 3, 19
MI. *See* Myocardial infarction (MI)
Midodrine, in vasovagal syncope, 6, 22
Milrinone
  chronic use of, 221, 235
  indications for, 171–172, 184, 226, 236
Mitral regurgitation, 72–73, 73f, 94
  in acute myocardial infarction, 86, 100
  comorbidity of, 243, 257
  diagnosis of, 33–34, 58
  echocardiographic images of, 34f, 330f, 337
  etiology of, 194–195, 210
  ischemic, 38, 60
Mitral stenosis, 40–41, 50, 61–62, 65
  complications of, 46, 64
  echocardiographic images of, 31–32, 57, 321, 321f, 329f, 334, 336–337
  management of, 32, 57
  percutaneous intervention for, 38, 60
  prosthetic, 52, 52f, 66
  rheumatic, 37–38, 60
  stress echocardiogram for, 32, 57–58
Mitral valve
  cleft leaflet of
    associated disease conditions of, 252, 263
    echocardiographic images of, 324, 324f, 335
  indications for repair of, 49, 64–65
  replacement of
    with bi-leaflet tilting-disk valve, reoperation on, 53, 66
    indications for, 49, 64–65
    sounds from, 44, 63
    with tricuspid annuloplasty, 35, 35f, 58–59
  surgery, 34, 58
Mitral valve prolapse, 50, 65
Mitral valve regurgitation
  management of, 50, 65
  with rheumatic etiology, 49–50, 65
Multifocal atrial tachycardia, 7, 23–24
Mustard procedure, 248, 261
Myocardial infarction (MI)
  acute, 71–102
    beta-blockers for, 80, 83, 96, 98
    diabetes mellitus in, 83, 98
    dofetilide in, 83, 98
    effect of gender on outcome of, 93, 101–102
    etiology of, 93, 102
    ICDs for, 81, 97
    intravenous lidocaine in, 83, 98
    intravenous magnesium in, 83, 98
    management of, 80, 96
    morbidity of, 80, 96
    mortality of prior bypass and, 114, 149
    new systolic murmur after, 115, 150

nitrates in, 83, 98
non–ST segment elevation. *See* Non–ST segment elevation myocardial infarction (NSTMI)
premature ventricular contraction after, 82, 97
recommended emergency room therapies for, 80, 96
reperfusion for, 93, 101
right ventricular. *See* Right ventricular infarction
ST segment–elevation, management of, 74, 80, 94, 96
triggers for, 79, 95
ventricular fibrillation after, 82, 97
warfarin in, 84, 98
anterior wall, 85, 99
diagnosis of, 44, 63
inferior wall
with right ventricle infarction, 107, 133
therapy for, 86, 100
perioperative, decrease in risk of, 94, 102
Myocardium, failing, downregulation of signaling along adrenergic pathway in, 265, 267–268
Myxedema, due to hypothyroidism, 308, 313

Narrow complex tachycardia, 4, 20
adenosine reduction for, 1, 18
Natriuretic peptide, B-type
effects of, 223, 235
properties of, 223, 235
Nesiritide, side effects of, 223, 235
Nimodipine, indications for, 164, 177
Nitrates, in acute myocardial infarction, 83, 98
Nitroglycerin, 164, 177
Nitroprusside, 164–177, 224, 236
Nondihydropyridine calcium antagonist, indications for, 109, 135
Non-Hodgkin's lymphoma, congenital absence of pericardium in, 300, 300f, 311
Non–ST segment elevation myocardial infarction (NSTMI), 70, 101
antiischemic therapy for, 109, 135
antiplatelet and anticoagulant therapy for, 109–110, 136, 137f
cardiac catheterization in, 90, 101
early risk stratification for, 108, 135
follow-up for, 91, 101
immediate management of, 109, 135
treatment of, 167, 179

Osteogenesis imperfecta, diagnosis of, 195, 210
Oxygen, myocardial, determinants of, 106, 133

Pacemaker, implanted, 8, 24
dual-chamber
background atrial fibrillation and, 11–12, 12f, 26
complications of, 10–11, 26
lead position of, 11f, 13, 27
for vasovagal syncope, 6, 22
infection from placement of, 15, 28

Pacemaker syndrome, 8, 24
Papillary fibroelastoma, echocardiographic images of, 319–320, 320f, 333–334
Papillary muscle rupture, echocardiographic images of, 316–317, 317f, 333
Patent ductus arteriosus, 242, 247, 256, 260
cardiac catheterization image of, 251f, 262
characteristic chest radiography findings in, 253, 263
management of, 246, 259
physical findings in, 252, 262
symptoms of, 197, 212
Percutaneous coronary intervention (PCI), 106, 131–132
abciximab in, 113, 145
indications for, 110, 138
Percutaneous peripheral vessel angioplasty, prognosis of, 200, 215
Percutaneous transluminal coronary angioplasty (PTCA)
in diabetic patients, 112, 143
effect of exercise training on, 105, 131
mortality and, 84–85, 99
Percutaneous transluminal renal angioplasty (PTRA), 201, 216
Pericardial cyst, 294–295, 295f, 310
Pericardial disease, 289–313
calcific, diagnosis of, 290f, 309–310
constrictive
cardiac catheterization in, 290–291, 291f, 310
differential diagnosis of, 295, 310
restrictive, differential diagnosis of, 295, 310
right ventricle filling and, 292–293, 293f, 310
Pericardial effusion
diagnosis of, 84, 99, 190, 206, 206f
echocardiographic images of, 316, 316f, 322–323, 323f, 332, 335
rheumatoid arthritis–related, 303–304, 312
treatment of, 190, 207
Pericardial hematoma, 296–297, 296f, 297f, 311
Pericardial tumor, neoplastic, most common, 309, 313
Pericardial valve, bovine, for aortic stenosis, 51, 66
Pericardiectomy, surgical evaluation for, 304, 312
Pericardiocentesis, indications for, 304–305, 312–313
Pericarditis
in acute myocardial infarction, 85, 99
acute viral, 300, 311
constrictive
echocardiographic images of, 302–303, 303f, 312, 326, 326f, 336
prognostic factors for, 303, 312
early postinfarction, 293–294, 294f, 310
echocardiographic imaging of, 289f, 309
granulomatous, 307, 307f, 313
management of, 289–290, 309
post-myocardial infarction, 300–301, 311
treatment of, 85, 99
uremia-related
management of, 297–298, 297f, 311
treatment of, 307–308, 307f, 313

Pericardium, congenital absence of, 300, 300f, 311
   common findings in, 305, 313
Peripheral vascular disease
   arteries affected by, 198, 213
   in diabetes, 200, 202, 215, 217
   diagnosis of, 201, 215–216
   management of, 199, 214
   risk factors for, 199, 214
   symptoms of, 202, 217–218
   in twins, 198, 213
Peripheral vessels, noncompliant, diagnosis of, 194, 210
Permanent junctional reciprocating tachycardia, 3, 19
PET, indications for, 223, 235
Pharmacodynamics, 160, 173
Pindolol, properties of, 163, 176
Plaque rupture, pathogenesis of, 81, 96
Platelet aggregation, mediation of, 267
Platelet glycoprotein IIb/IIIa inhibitor, effects of, 115,
      150–151
Platelet glycoprotein IIb/IIIa receptor antagonist, indications
      for, 109–110, 136, 137f
Pleural effusion, echocardiographic images of, 322–323, 323f,
      335
Pneumohydropericardium, iatrogenic, 306, 306f, 313
Pneumopericardium, 305f
Positron emission tomography (PET), indications for, 223,
      235
Posterior leaflet prolapse, severe mitral regurgitation and, 47,
      47f–48f, 49, 63–64
Postpericardiotomy syndrome, echocardiographic images of,
      322–323, 335
Potassium channel blockade, sudden death and, 10, 25
Pravastatin, 111, 112, 140, 143, 165, 178
Pregnancy
   anticoagulation in, 56–57, 68
   aortic stenosis and, 247, 260
   Eisenmenger's syndrome and, 247, 248, 260
   Marfan's syndrome and, 247, 260
   severe pulmonary hypertension and, 247, 260
   valvular heart disease and, 56–57, 68
Procainamide
   dosage of, 159, 173
   for Wolff-Parkinson-White syndrome, 15, 28
Prodrugs, 161, 174
Propafenone, 1, 2, 18
Propranolol, properties of, 163, 176
Prospective Pravastatin Pooling (PPP) project, 111, 140
Prosthetic valve abscess, 40, 61
Protamine
   dosage of, 168, 180
   increased allergic reaction to, 168, 180
Prothrombin complex, for hirudin-related bleeding, 114,
      148–149
PTCA. See Percutaneous transluminal coronary angioplasty
      (PTCA)
PTRA, 201, 216

Pulmonary arteriovenous fistula, 244, 258
Pulmonary atresia
   with intact ventricular septum, gender preponderance of,
      249, 261
   surgical procedures for, 248, 261
Pulmonary hypertension, severe, pregnancy and, 247, 260
Pulmonary stenosis, 54–55, 67, 242, 256
   cardiac catheterization image of, 249f, 262
   cardiac defects in, 244, 257
   supravalvular, associated disease conditions of, 252, 263
   treatment of, 55, 67
Pulmonary venous drainage, anomalous, 245, 258
   associated disease conditions of, 252, 263
Pulsus paradoxus, causes of, 306, 313

Quinidine, 2, 3, 18, 19

Ramipril, 106, 132
   aspirin and, 228, 237
   indications for, 106, 132
Rashkind procedure, 248, 261
RCA. See Right coronary artery (RCA)
Renal artery stenosis
   cause of, 202, 217
   diagnosis of, 201, 216
Reteplase, risk of stroke with, 81, 96
Revascularization, indications for, 199, 214
Rhabdomyolysis, 166, 178
Right coronary artery (RCA)
   anomalous origin of, 124f, 153
   occlusion of, 88, 92–93, 92f, 100
   perforation of, 125f, 153
   severe restenosis of, 91f, 101
   severe stenosis of, 122f, 128f, 152, 153
   stent in, 90–91, 101
Right ventricle dysplasia, arrhythmogenic, 16, 29
Right ventricle failure, acute, diagnosis of, 224, 236
Right ventricular infarction, 76, 95, 115, 150
   survival factors for, 115, 150
   treatment of, 77, 95
Ross procedure, 248, 261
Rubella, congenital, cardiovascular malformations associated
      with, 244, 257

S_2, decreased A_2 component of, 197, 213
S_4, in acute myocardial infarction, 107, 133
Saphenous vein grafts, atherosclerosis progression in, 111,
      141
Sarcoplasmic-endoplasmic reticulum calcium ATPase type 2
      (SERCA2), 265, 267
Scandinavian Simvastatin Survival Study (4S), 112,
      141–142
Sclerae, blue, 195, 210
Scleroderma, 130, 154
Senning procedure, 248, 261
SERCA2, 265, 267

SHOCK (Should we Emergently Revascularize Occluded Coronaries for Cardiogenic Shock) trial, 93, 102, 113, 144
Sick sinus syndrome, 8–9, 24–25
Sildenafil acetate, adverse interactions of, 82, 97
Simvastatin, 112, 141–142
Sixth Report of the Joint National Committee on Prevention, Detection, Evaluation, and Treatment of High Blood Pressure (JNC VI), 277, 285
Smoking
    cessation of, 79, 96
        in peripheral vascular disease, 199, 214
    effect of on ischemic heart disease, 112, 143–144
Smooth muscle cell, inducing proliferation of, 267, 269
Sodium channel blockers, 3
Spironolactone
    benefits of, 230, 238
    side effects of, 276, 284
Stable angina
    risk stratification in, 111, 139–140
    survival rates for, 113, 144
Staphylococcus epidermidis, in prosthetic valve endocarditis, 56, 68
Stenting
    in acute coronary syndrome, 76, 95
    in acute myocardial infarction, 80, 96
Stent thrombosis, 111, 140
Streptococcus viridans, in native valve endocarditis, 55, 68
Streptokinase
    risk of stroke with, 81, 96
    for ST segment–elevation myocardial infarction, 80, 96
    and t-PA compared, 84, 99
Stroke
    etiology of, 196, 211
    examination of, 196, 211
    reduction of with pravastatin, 111, 140
ST segment–elevation myocardial infarction (STMI), management of, 74, 80, 94, 96
Subaortic membrane, management of, 244, 258
Subaortic stenosis
    characteristic echocardiography findings in, 255f, 263
    with severe aortic valve insufficiency, 244, 258
Subarachnoid hemorrhage, nimodipine for, 164, 177
Subendocardium, vulnerability of, 106, 133
Subvalvular membrane, diagnosis of, 42, 42f, 62
Sudden cardiac death
    causes of, 7, 23
    primary prevention of, 6, 23
    rhythms associated with, 6, 22
    risk of, from aortic insufficiency, 37, 59
Sulfonamide, allergies to, 170, 182
Superior vena cava
    partial obstruction of, differential diagnosis of, 303, 312
    persistent left, associated disease conditions of, 252, 263
Syncope
    evaluation of, 7, 9, 23, 25

    in pulmonic stenosis, 55, 67
    vasovagal
        response during, 7, 23
        treatment of, 6, 22

Tachycardia
    atrioventricular nodal reentrant. See Atrioventricular nodal reentrant tachycardia
    multifocal atrial, 7, 23–24
    narrow complex. See Narrow complex tachycardia
    pacemaker-mediated, 10–11, 11f, 26
    permanent junctional reciprocating, 3, 19
    ventricular, 4–5, 21
    wide complex. See Wide complex tachycardia
Takayasu's arteritis, diagnosis of, 193, 209–210
Terfenadine, sudden death and, 10, 25
Tetralogy of Fallot
    characteristic chest radiography findings in, 252, 263
    echocardiographic images of, 332f, 337
    physical findings in, 252, 262
    surgical repair of, 242, 256
Thiazide, 170, 182
Thienopyridines, 166–167, 179
Thrombocytopenia, heparin-induced, 168, 181
Thrombolysis in Myocardial Infarction (TIMI), 78, 95, 115, 149–150
Thrombolytic agents
    contraindications for, 169
    as predictor of mortality, 107, 134
Ticlopidine
    in acute coronary syndrome, 75–76, 95
    antiplatelet effects of, 166–167, 179
    side effects of, 166, 179
Tilt table testing, head-upright, 7, 23, 24
TIMI, 78, 95, 115, 149–150
Tissue plasminogen activator (t-PA)
    accelerated, for acute myocardial infarction, 82, 97
    for inferior wall myocardial infarction, 85, 99
    reversal of, 85, 99
    risk of stroke with, 81, 96
    survival benefits of, 107, 133
Torsades de pointes, in long-QT syndrome, 14, 27
t-PA. See Tissue plasminogen activator (t-PA)
Transesophageal echocardiography, 33, 38, 58
    in diagnosis of subvalvular membrane, 42, 62
    indications for, 193, 209f
    after myocardial infarction, 44, 63
Transient ischemic attack, 45–46, 64
Transposition of great vessels
    congenitally corrected, 194, 210, 245, 259
    surgical procedures for, 248, 261
Tricuspid atresia, surgical procedures for, 248, 261
Tricuspid regurgitation
    diagnosis of, 234, 239
    etiology of, 55, 67–68
Tricuspid stenosis, 50, 65

Tricuspid valve replacement, 55, 67–68

Unstable angina
  antiischemic therapy for, 109, 135
  antiplatelet and anticoagulant therapy for, 109–110, 136, 137f
  early risk stratification for, 108, 135
  failure of medical therapy in, 114, 146–147
  hospitalization for, 106, 132
  immediate management of, 109, 135
Urosepsis, evaluation of, 40, 61

Valvular heart disease, 31–67. *See also specific disorders*
Valvuloplasty, percutaneous, 41, 61
  consideration for, 32, 58
  for mitral stenosis, 41
  for pulmonic stenosis, 55, 67
Vasculopathy, allograft, prevention of, 222, 235
Vasodilator therapy
  for aortic insufficiency, 37, 59
  effects of on left ventricular volume loop, 232f, 239
  for severe aortic insufficiency, 43, 62
Vasopressors, 171–172, 183–184
Ventricular fibrillation, morbidity of, 6, 21
Ventricular function, predictors of, 113, 145–146
Ventricular preexcitation, intermittent, treatment of, 7, 23–24
Ventricular septal defect, 78–79, 78f
  cardiac catheterization image of, 250f, 262
  echocardiographic images of, 321–322, 321f, 334
  gender preponderance of, 249, 261
  in pulmonary stenosis, 244, 257

Ventricular septal rupture, 86, 100
Ventricular tachycardia, treatment of, 4–5, 21
Verapamil
  contraindications for, 2, 18
  intravenous
    for chronic obstructive pulmonary disease, 10, 25
    in regular narrow complex tachycardia, 4, 20
  mechanisms of, 163, 177
Vesnarinone, chronic use of, 221, 235
Vitamin E, in acute myocardial infarction, 81, 97

Warfarin, 166, 169, 178, 181
  in acute myocardial infarction, 84, 98
  appropriate use of, 16, 29
  versus aspirin, 116, 151
  contraindications for, 35, 59
  and ethanol, 160–161, 174
  for mitral stenosis, 46, 64
  after transient ischemic attack, 45, 64
Weber-Osler-Rendu syndrome, 244, 258
West of Scotland Coronary Prevention Study (WOSCOPS), 112, 143
Wide complex tachycardia
  evaluation of, 14, 28
  treatment of, 14–15, 28
Williams syndrome, 197, 213
Wolff-Parkinson-White syndrome
  antiarrhythmic drug use in, 4, 20
  treatment of, 15, 28

Xamoterol, chronic use of, 221, 235